# Clinical Case Studies in Orthopedics

Editor: Cheryl Wilson

AMERICAN
MEDICAL PUBLISHERS
www.americanmedicalpublishers.com

AMERICAN
MEDICAL PUBLISHERS
www.americanmedicalpublishers.com

**Cataloging-in-Publication Data**

Clinical case studies in orthopedics / edited by Cheryl Wilson.
p. cm.
Includes bibliographical references and index.
ISBN 979-8-88740-625-1
1. Orthopedics. 2. Orthopedics--Diagnosis. 3. Orthopedics--Treatment.
I. Wilson, Cheryl.
RD731 .C55 2023
617.3--dc23



American Medical Publishers,
41 Flatbush Avenue,
1st Floor, New York,
NY 11217, USA

ISBN 979-8-88740-625-1 (Hardback)

# Clinical Case Studies in Orthopedics

# Contents

# Preface

The main aim of this book is to educate learners and enhance their research focus by presenting diverse topics covering this vast field. This is an advanced book which compiles significant studies by distinguished experts in the area of analysis. This book addresses successive solutions to the challenges arising in the area of application, along with it; the book provides scope for future developments.

Orthopedics is a medical specialty that deals with the diagnosis, treatment and prevention of disorders and injuries of the musculoskeletal system. This system includes bones, joints, muscles, ligaments, tendons, and nerves that allow the body to move and function. Orthopedics deals with the management of conditions ranging from fractures and sports injuries to degenerative diseases like arthritis. It employs various methods, including non-surgical and surgical interventions. The non-surgical interventions encompass physical therapy, medication and injections, while prominent surgical procedures include joint replacements or spinal surgeries. The goal of orthopedics is to restore mobility, reduce pain, and improve overall quality of life for patients. This book provides comprehensive insights into the field of orthopedics. It will serve as a valuable source of reference for graduate and postgraduate students.

It was a great honour to edit this book, though there were challenges, as it involved a lot of communication and networking between me and the editorial team. However, the end result was this all-inclusive book covering diverse themes in the field.

Finally, it is important to acknowledge the efforts of the contributors for their excellent chapters, through which a wide variety of issues have been addressed. I would also like to thank my colleagues for their valuable feedback during the making of this book.

**Editor**

# 1

# Traumatic Closed Proximal Muscle Rupture of the Biceps Brachii in Military Paratrooper

**Georgios Kalinterakis,[1] Emmanouil Antonogiannakis,[1] Ioannis Rampakakis,[1] Evangelos Tsialogiannis,[1] Athanasios Syllaios,[2] and Miltiadis Ziogas[1]**

[1]*First Department of Orthopedics, 401 General Military Hospital Of Athens, Athens 11525, Greece*
[2]*First Department of Surgery, General Hospital of Athens "Laiko", National and Kapodistrian University of Athens, Athens 11527, Greece*

Correspondence should be addressed to Georgios Kalinterakis; gkalinterakis@gmail.com

Academic Editor: Dimitrios S. Karataglis

Traumatic closed proximal muscle rupture of the biceps brachii has been infrequently cited in the medical bibliography. Early reports of this injury derived from US military during parachute jumps, and it may compromise >4% of injuries at altitude. The mechanism is a direct blow to the upper extremity by static lines. We report a case of traumatic closed proximal rupture of the biceps brachii in a healthy 25 years of age military paratrooper. He was managed with primary surgical repair, and after three years of follow-up, the patient has excellent functional results.

## 1. Introduction

Traumatic closed proximal muscle rupture of the biceps brachii has been infrequently cited in the medical bibliography. This injury is chiefly associated with military static line parachute jumps where the paratrooper orients the static line incorrectly around his arm at the onset of jumping causing a straight blunt force on the biceps brachii [1]. Moreover, United States of America is the only country which has reported this specific static line injury [2].

We report a case of traumatic closed proximal rupture of the biceps brachii in a healthy 25 years of age military paratrooper.

## 2. Case Report

A 25-year-old right-handed paratrooper was presented to orthopedic emergency department because he felt a sudden sharp pain in his right upper extremity after attempting a parachute jump.

On physical examination, there was pain around the right shoulder and upper arm. Open trauma was not observed. Furthermore, extensive ecchymosis and edema were presented due to subcutaneous hemorrhage with spreading in the forearm. The muscle defect was palpable, and Popeye's deformity was noticed as shown in Figure 1. Additionally, supination of the forearm and elbow flexion strength was evaluated in comparison with the uninjured limb. Both decrease in motor strength and weakness in elbow flexion were noted. Manual strength testing revealed 4/5 strength of elbow flexion and supination. Neurovascular examination of the afflicted upper extremity was negative.

Simple radiographs did not reveal bony pathology. Magnetic resonance imaging (MRI) of the right upper limb disclosed the proximal rupture of the biceps brachii at the musculotendinous junction (Figures 2(a) and 2(b)).

On the grounds that the patient was both active and young, operative treatment was decided in order the deformity be diminished and the strength be restored. The latter plays a prominent role in case of highly demanded occupation. The surgical intervention was undergone 10 days after the injury. Under general anesthesia, the patient was placed in beach chair positioning and an anterior approach was preferred. A lazy "S" 10-12 cm incision was made with a

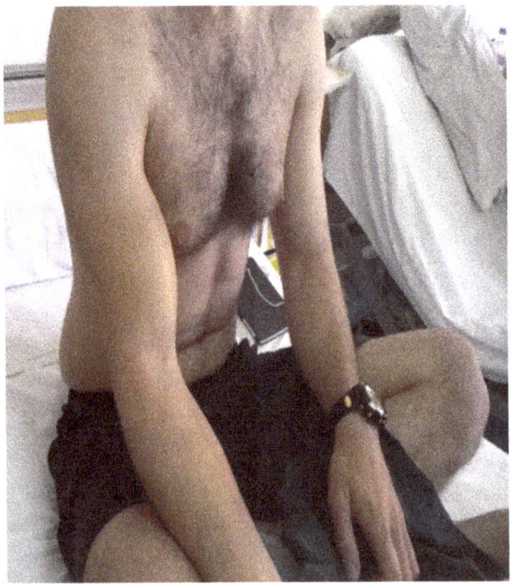

Figure 1: Acute biceps rupture in a military parachutist. Popeye deformity is noted.

proximal medial edge on the deltopectoral groove and ending with a distal midline edge on the lateral aspect of the humerus, about halfway down its shaft. When the subcutaneous fascia was opened, a great hematoma of roughly 300 cc was moved out. As a result, better visualization and mobilization of the muscle was achieved. After that, damaged tissue was carefully removed and muscle belly ends were thoroughly inspected. On observation, the long head of the biceps brachii was almost ruptured beneath the myotendinous junction and the short head was completely transected within the intramuscular substance (Figure 3). The musculocutaneous nerve was identified in the interval between the biceps and the brachialis muscles and carefully protected. Then, the gap was bridged with locking intramuscular nonabsorbable sutures (number 2, ETHIBOND EXCEL braided polyester on a tapered needle) (Figure 4). During that process, the elbow flexed to 90° and the forearm positioned in neutral. With the upper extremity in that position, the defect was diminished and the surgical repair was aptly facilitated. Lastly, the trauma was closed in layers.

Postoperatively, a posterior splint with the elbow at 90° was used for a period of 4 weeks. When the splint was removed, active ROM exercises based on gravity were started. The DASH score when the splint was removed was 64.2. At 8 weeks, physiotherapy was begun emphasizing on strengthening exercises. Altogether, 20 sessions were done and reevaluation was followed after one month. The DASH score was 16.7. The patient was able to fully return to former activities in six months' time. The DASH score was 0.0. The next follow-up was scheduled one year after the injury. After that, it was recommended that he should be examined once a year. The last follow-up that took place 3 years after the injury revealed great functional results with a full return of strength as well as satisfactory cosmetic results (Figures 5(a) and 5(b)). The patient did not mention any difficulties in his labor and everyday life activities.

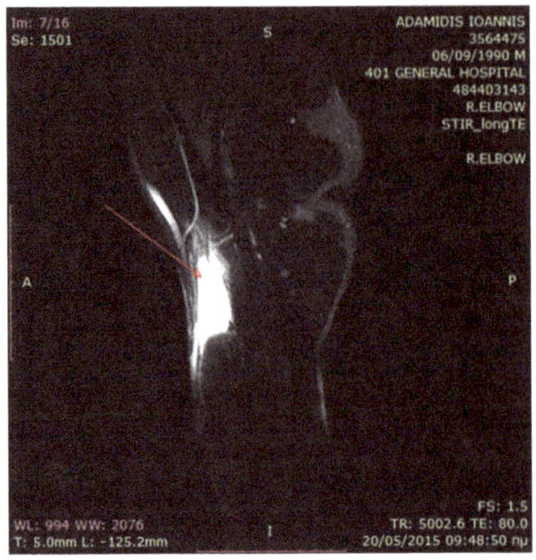


(a)

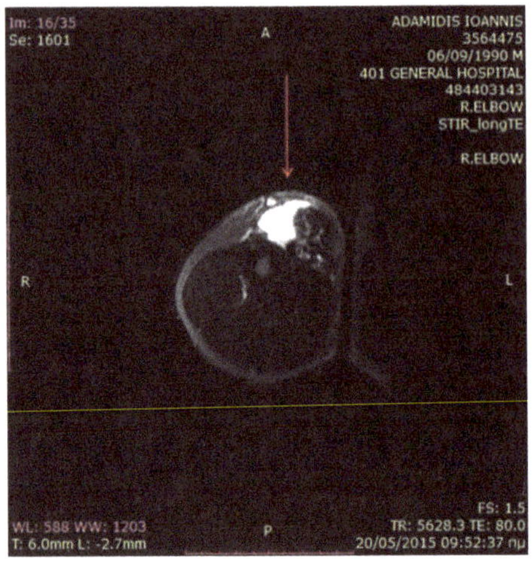


(b)

Figure 2: (a, b) MRI images showing an intrasubstance tear of the biceps brachii (arrows) with a large hematoma filling the defect.

## 3. Discussion

Closed proximal ruptures of the biceps brachii muscle are rare incidents, and they usually involve the long head of the biceps. Early reports of this injury derived from US military during parachute jumps, and it may compromise >4% of injuries at altitude [3].

The most common mechanism is a direct blow to the upper extremity by static lines. It is claimed that the static line becomes misrouted under the arm at the time of exit from the aircraft, and this in turn ends up with a blunt trauma to the biceps belly [4]. In our case, the jump platform was a C130 military aircraft. The parachute used was a MC1-1C maneuverable parachute assembly designed by the United States Army in 1988 for military static line airborne operations. This type of injury occurs in the phase of the exit. As the paratroopers approach the door, they hold the static line in their right hand in the case of exiting the right door (as in our case) or in their left hand in the case of exiting the left door. When they reach the door, the paratroopers hand off the static line to the jumpmaster and forcefully adduct their

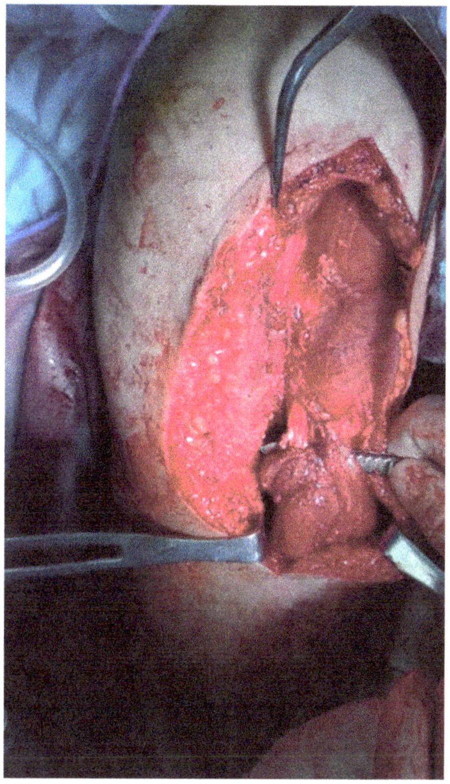

FIGURE 3: Intraoperative photograph showing the intramuscular biceps tear (yellow arrows).

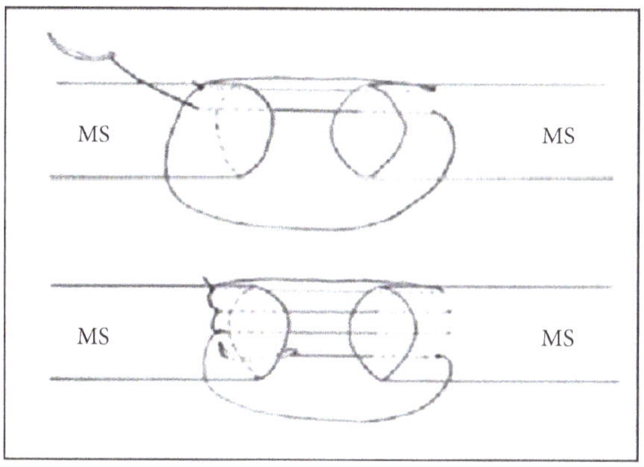


FIGURE 4: Locking intramuscular sutures secure both the proximal and distal muscle segments (MS).

arms holding the reserve parachute. During the free fall, the body of the paratrooper is in a horizontal position for some seconds because of the speed and direction of the aircraft. At the same time, the static line unfolds and finally becomes taut, pulling the deployment bag, in which the parachute is packed, and allowing the canopy to inflate. In the unfortunate event of misrouting of the static line, a localized force may be exerted on the anterior surface of the arm and cause injuries to the upper extremity. This is exactly what happened in our case, according to the description of the patient. The onset of the pain was in the first seconds of the exit and continued to exist for the rest of the fall [3, 5].

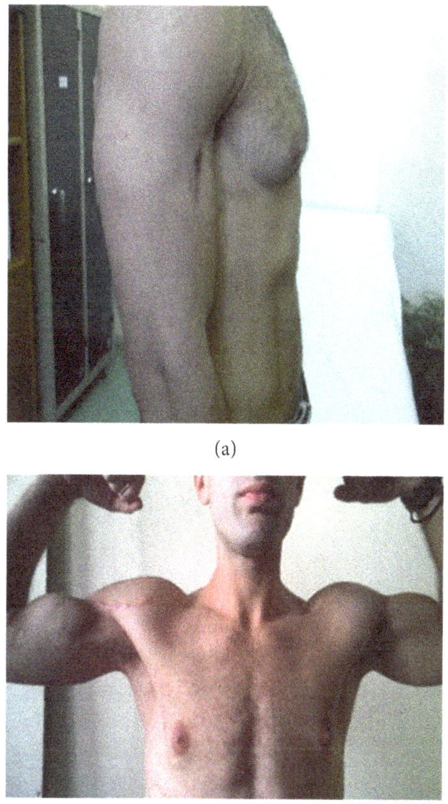

(a)

(b)

FIGURE 5: Postoperative images three years after the surgery.

The largest series biceps muscle belly tears have come from Womack Army Medical Center in Fort Bragg, NC. Heckman and Levine reported 48 patients in 1978 [1] and Kragh and Basamania reported 12 patients in 2002 [6]. Outside of military parachutists, biceps muscle belly tears are only reported as individual cases [7 9]. Imaging may include ultrasonography and magnetic resonance imaging (MRI). The latter seems to be useful for the detection and characterization of this injury while ultrasound has been reported as an adjunct to MRI in both diagnosis and determination of injury severity [4]. In this case, MRI of the right upper limb revealed the injury confirming its essential role in diagnosis.

Treatment can be either operative or nonoperative. Early reports suggested operative exploration and primary repair [10]. Currently, there is a scarcity of randomized, controlled studies to support standardized operative or nonoperative treatment while few treatment comparison studies have been performed (Table 1). Heckman and Levine compared operative repair vs. early percutaneous hematoma evacuation and immobilization, but no significant difference in clinical outcomes was found [1]. On the contrary, Kragh and Basamania demonstrated better results with operative repair when it comes to strength, appearance, and patient satisfaction [6]. Although no comprehensive data exists to support operative vs. nonoperative treatment, the present case was treated surgically with excellent postoperative results. With regard to postoperative immobilization and rehabilitation,

Table 1: The table demonstrates the published studies regarding the traumatic intrasubstance rupture of the biceps brachii, the type of treatment, and their results.

| Study | Treatment | Outcome |
|---|---|---|
| Conwell [11] | Open, debridement, no repair, splinting | Good outcome reported |
| Gilcrest [10] | Surgical repair with primary reattachment using catgut suture and fascial flap | Unreported |
| Tobin et al. [12] | Unreported | Unreported |
| Heckman & Levine [1] | Nonoperative group: hematoma aspiration, splinting for 6 weeks in acute flexion. Operative group: open, debridement, primary repair, splinted in acute flexation for 4 weeks, then 90° flexation for 2 weeks, followed by gentle ROM | 53% return of elbow flexion in the nonoperative group vs. 76.5% in the operative group. One wound infection was reported. No complications in the nonoperative group |
| Mellen [13] | Open, exploration, hematoma evacuation, excision of intraluminal thrombus, brachial artery grafting and repair, no biceps repair performed | Skin breakdown and superficial wound infection reported. Visible and palpable defect persisted |
| DiChristina & Lustig [7] | Open, primary repair, 3 weeks in splint | Full ROM, 5/5 strength at 4 months |
| Bricknell [14] | Closed, 4 weeks in sling | Visible and palpable defect persisted, no functional deficit compared to contralateral side |
| Balkissoon et al. [15] | Nonoperative | Unreported |
| Craig & Lee [3] | Unreported | Unreported |
| Kragh & Basamania [6] | Nonoperative: sling & NSAIDs. Operative: open, debridement, primary repair, 3-5 day immobility followed by dynamic splinting with extension limited to 30° with early active ROM | All patients returned to full ROM. No complications, job changes, or poor functional outcomes reported. Patients disliked the Popeye deformity. Nonoperative patients regained 65% of contralateral supination/flexion compared with 89% of those repaired operatively |
| Shah & Pruzansky [9] | Open, debridement, primary repair, postoperative splinting for 4 weeks, followed by hinged bracing for 6 weeks | Full ROM, 5/5 strength at 5 months |
| Carmichael et al. [8] | Open, debridement, no repair | Full ROM, 5/5 strength at 8 months |
| Chen & Chew [16] | Nonoperative, cast immobilization for 6 weeks in hyperflexed supinated position | Satisfactory cosmetic and functional results were reported |

NSAIDs: nonsteroidal anti-inflammatory drugs, ROM: range of motion.

recommendations have varied including elbow immobilization at ≥90° of flexion from 3 days to 3 weeks postoperatively, followed by the use of a dynamic splint for early motion [6, 7]. Although in this case a posterior splint with the elbow at 90° was used for a period of 4 weeks, there were no problems in terms of the rehabilitation program with good functional outcomes in the long term. Finally, the duration of follow-up in most of the studies was short while in some of them the outcome was completely omitted [4].

In conclusion, closed proximal tears of the biceps brachii comprise a rare injury. Military static line parachute jumps seem to be the predominant mechanism. As a result, orthopaedic surgeons must be aware of this clinical feature especially if they work in military hospitals. This study corroborates the superiority of surgical repair in a long term basis and acts as a contributory factor in medical literature in terms of guiding treatment.

## Consent

Consent was obtained.

## References

[1] J. D. Heckman and M. I. Levine, "Traumatic closed transection of the biceps brachii in the military parachutist," *The Journal of Bone & Joint Surgery*, vol. 60, no. 3, pp. 369–372, 1978.

[2] M. C. M. Bricknell and S. C. Craig, "Military parachuting injuries: a literature review," *Occupational Medicine*, vol. 49, no. 1, pp. 17–26, 1999.

[3] S. C. Craig and T. Lee, "Attention to detail: injuries at altitude among U.S. Army Military static line parachutists," *Military Medicine*, vol. 165, no. 4, pp. 268–271, 2000.

[4] D. J. Wilson, S. A. Parada, J. M. Slevin, and E. D. Arrington, "Intrasubstance ruptures of the biceps brachii: diagnosis and management," *Orthopedics*, vol. 34, no. 11, pp. 890–896, 2011.

[5] US Army, *FM 3-21.220 Static Line Parachuting Techniques and Tactics: Training Handbook On Parachute Jumping, Jumpmaster, Drop Zone, Airborne Operations, Military Team, Aircraft, and Combat Equipment Loads*, Field Manual Reference Guide, Washington, 2003, Chapter 3.

[6] J. F. Kragh Jr. and C. J. Basamania, "Surgical repair of acute traumatic closed transection of the biceps brachii," *The Journal of Bone and Joint Surgery-American Volume*, vol. 84, no. 6, pp. 992–998, 2002.

[7] D. G. DiChristina and K. A. Lustig, "Rupture Through the Short Head of the Biceps Muscle Belly: A Case Report," *Clinical Orthopaedics and Related Research*, vol. 277, pp. 139–141, 1992.

[8] K. D. Carmichael, L. Foster, and J. P. Kearney, "Biceps muscle rupture in a water skier," *Orthopedics*, vol. 28, no. 1, pp. 35–37, 2005.

[9] A. K. Shah and M. E. Pruzansky, "Ruptured biceps brachii short head muscle belly: a case report," *Journal of Shoulder and Elbow Surgery*, vol. 13, no. 5, pp. 562–565, 2004.

[10] E. I. Gilcrest, "The common syndrome of repture dislocation and elongation of the long head of the biceps brachii: An analysis of one hundred cases," *Surgery, Gynecology & Obstetrics*, vol. 58, pp. 322–340, 1934.

[11] H. Conwell, "Subcutaneous rupture of the biceps flexor cubiti: report of one case," *The Journal of Bone and Joint Surgery*, vol. 10, pp. 788–790, 1928.

[12] W. J. Tobin, L. J. Cohen, and J. T. Vandover, "Parachute injuries," *JAMA: The Journal of the American Medical Association*, vol. 117, no. 16, p. 1318, 1941.

[13] P. F. Mellen, "Parachute static line injury with vascular compromise," *Military Medicine*, vol. 154, no. 7, pp. 364-365, 1989.

[14] M. C. M. Bricknell, "Traumatic Rupture of Bicepts Brachii - a Hazard of Military Parachuting," *Journal of the Royal Army Medical Corps*, vol. 137, no. 3, pp. 144-145, 1991.

[15] A. R. Balkissoon, C. F. Snyder, and C. Basmanian, "MR imaging of traumatic closed injuries of the biceps brachii muscle in military parachutists," *American Journal of Roentgenology*, vol. 170, no. 5, pp. 1400-1401, 1998.

[16] H. W. Chen and F. S. Chew, "Complete rupture of both heads of the biceps brachii muscle belly by blunt trauma," *Radiology Case Reports*, vol. 1, no. 4, pp. 145–148, 2006.

# 2

# Rare Isolated Pectoralis Minor Tear from a Noncontact Injury: Case Report and Review of the Literature

**Danica D. Vance, Usama Qayyum, and Charles M. Jobin**

*The Center for Shoulder, Elbow and Sports Medicine, Columbia University Medical Center, New York, NY, USA*

Correspondence should be addressed to Danica D. Vance; ddv305@gmail.com

Academic Editor: Koichi Sairyo

Isolated pectoralis minor tears are rare orthopedic injuries often in weightlifters or contact sports and should be included in the differential when evaluating athletes with anterior shoulder pain. These injuries are often mistaken for pectoralis major muscle stains and tears. Advanced imaging with MRI helps define the anatomic location and grade of injury. Treatment is usually conservative with full return to activity after a brief period of rest for a few weeks. The purpose of this article is to present a case report and review of the literature on the clinical evaluation, imaging, and treatment of an isolated pectoralis minor tears.

## 1. Introduction

Isolated pectoralis minor tears are rare orthopedic injuries with only a handful of cases reported in the literature. Musculoskeletal shoulder pain localized to the anterior chest and shoulder can be a diagnostic dilemma. The differential diagnosis includes contusion from trauma, costochondritis, muscle strain, pectoralis major tendon tear, and internal derangements of the shoulder. Pectoralis major tears occur from a forced adduction and internal rotation injury often in weightlifters or contact sports [1]. Although rare, isolated pectoralis minor tears may occur from abnormal scapular forces or fatigue of scapular stabilizing musculature and should be included in the differential when evaluating patients with anterior shoulder pain, especially those with tenderness over the coracoid, or lateral chest wall pain near the shoulder [2].

Previous case reports of isolated pectoralis minor tears have described injuries occurring during a contact sport such as American football [2, 3] and ice hockey [4]. In contrast, our case report describes an isolated pectoralis minor tendon tear sustained in a 24-year-old female while she was performing a side plank exercise presumably from loss of endurance and an eccentric loading of her pectoralis minor tendon. These injuries are often mistaken for the more common pectoralis major muscle stains and tears. The purpose of this article is to present the clinical evaluation, imaging, and treatment of an isolated pectoralis minor tear in a young healthy individual sustained from a noncontact injury.

## 2. Case History

A 24-year-old left hand dominant female, smoker for the last five years without a significant medical history, presented one day after an injury at the gym with left shoulder pain. She reports, while preforming a side plank, a maneuver where her body weight is supported by her arm in a side pushup-like position; she felt a pop and snap in her front shoulder and chest area. At the time of injury, the patient had her complete body weight on her fully extended left arm. She had immediate pain without any associated numbness and tingling. The pain did not improve and started to radiate to the neck and down her anterior chest and arm.

Initial physical examination revealed mild asymmetry of the left anterior axillary crease without any gross deformity or ecchymosis. She had tenderness over the left biceps groove and pectoralis major tendon with pain on resisted arm internal rotation. Her brachial plexus and axilla were nontender. Active scapular protraction and retraction were painful. Her coracoid tip was tender to palpation. The remainder of

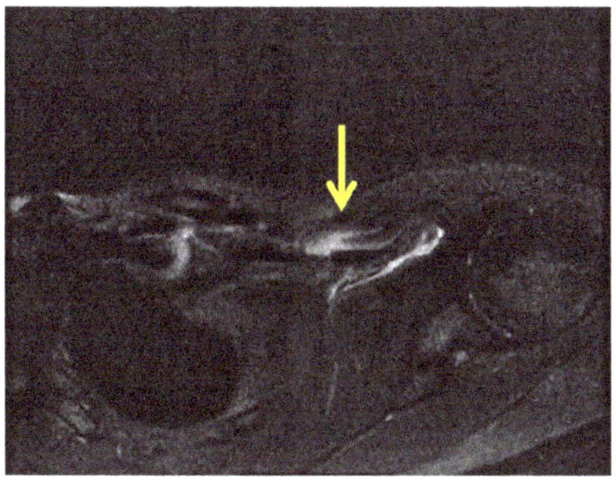

FIGURE 1: Axial T2-weighted magnetic resonance imaging showing disruption of the pectoralis minor myotendinous junction with surrounding edema and associated intramuscular edema.

the shoulder exam, including range of motion and neurovascular exam, was unremarkable.

## 3. Imaging

Radiographs of her shoulder were unremarkable. Due to the abnormal exam findings and concern for a pectoralis major high-grade muscle strain, a magnetic resonance imaging (MRI) study was ordered. The MRI revealed a grade 3 myotendinous tear of the pectoralis minor with complete disruption of the muscle fibers and visible gaping of the tissue. Additionally, imaging demonstrated surrounding fluid at the myotendinous junction of the pectoralis minor with adjacent muscular edema (Figure 1). The pectoralis major myotendinous complex and rest of the surrounding soft tissue showed no injury.

## 4. Treatment

This injury was managed with conservative treatment including rest, icing, anti-inflammatories, and activity modification. After 2 weeks, the patient recovered to 90 percent without complaints. By 3 weeks, the patient had resumed light workouts with aerobics and dance. At 3-month follow-up, the patient reported no residual disability with full return to all sporting activities. At six-month follow-up, the clinical exam demonstrated an excellent outcome with a physical exam symmetric to the uninjured arm and shoulder. Patient subjective pain score and shoulder assessment scores were as follows: ASES = 100, SST = 12, and constant score = 95. Patient SF-36 scores following nonoperative treatment were high for all categories (physical function = 100%, physical health = 100%, emotional role = 100%, energy/fatigue = 75%, emotional well-being = 88%, social functioning = 100%, pain = 90%, general health 86%, and health change 75%). The patient had a full painless range of motion of 175° of forward elevation, 65° of external rotation (ER), T5 internal rotation (IR), and strength that was 5/5 and symmetric to the contralateral shoulder. She had no scapular winging or weakness in scapular protraction and retraction.

## 5. Discussion

Pectoralis minor injuries are rare and may be caused by both contact and noncontact traumatic events. The mechanism of injury can be characterized by an eccentric load in a fatigued pectoralis minor muscle. Conservative treatment has been successful in the few case reports of this unique injury.

The pectoralis minor tendon originates from the outer surface of the third through the fifth ribs. Its fibers pass superiorly and laterally and converges to a flat tendon that inserts on the medial superior border of the coracoid process, adjacent to the conjoint tendon [2]. The primary role of the pectoralis minor tendon is to stabilize the scapula by drawing it anteriorly and inferiorly over the thoracic wall [5].

The exact mechanism of pectoralis minor tendon rupture is unknown. Various factors such as excessive strain, abnormal loading, and eccentric forces on the muscle play crucial roles. Injury to the pectoralis minor can occur with direct force to the shoulder or forced ER of the arm [3]. Skeletal muscle is a continuous adapting tissue that responds to stress by changing its physiological function and mass. However, acute stresses that exceed the adaptability leads to injury [6].

Injury to the pectoralis minor tendon can occur through contact injuries in athletes either by direct blows to the anterior shoulder or forced ER of the arm while abducted. The myotendinous junction is the most common sight of injury amongst the current experimental models demonstrating muscle strains [7]. To our knowledge, our case report is the first to describe an injury to the pectoralis minor without contact, as the injury in this case was sustained while the patient was preforming a side plank at the gym. The mechanism of injury was likely due to fatigue of the anterior scapular stabilizers during the eccentric loading of the pectoralis muscles, causing the scapular to be eccentrically forced into retraction.

Physical examination is critical as soft tissue injuries of musculoskeletal origin are elicited by palpating on active trigger points and demonstrating pain or weakness with resisted muscle function. Pec minor injuries present as anterior shoulder pain and tenderness to palpation over the coracoid [3]. Shoulder extension and ER also generate pain [4]. Evaluation of the shoulder at 90° and 150° of horizontal abduction generates tension across the pectoralis minor most effectively [8].

Advanced imaging is recommended if a significant injury is suspected to the pectoralis complex, but no obvious deformity is discovered. A grade 1 strain on imaging is defined as having edema without laxity in any fibers or gapping within the myotendinous complex. Pectoralis minor grade 1 strains have been confused in the past with symptoms of angina [9]. Grade 2 stains demonstrate laxity in fibers indicating significant strain but without tissue gapping. Grade 3 myotendinous tears are defined as a complete disruption of muscle fibers with a visible tissue defect. Other reports of pectoralis minor tears in the literature have revealed tears in the tendon with edema in the muscle mass [3], complete absence of pec minor tendon attachment over the coracoid, and high intensity signal across the entire muscle [4].

Sports medicine literature demonstrates the use of slings, pendulum exercises, and physical therapy for postinjury rehabilitation. A detailed physical clinical exam to exclude any residual injury or disability is performed before athletes start dynamic sport-specific exercises [4]. Conservative treatment has been successful in nearly every patient reported with pectoralis minor injury. Reports of recalcitrant pectoralis tendinopathy have been successfully treated with corticosteroid injections [10]. The patient in this report made a full recovery with a complete normal shoulder with conservative management that included rest, ice, NSAIDs, and activity modification for 2 to 4 weeks.

Pectoralis minor myotendinous injuries are uncommon. When they do occur, the patients are often healthy active individuals, including professional athletes and those who play contact sports. However, pectoralis minor injuries should always be considered when a patient presents with atypical anterior musculoskeletal shoulder and chest wall pain as noncontact mechanisms of injury do occur. Pain and tenderness near the coracoid along with physical exam findings of painful resisted scapular protraction should alert the orthopedist to a possible pectoralis minor injury. Advanced imaging with MRI helps define the anatomic location and grade of injury. Treatment is usually conservative with full return to activity after a brief period of rest for a few weeks.

## Disclosure

The author, Charles M. Jobin, has the following disclosures: Acumed, LLC: paid consultant and paid presenter or speaker; American Shoulder and Elbow Surgeons: board or committee member; CFO LLC: paid consultant; DePuy, a Johnson & Johnson Company: paid consultant; Journal of the American Academy of Orthopaedic Surgeons: editorial or governing board; Tornier: paid presenter or speaker; Wright Medical Technology Inc.: paid consultant; and Zimmer: paid consultant and paid presenter or speaker.

## References


[1] P. D. Metzger, J. R. Bailey, R. D. Filler, R. A. Waltz, M. T. Provencher, and C. B. Dewing, "Pectoralis major muscle rupture repair: technique using unicortical buttons," *Arthroscopy Techniques*, vol. 1, no. 1, pp. e119–e125, 2012.

[2] J. E. Zvijac, B. Zikria, and A. Botto-van Bemden, "Isolated tears of pectoralis minor muscle in professional football players: a case series," *American journal of orthopedics*, vol. 38, no. 3, pp. 145–147, 2009.

[3] X. Li, M. T. Gorman, J. S. Dines, and O. Limpisvasti, "Isolated tear of the pectoralis minor tendon in a high school football player," *Orthopedics*, vol. 35, no. 8, pp. e1272–e1275, 2012.

[4] K. Kalra and B. Neri, "Isolated pectoralis minor tendon tear in a professional ice hockey player—radiographic findings and presentation," *Skeletal Radiology*, vol. 39, no. 12, pp. 1251–1253, 2010.

[5] C. J. Mehallo, "Isolated tear of the pectoralis minor," *Clinical Journal of Sport Medicine*, vol. 14, no. 4, pp. 245-246, 2004, discussion 247.

[6] J. G. Tidball, "Mechanisms of muscle injury, repair, and regeneration," *Comprehensive Physiology*, vol. 1, no. 4, pp. 2029–2062, 2011.

[7] J. G. Tidball, "Myotendinous junction injury in relation to junction structure and molecular composition," *Exercise and Sport Sciences Reviews*, vol. 19, pp. 419–445, 1991.

[8] J. Umehara, M. Nakamura, K. Fujita et al., "Shoulder horizontal abduction stretching effectively increases shear elastic modulus of pectoralis minor muscle," *Journal of Shoulder and Elbow Surgery*, vol. 26, no. 7, pp. 1159–1165, 2017.

[9] G. E. Lawson, L. Y. Hung, G. D. Ko, and M. A. Laframboise, "A case of pseudo-angina pectoris from a pectoralis minor trigger point caused by cross-country skiing," *Journal of Chiropractic Medicine*, vol. 10, no. 3, pp. 173–178, 2011.

[10] D. N. Bhatia, J. F. de Beer, K. S. van Rooyen, F. Lam, and D. F. du Toit, "The "bench-presser's shoulder": an overuse insertional tendinopathy of the pectoralis minor muscle," *British Journal of Sports Medicine*, vol. 41, no. 8, p. e11, 2007.

# 3

# Knee Sepsis after Suprapatellar Nailing of an Open Tibia Fracture: Treatment with Acute Deformity and External Fixation

**Chelsea E. Minoughan**,[1] **Adam P. Schumaier,**[1] **and Frank R. Avilucea**[2]

[1]*University of Cincinnati Department of Orthopaedics and Sports Medicine, Cincinnati, OH, USA*
[2]*Orlando Health Orthopedic Institute Orthopedic and Sports Medicine Group, Orlando, FL, USA*

Correspondence should be addressed to Chelsea E. Minoughan; voelklce@mail.uc.edu

Academic Editor: Werner Kolb

*Case.* A 31-year-old male was involved in a dirt bike accident and sustained an isolated type II open mid-distal tibia fracture. The patient underwent suprapatellar intramedullary nailing and subsequently developed knee sepsis. *Conclusion.* This patient was managed with irrigation and debridements of the knee, fracture site, and intramedullary canal. A resultant soft-tissue defect over the fracture site obviated primary closure. Creation of an acute deformity stabilized by a Taylor spatial frame allowed primary wound closure. After soft tissue healing occurred, the frame was used to correct the intentional deformity and maintain reduction until full healing occurred.

## 1. Introduction

Open tibia fractures are relatively common injuries [1, 2] that can be challenging to treat [3, 4]. Stabilization of these fractures is often performed with intramedullary nailing (IMN), a technique that involves implant placement through either a suprapatellar or infrapatellar portal. Comparison of the two approaches demonstrates that suprapatellar nailing (SPN) facilitates improved alignment, particularly in distal or proximal fractures, [5, 6] and less fluoroscopic usage [7, 8]; however, a potential drawback to SPN of open fractures is iatrogenic knee sepsis as the technique requires intra-articular passage of instruments and the final implant. A 2017 study suggested that knee sepsis following suprapatellar nailing of open fractures does not occur [6], but a 2018 retrospective analysis reported two cases, suggesting a small but present risk for joint contamination [9].

We report the case of a 31-year-old male involved in a dirt bike accident who sustained a type II open tibia fracture and developed knee sepsis following irrigation and debridement (I&D) and suprapatellar nailing. To the best of our knowledge, this is the third documented case of knee sepsis following suprapatellar nailing of an open tibia fracture. Also unique to this case, the patient was definitively treated with a Taylor spatial frame to treat the fracture and also a resultant anteromedial soft-tissue defect at the fracture site following debridement; the frame enabled an intentional deformity to permit primary soft-tissue closure followed by deformity correction. This patient was informed that data pertaining to the case would be submitted for publication, and he provided consent.

## 2. Case Presentation

An otherwise healthy, nonsmoking, 31-year-old male ($25.0\,kg/m^2$) was involved in a dirt bike accident and sustained an isolated type II distal diaphyseal tibia fracture with an associated segmental fibula fracture (Figure 1). Neurovascular assessment demonstrated no deficits, and inspection of the leg revealed a 1 cm transverse wound contaminated with grass. The patient initially underwent bedside irrigation and received intravenous (IV) cefazolin, gentamicin, and penicillin G. A splint was applied. Intraoperative irrigation and debridement (I&D) followed by placement of a suprapatellar IMN was completed within the first 24 hours after the patient's arrival. The patient received two doses of IV Ancef postoperatively and was uneventfully discharged with nonweightbearing status on the affected extremity. The patient developed progressive knee discomfort and by week four reported severe pain; examination at that juncture

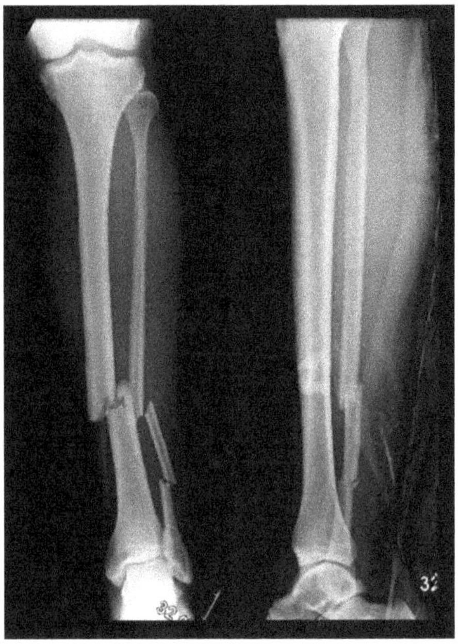

Figure 1: Anteroposterior (AP) and lateral radiographs of the left leg demonstrating a transverse distal diaphyseal tibial fracture and segmental fibular fracture.

identified a large knee effusion, erythema, and minimal tolerance for knee range-of-motion (ROM). Inspection of the fracture site showed mild erythema with serosanguinous drainage. Aspiration of the knee demonstrated cloudy yellow fluid and, its analysis, a white cell count >100,000 with 96% neutrophils; cultures grew gram-negative rods. At this time, patient care was transferred to the senior author.

I&D of the knee, fracture site, and intramedullary canal was completed following the removal of hardware. Discolored fluid was noted in the knee with palpable loculations in the suprapatellar pouch. Grass was identified in the knee and at the fracture site. A synovectomy of the loculated tissue in the knee was completed, and the surgical footprint at the fracture site was extended proximally and distally to permit local debridement of the bone and soft tissue; nonviable skin was excised resulting in a 1 × 3 cm soft-tissue defect directly over anteromedial tibial fracture site. A reamed irrigator aspirator (RIA) was used to debride the entirety of the intramedullary canal. A total of two separate debridements were performed. Following the second debridement, the soft-tissue defect was too large for primary closure and discussion with the patient included a flap for soft-tissue coverage or use of a Taylor spatial frame with induced deformity to allow primary soft-tissue closure. The patient opted for a frame.

A three-ring frame was applied to the tibia followed by application of Fast-Fx (Smith & Nephew, Memphis, TN) struts between the rings above and below the fracture site. An anatomic reduction of the tibia was completed prior to wound closure, and the strut lengths were recorded; baseline pulses were monitored with a Doppler, and capillary refill was noted. The fracture site was shortened and varus recurvatum deformity was induced until tension-free primary closure of the wound was possible; the struts were fastened, vascular status reassessed, and wound closed (Figures 2 and 3(a)). Postoperatively, the patient had no change in neurovascular status.

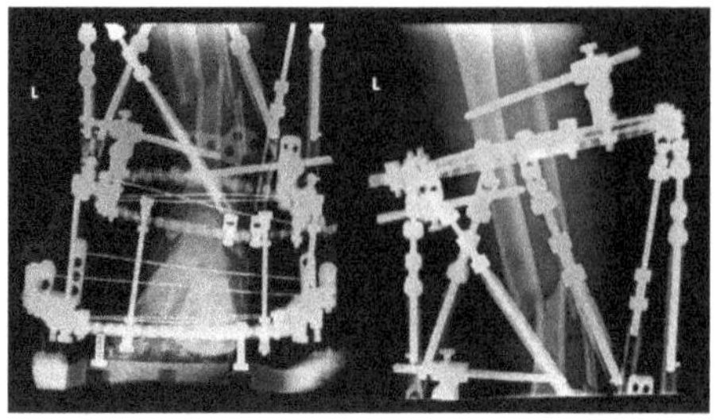

Figure 2: AP and lateral radiographs of the left leg illustrating the induced deformity created with the Taylor spatial frame to allow for primary soft-tissue wound closure.

Patient's sutures were maintained for four weeks (wound healed) at which point deformity correction commenced at a rate of 0.75 mm per day for a 27-day period (Figure 4). Throughout the 27-day period, the patient was evaluated weekly, the soft tissues remained intact, near-anatomic alignment was achieved, there were no signs or symptoms of infection, and the patient completed parenteral antibiotics prescribed by the infectious disease team to treat Enterobacter cloacae and Enterococcus faecalis. Once anatomic alignment was achieved, the fracture site was compressed, the foot ring was removed, the patient initiated weightbearing, and the patient was evaluated monthly. At week 24, the frame was removed as radiographic fracture union was achieved (Figure 5). At final follow-up (postoperative month 16), the patient displayed a nonantalgic gait, fully healed surgical sites (Figure 3(c)), and no signs of infection and was working full-time as an auto mechanic.

## 3. Discussion

This report demonstrates a confirmed case of septic arthritis following SPN of an open tibia fracture. Additionally, the patient's soft-tissue defect was closed primarily without a tissue transfer, and the fracture united without internal implants. External fixation following infection and soft tissue loss requires a significant compliance, but this report demonstrates that a desirable result may be achieved. Recently, definitive fixation via suprapatellar IMN has gained favor [5, 6, 9] due to stationary limb positioning resulting in improved fracture alignment and reduced fluoroscopy time [7, 8]. However, the risk of knee sepsis associated with an intra-articular starting point has not been defined in the setting of contaminated open fractures.

In 2017 and 2018, two studies evaluated the rates of knee sepsis associated with suprapatellar nailing of open tibia fractures [6, 9]. Mitchell et al. evaluated 139 open tibia fractures (type II (41%); type III (46%)) treated with suprapatellar nailing and only identified one case of knee sepsis which was attributed to an ascending necrotizing soft tissue infection that ultimately involved the knee joint [6]. Marecek et al. evaluated 289 fractures (type II (31%); type III (56%)) treated with either suprapatellar nailing

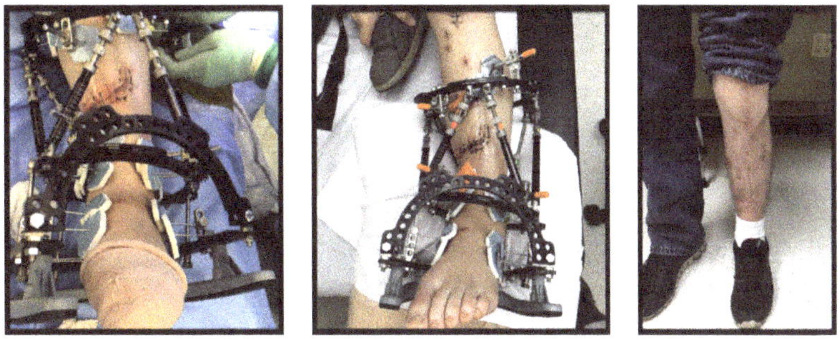

(a) (b) (c)

FIGURE 3: Clinical images demonstrating the acute deformity and soft-tissue closure (a) intraoperatively, (b) 1-week postoperatively, and (c) at final follow-up.

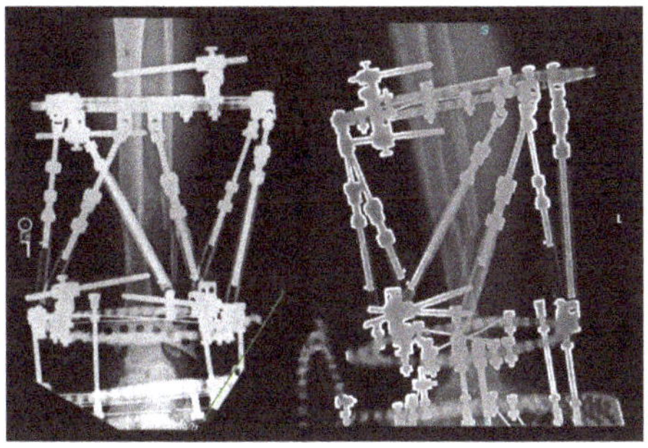

FIGURE 4: AP and lateral radiographs of the left leg demonstrating deformity correction after a 27-day period.

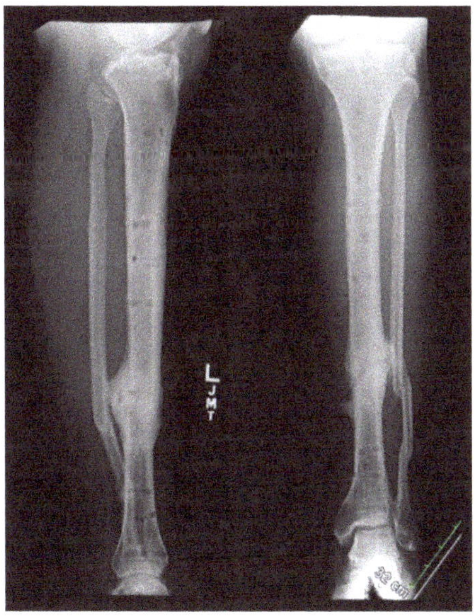

FIGURE 5: AP and lateral radiographs of the left leg show a united fracture at week 24.

($n = 147$) or infrapatellar nailing ($n = 142$). The authors reported two cases (1.4%) of knee sepsis in the suprapatellar group and zero cases (0%) in the infrapatellar group. It was concluded that the risk of knee sepsis following suprapatellar nailing is small but present [9]. Notably, both studies defined knee sepsis by positive aspiration. Marecek et al. reported two patients with "superficial infections" who presented with knee pain, swelling, and erythema. They were treated with antibiotics for presumed septic arthritis but were not included in the knee sepsis category because an aspiration was not obtained. As such, the incidence of knee sepsis following suprapatellar nailing of open fractures may be underestimated.

A common treatment for open tibia fractures with significant soft-tissue defects is the "fix and flap," which utilizes internal fixation and a rotational or free flap to close the soft-tissue defect [10, 11]. In our patient, there was a concern that placing an internal implant in the setting of knee sepsis contaminated intramedullary space, and soft tissue infection might create another substrate for microorganism colonization. While there is evidence supporting the maintenance of internal hardware in the setting of an acute postoperative infection [12], predictors of failure included the presence of an IMN or gram-negative infection, variables that were both present in our patient. Others suggest that external fixation for severe open tibial fractures may reduce the risk of infections when compared to internal fixation because no hardware is placed at the fracture site [13, 14]. In our patient, ring fixation ultimately permitted fracture stabilization in the setting of a postoperative infection and also enabled a concomitant soft-tissue reconstruction.

The use of intentional deformity to facilitate soft-tissue reconstruction has been described for a variety of posttraumatic conditions [15–17] including its combined use with local rotational flaps for large soft-tissue defects of the leg [18]. While the use of either a rotational flap or free-tissue transfer remains the standard of care, the factors that may limit its use include lack of access to a microvascular surgeon, patient preference, or patient is not a candidate for such a soft-tissue procedure. The current report further highlights that acute shortening with angular deformity can be effective and avoid the need for flap. In our case, the factors that permitted the technique to work included a soft-tissue void that could be primarily closed without compromising vascularity to the foot and having a fibula fracture at a level near that of the tibial injury to allow deformity in the direction of soft tissue loss.

Finally, given the intraoperative findings in our case, it is important to highlight the importance of meticulous debridement with wide excision of the involved soft tissue and bone in the surgical management of any open fracture.

## Disclosure

Dr. Frank Avilucea has the following disclosures: Zimmer Biomet: paid consultant; Orthopaedic Trauma Association: committee member.

## References


[1] C. M. Court-Brown, S. Rimmer, U. Prakash, and M. M. McQueen, "The epidemiology of open long bone fractures," *Injury*, vol. 29, no. 7, pp. 529–534, 1998.

[2] C. D. Weber, F. Hildebrand, P. Kobbe et al., "Epidemiology of open tibia fractures in a population-based database: update on current risk factors and clinical implications," *European Journal of Trauma and Emergency Surgery*, 2018.

[3] R. Gustilo and J. Anderson, "Prevention of infection in the treatment of one thousand and twenty-five open fractures of long bones: retrospective and prospective analyses," *The Journal of Bone & Joint Surgery*, vol. 58, no. 4, pp. 453–458, 1976.

[4] C. Papakostidis, N. K. Kanakaris, J. Pretel, O. Faour, D. J. Morell, and P. V. Giannoudis, "Prevalence of complications of open tibial shaft fractures stratified as per the Gustilo-Anderson classification," *Injury*, vol. 42, no. 12, pp. 1408–1415, 2011.

[5] D. S. Chan, R. Serrano-Riera, R. Griffing et al., "Suprapatellar versus infrapatellar tibial nail insertion: a prospective randomized control pilot study," *Journal of Orthopaedic Trauma*, vol. 30, no. 3, pp. 130–134, 2016.

[6] P. M. Mitchell, B. M. Weisenthal, and C. A. Collinge, "No incidence of postoperative knee sepsis with suprapatellar nailing of open tibia fractures," *Journal of Orthopaedic Trauma*, vol. 31, no. 2, pp. 85–89, 2017.

[7] Q. Sun, X. Nie, J. Gong et al., "The outcome comparison of the suprapatellar approach and infrapatellar approach for tibia intramedullary nailing," *International Orthopaedics*, vol. 40, no. 12, pp. 2611–2617, 2016.

[8] P. M. Courtney, A. Boniello, D. Donegan, J. Ahn, and S. Mehta, "Functional knee outcomes in infrapatellar and suprapatellar tibial nailing: does approach matter?," *American Journal of Orthopedics*, vol. 44, no. 12, pp. E513–E516, 2015.

[9] G. S. Marecek, L. T. Nicholson, F. H. Broghammer et al., "Risk of knee sepsis after treatment of open tibia fractures: a multicenter comparison of suprapatellar and infrapatellar approaches," *Journal of Orthopaedic Trauma*, vol. 32, no. 2, pp. 88–92, 2018.

[10] M. Godina, "Early microsurgical reconstruction of complex trauma of the extremities," *Plastic and Reconstructive Surgery*, vol. 78, no. 3, pp. 285–292, 1986.

[11] S. Gopal, P. V. Giannoudis, A. Murray, S. J. Matthews, and R. M. Smith, "The functional outcome of severe, open tibial fractures managed with early fixation and flap coverage," *The Bone & Joint Journal*, vol. 86-B, no. 6, pp. 861–867, 2004.

[12] M. Berkes, W. T. Obremskey, B. Scannell, J. K. Ellington, R. A. Hymes, and M. Bosse, "Maintenance of hardware after early postoperative infection following fracture internal fixation," *The Journal of Bone and Joint Surgery*, vol. 92, no. 4, pp. 823–828, 2010.

[13] M. Inan, M. Halici, I. Ayan, M. Tuncel, and S. Karaoglu, "Treatment of type IIIA open fractures of tibial shaft with Ilizarov external fixator versus unreamed tibial nailing," *Archives of Orthopaedic and Trauma Surgery*, vol. 127, no. 8, pp. 617–623, 2007.

[14] J. J. Keeling, D. E. Gwinn, S. M. Tintle, R. C. Andersen, and F. X. McGuigan, "Short-term outcomes of severe open wartime tibial fractures treated with ring external fixation," *The Journal of Bone and Joint Surgery-American Volume*, vol. 90, no. 12, pp. 2643–2651, 2008.

[15] K. G. Bundgaard and K. S. Christensen, "Tibial bone loss and soft-tissue defect treated simultaneously with Ilizarov-technique–a case report," *Acta Orthopaedica Scandinavica*, vol. 71, no. 5, pp. 534–536, 2009.

[16] A. Lerner, L. Fodor, M. Soudry, I. J. Peled, D. Herer, and Y. Ullmann, "Acute shortening: modular treatment modality for severe combined bone and soft tissue loss of the extremities," *The Journal of Trauma*, vol. 57, no. 3, pp. 603–608, 2004.

[17] A. Lerner, L. Fodor, H. Stein, M. Soudry, I. J. Peled, and Y. Ullmann, "Extreme bone lengthening using distraction osteogenesis after trauma: a case report," *Journal of Orthopaedic Trauma*, vol. 19, no. 6, pp. 423–427, 2005.

[18] M. J. Beltran, J. A. Blair, C. R. Rathbone, and J. R. Hsu, "The gradual expansion muscle flap," *Journal of Orthopaedic Trauma*, vol. 28, no. 1, pp. e15–e20, 2014.

# 4

# Complex Case of Open Fracture-Dislocation of the Elbow

**Tommy Primeau,[1,2] Philippe Beauchamp-Chalifour,[1,2] and Stéphane Pelet[1,2]**

[1]*Centre de Recherche FRQS du CHU de Québec—Hôpital Enfant-Jésus, 1401, 18ème Rue, (Québec), Québec, Canada G1J 1Z4*
[2]*Department of Orthopedic Surgery, CHU de Québec—Hôpital Enfant-Jésus, 1401, 18ème Rue, (Québec), Québec, Canada G1J 1Z4*

Correspondence should be addressed to Stéphane Pelet; stephane.pelet.ortho@gmail.com

Academic Editor: Johannes Mayr

Complex elbow instability is difficult to surgically address. Careful consideration of the fractures and soft tissue injuries is required. We present the case of a patient who sustained an open fracture-dislocation of the elbow with significant loss of the external humeral condyle and partial loss of the olecranon. He was surgically treated with an iliac crest tricortical autograft fixed with a buttress plate and a lag screw. His lateral ulnar collateral ligament was reconstructed with tendinous autograft collected from his third and fourth extensor *digitorum longus* tendons. While the procedure complicated with a *Nocardia* infection and wound breakdown, the patient almost had full range of motion without instability at 11 months of follow-up.

## 1. Introduction

The elbow is one of the most commonly dislocated joints, with an incidence of acute dislocation of 5.21 per 100 000 person-years [1]. Complex elbow instability consists of one or many osteoarticular fractures associated with capsular, ligament, and musculotendinous injuries, resulting in a global elbow instability [2].

The radial head and the coronoid process are the most commonly fractured structures in these injuries [3]. Six main types of complex elbow instability have been described: (1) radial head fractures with ligament injuries with or without dislocation, (2) coronoid process fractures with medial collateral ligament injury, (3) terrible triad injuries, (4) posterior Monteggia lesions, (5) transolecranon fracture-dislocation, and (6) shear fractures of the humerus with collateral ligament injury with or without dislocation [2].

Open fracture-dislocation of the elbow is still a very rare entity, and few case reports have described such injuries [4]. Thus, the optimal treatment for those patients remains unclear.

Management of these types of injury is complex and requires consideration of the fractures and soft tissue components. Improper management increases the risk of chronic elbow instability and posttraumatic arthritis [5].

This report presents a case of a patient with an open fracture-dislocation of the elbow with significant loss of the external humeral condyle and partial loss of the olecranon. To our knowledge, little information is available about the management of such case, and no similar cases have been previously described.

## 2. Case Report

A 39-year-old man was involved in a high-velocity motor vehicle accident. He sustained an open fracture of the right elbow, with significant loss of the external humeral condyle and partial loss of the olecranon. This fracture was classified as a *Gustillo* type IIIA injury. There was no neurovascular compromise. The patient was treated in a community center, close to the accident, where he received surgical care (debridement and partial excision of the olecranon). The wound was fully closed. The upper arm was then immobilized in a splint (Figure 1). IV antibiotics (cefazolin-gentamicin) were started for 5 days.

The day following his elbow surgery, the patient fell in a staircase and sustained a C7-C8 and C8-T1 fracture-dislocation. This injury caused neurologic damage (quadriparesis), and his right arm became his only functional limb. Following this injury, the patient was moved to our tertiary

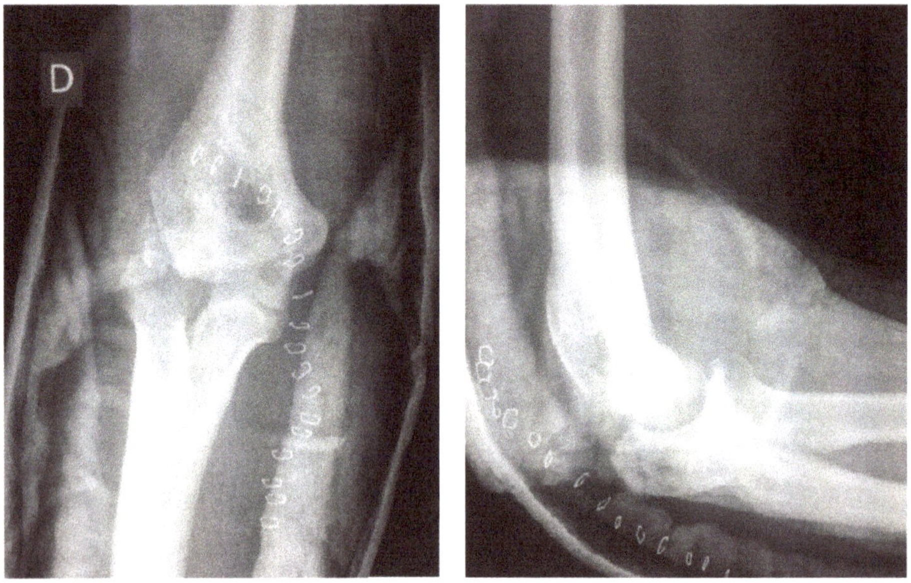


(a) (b)

Figure 1: (a) Anteroposterior view of the elbow and (b) lateral view of the elbow following surgical debridement and partial olecranon excision.

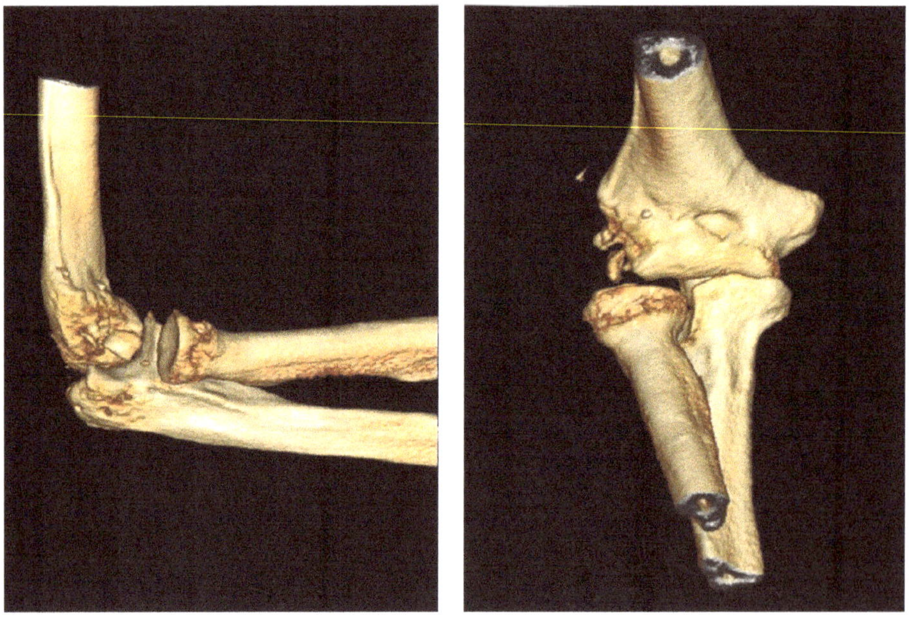

(a) (b)

Figure 2: (a) Lateral view and (b) anterior view of preoperative *3-D CT scan* reconstruction showing external condyle loss and radial head subluxation.

center to get spinal fusion. During the spinal surgery, the elbow was tested under fluoroscopy. The patient's elbow showed varus instability and a positive pivot shift test. A CT scan of the elbow was obtained the following day and showed bony loss from the external humeral condyle and subluxation of the radial head (Figure 2).

We decided to treat the patient's elbow surgically. The surgery underwent nine days after the initial trauma (after transfer from the community center, spine procedure and elbow imaging). A posterior approach to the elbow was used along with an extensive elbow debridement. A tricortical iliac crest graft was then collected from the patient's right side to replace the humeral condyle bone loss. A tendinous graft was collected from his third and fourth extensor *digitorum longus* tendons to reconstruct the lateral collateral ligament. The tendinous graft was fixed to the bone graft through two tunnels (anterior to posterior and lateral to medial). The iliac crest graft was then fixed to the humerus with a cancellous

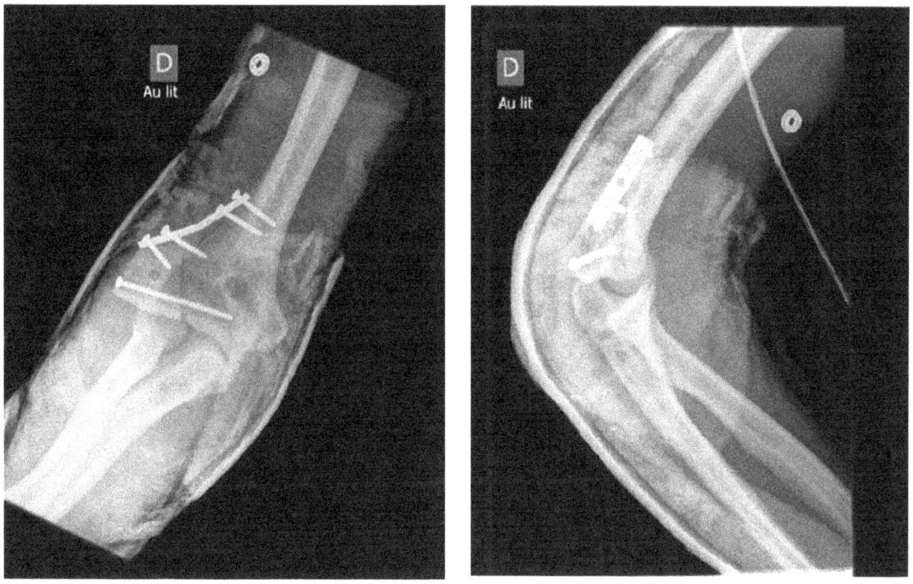


(a) (b)

FIGURE 3: (a) Anteroposterior and (B) lateral 14 days postoperative X-rays of the right elbow.

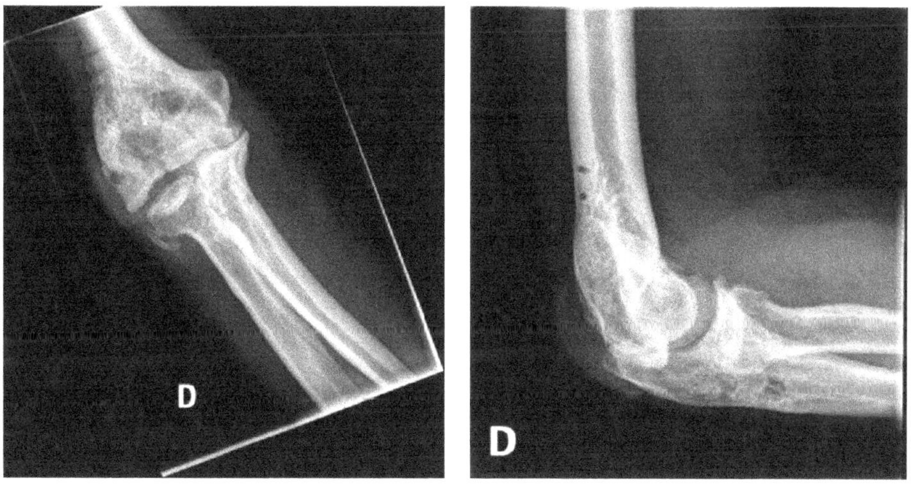


(a) (b)

FIGURE 4: (a) Anteroposterior and (b) lateral 11 months postoperative X-rays of the right elbow.

screw. A five-hole one-third tubular plate was used as buttress. The graft was left prominent on the lateral side to improve lateral stability of the elbow. The lateral collateral ligament was then reconstructed by fixing the tendinous graft to the proximal ulna with two bundles. We took care to preserve our reconstructed lateral collateral ligament's isometry during flexion and extension movements. Reduction and stability of the elbow joint were verified under fluoroscopy. The wound was closed with staples, and a posterior splint was applied for three weeks. 14 days postoperative X-rays are presented on Figure 3. At three weeks following the surgery, passive and active ranges of motion were initiated.

While wearing the splint, the patient developed a pressure wound on the lateral side of his elbow (at the site of the reconstruction). This wound later complicated into a *Nocardia* septic arthritis, which required surgical debridement. Four months after the reconstruction, range of motion was 30-120 degrees with full pronation and supination, without any evidence of instability.

Two months later, instrumentation was removed and a rotational flap was done to increase soft tissue coverage of the articulation. Five months after that procedure, the patient developed a *Nocardia* osteomyelitis of the humerus and was treated with 6 weeks of IV antibiotics (penicillin) and a surgical debridement. The patient responded well to our treatment. Eleven months after the initial intervention, range of motion of the joint ranged from 30 to 120 degrees of flexion, without clinical instability. Osteosynthesis was achieved according to X-rays of the elbow (Figure 4).

## 3. Discussion

Complex elbow instability is a very difficult pathology to surgically address. Morrey and An showed that the primary elbow stabilizers are the coronoid process, the olecranon, the humeral trochlea, and the collateral ligaments, while the secondary stabilizers are the radial head, the capitulum, the anterior capsule, the musculotendinous units, and the interosseous membrane [6]. Thus, it is essential to consider fractures as well as the soft tissue injuries in the treatment of complex elbow instability.

In our case, function restoration of the right elbow was especially important. The right arm was our patient's most useful limb considering his quadriparesis. As in every elbow injury, our main goals were to achieve stable osteosynthesis, correct and stable reduction, and to allow early range of motion.

Several options were possible for the bony reconstruction. Hattori et al. described a case of distal humeral fracture with significant bony loss treated with a tricortical iliac crest autograft [7]. They reported a good functional evolution at two years, despite the absence of articular cartilage [7]. Iliac crest autograft is also associated with a low risk of complications and allows surgeons to use a tricortical graft with a good amount of cancellous bone [8]. For those reasons, we choose this option for our bony reconstruction. As for other possible bone autografts, a case of bony reconstruction using a 1st metatarsophalangeal joint autograft for the elbow was described, but this technique resulted in important lateral instability following the surgery [9]. A total elbow arthroplasty or hemiarthroplasty is generally chosen in cases of low-demand elderly patients with osteoporosis [10, 11]. The high rate of complications associated with elbow arthroplasty, such as ulnar nerve injury, intraoperative fractures, triceps rupture, deep infection, and important functional limitations oriented our choice away from that option [10, 11]. As for arthrodesis, it is mainly considered a salvage procedure because of the complications and functional limitations associated [12]. In this case, since that arm needed to be the most functional one, we felt that arthrodesis was not the best solution. We also could have used allografts to reconstruct the bony defect, but the high rate of nonunion, resorption, and infection, especially in the case of an open fracture, led us away from that option [13].

O'Driscoll et al. have shown that the lateral ulnar collateral ligament is the main posterolateral stabilizer of the elbow, thus stressing the importance of its reconstruction [14]. Studies have shown that there is no advantage conferred by the use of a single or double-bundle reconstruction [15]. Classically, the *palmaris longus* is used, but was nonexistent in this patient [16]. The use of toe extensors has been described for collateral ligaments of the elbow but accounts for less than 2% of all autograft used according to a recent review of the literature and meta-analysis of 619 patients [17–19]. We although found the use of the third and fourth extensor *digitorum longus* tendons practical because of its easy retrieval and the fact that the patient would not be able to use his legs because of his spinal cord injury. *Gracilis* tendon, *semitendinous* tendon, triceps tendon, *plantaris* tendon, and extensor *carpi radialis longus* tendon have also been used for elbow ligament reconstruction [19]. However, we thought they would be harder to retrieve and add morbidity to the surgery. Allografts, especially the extensor *hallucis longus*, have also been used with good functional results [20]; although, they were used in chronic setting [20]. Synthetic grafts are still experimental options for elbow ligament reconstruction but have shown promising results [21]. Ten consecutive cases of chronic elbow instability have been surgically treated with a synthetic polyester ligament [21]. They were all stable at 27 months following surgery [21]. Many techniques have been described to reconstruct the lateral ulnar collateral ligament, but none was shown to be superior to the other (single versus double-stranded reconstruction) [15]. As for the tunnel to fix the ligament, its ideal location remains unclear due to prominence variability of the tubercule of the supinator crest [22]. A recent cadaveric study of seven patients comparing the stability of 70 tunnels using a double-stranded lateral ulnar collateral ligament found that reasonable elbow stability could be achieved as long as 1 of the 2 ulnar tunnels was located at or distal to the radial head-neck junction [23].

Following the surgery, the patient developed a pressure wound followed by infection because of the use of a splint. To avoid such complications, an elbow joint-overlapping external fixation as a first-staged fixation could have been used. Although a retrospective comparative study of 24 patients with an open or closed distal humerus fracture compared the use of primary external fixation and second-staged open reduction and internal fixation (ORIF) versus initial definitive ORIF [24]. With a median follow-up of 37 months, the study demonstrated higher complication rate and greater loss of extension for patients in the external fixation group (39 versus 17 degrees, $p = 0.048$, [24]. In our case, the reconstruction of the lateral epicondyle with an iliac crest autograft added to the complexity of the fracture, which drew us away from external fixation.

Complex elbow instability is a very challenging pathology for orthopaedic surgeons, especially in the case of an open fracture-dislocation. To our knowledge, no such case has been reported and makes the management of such injury difficult. We feel that the use of a tricortical iliac crest autograft to restore the bony architecture and the use of the third and fourth extensor *digitorum longus* tendons gave us the best chance to achieve good functional outcome for our patient. This was confirmed by the autograft osteointegration, the maintained reduction, the absence of instability, and the acceptable range of motion obtained at the eleven-month follow-up.

## References


[1] J. W. Stoneback, B. D. Owens, J. Sykes, G. S. Athwal, L. Pointer, and J. M. Wolf, "Incidence of elbow dislocations in the United States population," *The Journal of Bone and Joint Surgery-American Volume*, vol. 94, no. 3, pp. 240–245, 2012.

[2] G. Giannicola, F. M. Sacchetti, A. Greco, G. Cinotti, and F. Postacchini, "Management of complex elbow instability," *Musculoskeletal Surgery*, vol. 94, no. S1, pp. 25–36, 2010.

[3] K. A. Hildebrand, S. D. Patterson, and G. J. W. King, "Acute elbow dislocations : simple and complex," *Orthopedic Clinics of North America*, vol. 30, no. 1, pp. 63–79, 1999.

[4] D. Shivanna, B. Aski, D. Manjunath, and A. Bhatnagar, "A rare combination open fracture dislocation of elbow with open fracture both bones forearm with radial nerve palsy," *Journal of Orthopaedic Case Reports*, vol. 4, no. 2, pp. 13–16, 2014.

[5] M. A. Broberg and B. F. Morrey, "Results of treatment of fracture-dislocations of the elbow," *Clinical Orthopaedics and Related Research*, no. 216, pp. 109–119, 1987.

[6] B. F. Morrey and K. N. an, "Articular and ligamentous contributions to the stability of the elbow joint," *The American Journal of Sports Medicine*, vol. 11, no. 5, pp. 315–319, 1983.

[7] Y. Hattori, K. Doi, J. M. Pagsaligan, S. Takka, and K. Ikeda, "Arthroplasty of the elbow joint using vascularized iliac bone graft for reconstruction of massive bone defect of the distal humerus," *Journal of Reconstructive Microsurgery*, vol. 21, no. 5, pp. 287–291, 2005.

[8] P. C. Cavadas, L. Landin, A. Thione, J. Ibañez, P. Nthumba, and I. Roger, "Reconstruction of massive bone losses of the elbow with vascularized bone transfers," *Plastic and Reconstructive Surgery*, vol. 126, no. 3, pp. 964–972, 2010.

[9] M. Shibata, "Elbow joint reconstruction using metatarsophalangeal joint of the great toe," in *Experimental and Clinical Reconstructive Microsurgery*, pp. 496–501, Springer, Tokyo, Japan, 1st edition, 2003.

[10] L. P. Müller, S. Kamineni, P. M. Rommens, and B. F. Morrey, "Primary total elbow replacement for fractures of the distal humerus," *Operative Orthopädie und Traumatologie*, vol. 17, no. 2, pp. 119–142, 2005.

[11] K. J. Burkhart, S. Nijs, S. G. Mattyasovszky et al., "Distal humerus hemiarthroplasty of the elbow for comminuted distal humeral fractures in the elderly patient," *The Journal of Trauma: Injury, Infection, and Critical Care*, vol. 71, no. 3, pp. 635–642, 2011.

[12] L. M. Reichel, B. P. Wiater, J. Friedrich, and D. P. Hanel, "Arthrodesis of the elbow," *Hand Clinics*, vol. 27, no. 2, pp. 179–186, 2011.

[13] A. Ehsan, B. Lee, and J. M. Itamura, "Total elbow allografts with collateral ligament reconstruction for posttraumatic elbow injuries," *Journal of Orthopaedic Science*, vol. 15, no. 6, pp. 795–803, 2010.

[14] S. W. O'Driscoll, D. F. Bell, and B. F. Morrey, "Posterolateral rotatory instability of the elbow," *The Journal of Bone and Joint Surgery American Volume*, vol. 9, no. 2, pp. 240–246, 1991.

[15] G. J. W. King, C. E. Dunning, Z. D. S. Zarzour, S. D. Patterson, and J. A. Johnson, "Single-strand reconstruction of the lateral ulnar collateral ligament restores varus and posterolateral rotatory stability of the elbow," *Journal of Shoulder and Elbow Surgery*, vol. 11, no. 1, pp. 60–64, 2002.

[16] B. J. Erickson, J. D. Harris, P. N. Chalmers et al., "Ulnar collateral ligament reconstruction: anatomy, indications, techniques, and outcomes," *Sports Health*, vol. 7, no. 6, pp. 511–517, 2015.

[17] F. M. Azar, "Operative treatment of ulnar collateral ligament injuries of the elbow in athletes," *Operative Techniques in Orthopaedics*, vol. 11, no. 1, pp. 63–67, 2001.

[18] J. T. Rohrbough, D. W. Altchek, J. Hyman, R. J. Williams, and J. D. Botts, "Medial collateral ligament reconstruction of the elbow using the docking technique," *The American Journal of Sports Medicine*, vol. 30, no. 4, pp. 541–548, 2002.

[19] N. C. Hagemeijer, F. M. A. P. Claessen, R. de Haan, R. Riedijk, D. E. Eygendaal, and M. P. van den Bekerom, "Graft site morbidity in elbow ligament reconstruction procedures: a systematic review," *The American Journal of Sports Medicine*, vol. 45, no. 14, pp. 3382–3387, 2017.

[20] M. Conti Mica, P. Caekebeke, and R. van Riet, "Lateral collateral ligament injuries of the elbow—chronic posterolateral rotatory instability (PLRI)," *EFORT Open Reviews*, vol. 1, no. 12, pp. 461–468, 2016.

[21] G. J. K. Tawari, T. Lawrence, and D. Stanley, "Surgical reconstructions for posterolateral rotatory instability of elbow using a synthetic ligament," *Shoulder & Elbow*, vol. 5, no. 4, pp. 251–255, 2013.

[22] O. A. Anakwenze, K. Khanna, W. N. Levine, and C. S. Ahmad, "Characterization of the supinator tubercle for lateral ulnar collateral ligament reconstruction," *Orthopaedic Journal of Sports Medicine*, vol. 2, no. 4, article 232596711453096, 2014.

[23] H. M. Kim, C. R. Andrews, E. P. Roush, G. I. Pace, and G. S. Lewis, "Effect of ulnar tunnel location on elbow stability in double-strand lateral collateral ligament reconstruction," *Journal of Shoulder and Elbow Surgery*, vol. 26, no. 3, pp. 409–415, 2017.

[24] C. Kösters, S. Lenschow, E. Schulte-Zurhausen, S. Roßlenbroich, M. J. Raschke, and B. Schliemann, "Management of comminuted fractures of the distal humerus: clinical outcome after primary external fixation versus immediate fixation with locking plates," *Archives of Orthopaedic and Trauma Surgery*, vol. 137, no. 12, pp. 1693–1698, 2017.

# 5

# Presumed Glenoid SLAP Tear in an Adolescent Football Player Belied the Presence of a Coracoid Growth Plate Fracture: A Diagnostic Conundrum

**John G. Skedros, J. Hunter Marshall, and John T. Cronin**

*Utah Orthopaedic Specialists, Salt Lake City, Utah, USA*

Correspondence should be addressed to John G. Skedros; jskedrosmd@uosmd.com

Academic Editor: George Mouzopoulos

We report the case of a 13-year-old male who sustained a right shoulder injury while playing quarterback in an American football game. A noncontrast MRI scan showed evidence of a possible grade 1 SLAP tear (SLAP = superior labral anterior-posterior), and surgery was recommended. However, at the preoperative visit, the surgeon was suspicious that the main source of pain had been missed. Bilateral shoulder radiographs taken for comparative analysis revealed a Salter-Harris type I coracoid growth-plate fracture. Therefore, the surgeon planned to manage the patient nonoperatively and postponed the proposed SLAP tear surgery. The patient was instructed to cease participation in athletic events and undergo physical therapy. Hoping to expedite his healing with platelet or stem cell injections, the parents sought an opinion from another physician who obtained a right shoulder MRI with intra-articular contrast. This confirmed that there was no SLAP tear. We concluded that the patient initially had glenohumeral and coracoclavicular ligament strains and a coracoid growth-plate fracture. The SLAP tear suggested by the initial MRI proved to be a red herring, belying an accurate diagnosis. The patient ultimately recovered fully with physical therapy and without surgery or other interventions.

## 1. Introduction

As participation in athletics increases among the pediatric population, reported cases of shoulder injuries are rising [1–3]. Therefore, the probability that a physician will see a patient with a relatively rare fracture or injury, such as a Salter-Harris type I fracture of the coracoid process, is also increasing. This case is presented to spotlight coracoid physeal injuries as a consideration when evaluating pediatric patients for shoulder pain.

Our patient is a 13-year-old male who was initially seen for a right shoulder injury after a fall. A SLAP tear was suggested on a noncontrast MRI scan. At the time of a preoperative evaluation for repair of this suspected lesion, the surgeon recognized the possibility that the patient might have a Salter-Harris type I fracture of the coracoid growth plate in addition to anterior glenohumeral capsular ligament and coracoclavicular ligament (CCL) strains. This fracture diagnosis was confirmed with bilateral axillary-lateral radiographs showing evidence of damage to the growth plate on the injured side and a nearly fused growth plate on the opposite side. He was managed conservatively.

## 2. Case Presentation

A healthy 13-year-old Caucasian male was referred to our clinic for persistent right shoulder pain after a fall in an American football game weeks earlier. At the time of the injury, he dove for a loose ball and fell on the lateral aspect of his right shoulder. He was unable to continue to play due to pain from the injury. There was no evidence of a shoulder dislocation. The patient was initially treated and monitored by his primary care physician, who felt after several weeks of persistent pain the patient should consult with an orthopedic surgeon.

The patient first visited our clinic 7.5 weeks after the injury. Physical examination revealed mild tenderness with palpation over and lateral to the coracoid process and with crossed body adduction and shoulder impingement maneuvers (Hawkin's and Neer). There was also a mild positive sulcus sign, and with the patient supine, there was mild anterior subluxation with passive abduction and external rotation of his right shoulder (i.e., positive apprehension test). Anterior-posterior, scapula-Y, and axillary-lateral radiographs of the right shoulder showed a patent growth plate that was not considered atypical at that time because of the patient's age. An MRI without contrast was ordered of the right shoulder for suspected injury to the joint capsule and/or labrum.

The parents were anticipating that the next appointment would be to schedule shoulder surgery because they had seen the MRI report that stated that there was "irregular linear increased T2 signal within the superior labrum directed away from the glenoid" (Figure 1(a)). At that time, neither the radiologist nor orthopedic surgeon recognized the increased T2 signal in the bone near the coracoid growth plate might represent injury. Recognizing the rarity of SLAP tears in adolescents who did not have a shoulder dislocation, we tried to identify other potential sources of the patient's pain that had not been considered at the first consultation. Consequently, at his second visit to our clinic, radiographs were taken of each shoulder and showed a nearly fused main (basilar) growth plate of the left (non-injured) coracoid, while the right coracoid growth plate was still patent and had mild heterogeneity in contour suggestive of a Salter-Harris type I fracture (Figure 2). Notably, the epiphyseal plate of the coracoid process in normal healthy adolescents mirrors the contralateral side and generally closes symmetrically by 18 years of age [4, 5]. But bilateral asymmetry of closure of the main coracoid growth plate has been described in 3 of 131 (2.3%) modern skeletons in a sample from Portugal [5]. In this context, we concluded that different radiographic appearances of our patient's coracoids also supported the diagnosis of a nondisplaced growth plate fracture. His pain persisted primarily because of his continued attempts to participate in athletic activities in the setting of concomitant ligament injuries. He was enrolled in a physical therapy program, and a three-month follow-up appointment was scheduled.

During the interim between this last clinical visit and the next follow-up appointment, the patient again strained his right shoulder after falling on the playground at school. His parents sought a second opinion at an outside clinic that specialized in managing pain with injections, especially stem cells and platelet-rich plasma (PRP). They expressed concern to us that we were not treating their son as aggressively as they deemed necessary, and they also hoped that such injections might help enhance healing. At that other clinic, an MRI with intra-articular contrast of the right shoulder was ordered. This second shoulder MRI was 3.5 months after the first MRI. The region of the superior labrum that previously appeared to show a tear did not fill with gadolinium, indicating the abnormality was not a SLAP tear but rather a vascular or developmental variant (Figure 2(b)).

At the third visit to our clinic (four months after the first visit), another radiograph of the right shoulder was taken that showed that the injured coracoid growth plate was fusing. Physical examination showed mild anterior shoulder subluxation with mild subacromial pain. Continued physical therapy was recommended to address what we ultimately considered to be the most significant lingering problem (anterior subluxation from ligament stretch injury). The patient did not receive any supplemental injections. Three months later, he had no pain and was able to play quarterback in football without pain or any other limitations.

## 3. Discussion

This case highlights nuances that are important to consider when evaluating a suspected glenoid SLAP tear in an adolescent patient. The incidence and epidemiology of SLAP tears in adolescents have not been systematically studied and reported in a large number of patients. A few studies from pediatric hospitals have published retrospective case data regarding glenohumeral labral pathologies and generally report relatively low prevalence rates in this demographic group [6–8]. For example, Zbojniewicz et al. [8] reviewed 205 shoulder arthroscopy cases of patients aged 8-18 years and compared MRI findings to the intraoperative arthroscopic findings and found only nine (4.4%) cases with labral tears. The prevalence of glenoid labral pathology is most likely much lower [9] because this sample was biased towards shoulder pathologies. However, as participation in athletics increases among the pediatric population, reported cases of shoulder injuries are rising [1–3].

Diagnosing glenoid labral tears requires a combination of clinical evaluation and proper imaging techniques. Based on the mild sulcus sign and mild anterior subluxation, further evaluation of our patient's glenohumeral joint was warranted. However, as evidenced in our case, standard MR imaging may not provide the level of specificity that is required to correctly identify nonpathological labrums. MR arthrography (MRA) provides a more optimal visualization of intra-articular structures [10].

In patients aged <18 years, scapular fractures account for 0.33% of all fractures, with a peak incidence at the age of 14 years in males and 11 years in females [11, 12]. It is estimated that coracoid fractures comprise less than <10% of scapular fractures [11]. Ogawa et al. [13] segregated coracoid fractures into two main categories: type-1 is any fractures proximal to the coracoclavicular ligament (CCL) attachments, and type-2 is fractures distal to the CCL attachments. In pediatric patients, Ogawa type-1 fractures of the coracoid process predominate due to the relative difference in strength between the CCLs (relatively stronger) and physeal cartilage (relatively weaker). This explains why adolescents who play sports are at a higher risk of sustaining a coracoid physeal injury [11, 14]. Due to the very low prevalence and typically nondisplaced nature of these fractures, they often go undiagnosed upon initial evaluation. This is what happened in our patient.

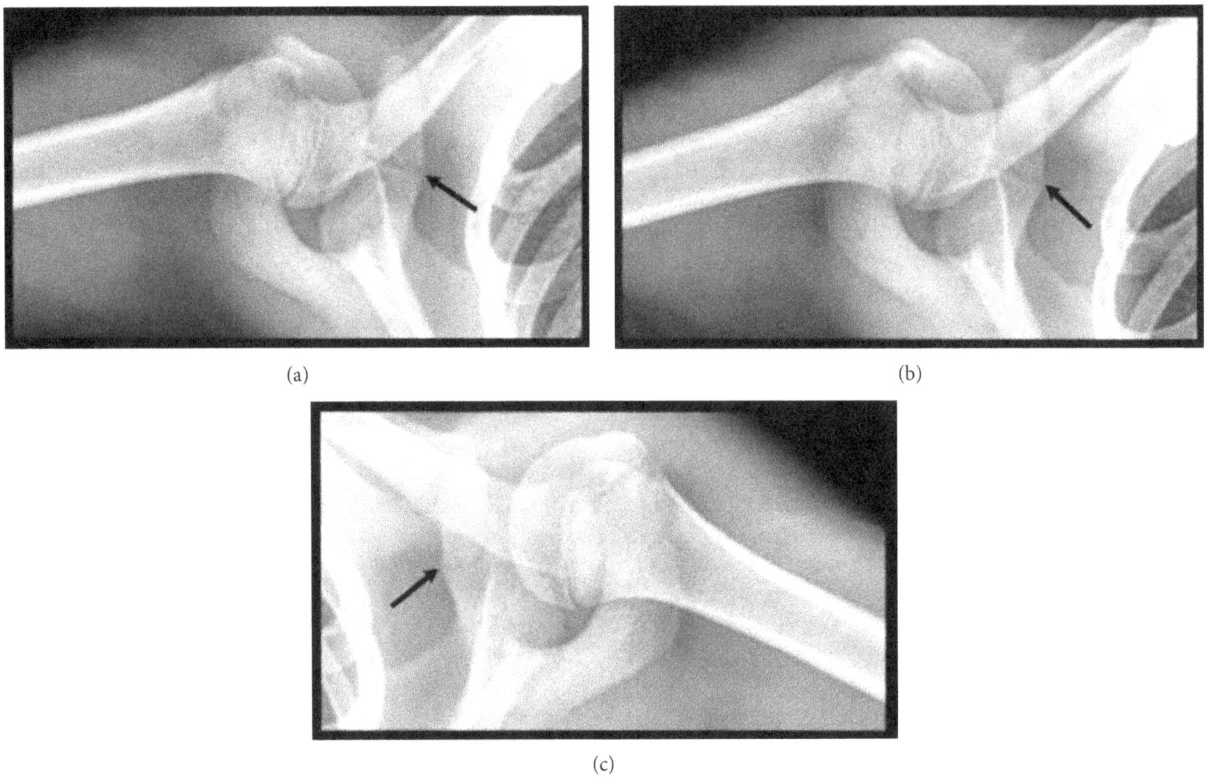


FIGURE 1: (a) Radiograph of injured shoulder taken at first clinical visit (12/27/2018) (7.5 weeks after the injury). (b) Radiograph of injured shoulder taken at the second clinical visit (1/31/2019) (approximately 11 weeks after the index injury). Note that the lucency extends across the entire coracoid. (c) Radiograph of contralateral (noninjured) shoulder taken at second clinical visit. Note that the lucency at the medial aspect of the coracoid is much less obvious when compared to the injured side.

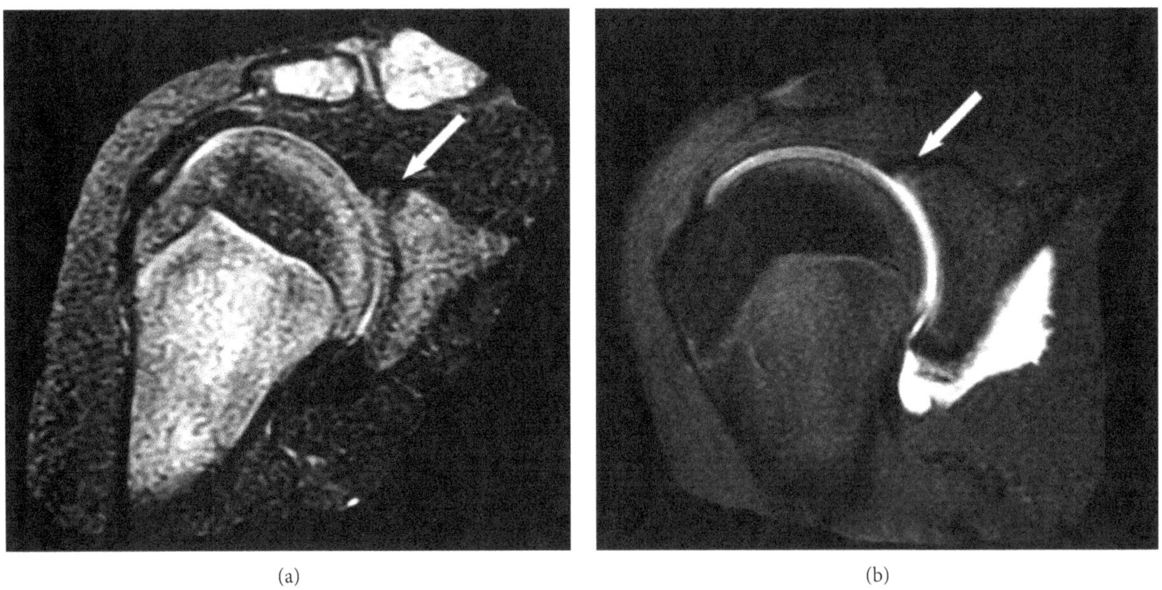


FIGURE 2: MR images of the patient's injured shoulder. Arrows point to the suspected SLAP tear in both images. (a) This image was taken approximately 11 weeks after the index injury. (b) This image is from the second MRI, which was approximately 27 weeks after the index injury. Because T2-weighted imaging was not performed during the second MRI scan, a direct comparison cannot be made to part (a). Also, the left (noninjured) shoulder was not evaluated with MRI.

Additionally, coracoid fractures are difficult to detect with typical radiographic views and require specific patient positioning for radiographic identification (e.g., angle-up view, anterior oblique view, or scapular-Y view) [11, 15–17]. When using these specialized views, radiography is usually sufficient for diagnosing acute coracoid physeal injuries [18].

Despite these potential diagnostic challenges, coracoid physeal injury should be considered when evaluating a pediatric patient for shoulder pain [19, 20]. As demonstrated by the clinical data reported by Mondori et al. [21], simultaneous fracture of the coracoid epiphysis and labral tear is not likely. Of the 37 patients that they describe with epiphyseal separation of the coracoid, none had injury to the glenohumeral labrum. Although these results are limited because only 10% of the cases reviewed underwent MRI examination, their findings are clear—the coexistence of a labrum tear and a coracoid growth plate is not likely in pediatric patients. They reported that the typical injury associated with a coracoid physeal injury is an acromioclavicular joint injury, which is what also occurred in our case. The grade 1 acromioclavicular strain that our patient had is also similar to the concomitant injury in the three additional case reports of patients 9, 13, and 14 years old [22–24]. These three additional cases also lacked evidence of significant labral injury. Generally, nondisplaced fractures of the coracoid are treated conservatively as are also most acromioclavicular injuries in adolescents [25–31]. Ogawa et al. [11] reported that 79% of pediatric patients with coracoid physeal injuries were successfully treated with conservative methods.

## 4. Conclusion

When evaluating a pediatric patient with posttraumatic shoulder pain, coracoid physeal injury should be considered in the differential diagnosis. This demographic is particularly susceptible to chondral shear injuries at the coracoid physis due to the relatively stronger CCLs pulling traction on the coracoid. The prevalence of SLAP tears in the pediatric population is exceedingly low, and the suspected presence of this injury in our patient's initial MRI scan belied an accurate diagnosis. He ultimately had a full recovery without surgery.

## Consent

The patient and his parents gave consent for the writing and publication of this case report.

## References

[1] T. W. Robinson, J. Corlette, C. L. Collins, and R. D. Comstock, "Shoulder injuries among US high school athletes, 2005/2006-2011/2012," *Pediatrics*, vol. 133, no. 2, pp. 272–279, 2014.

[2] J. E. Moyer and J. M. Brey, "Shoulder injuries in pediatric athletes," *The Orthopedic Clinics of North America*, vol. 47, no. 4, pp. 749–762, 2016.

[3] J. T. Aoyama, P. Maier, S. Servaes et al., "MR imaging of the shoulder in youth baseball players: anatomy, pathophysiology, and treatment," *Clinical Imaging*, vol. 57, pp. 99–109, 2019.

[4] J. Freyschmidt, J. Wiens, A. Sternberg, and J. Brossmann, *Freyschmidt's "Koehler/Zimmer" Borderlands of the Normal and Early Pathological Findings in Skeletal Radiography*, Thieme, Stuttgart, 5th edition, 2003.

[5] H. Coqueugniot and T. D. Weaver, "Brief communication: infracranial maturation in the skeletal collection from Coimbra, Portugal: new aging standards for epiphyseal union," *American Journal of Physical Anthropology*, vol. 134, no. 3, pp. 424–437, 2007.

[6] E. W. Edmonds, J. H. Roocroft, and S. N. Parikh, "Spectrum of operative childhood intra-articular shoulder pathology," *Journal of Children's Orthopaedics*, vol. 8, no. 4, pp. 337–340, 2014.

[7] E. A. Eisner, J. H. Roocroft, and E. W. Edmonds, "Underestimation of labral pathology in adolescents with anterior shoulder instability," *Journal of Pediatric Orthopedics*, vol. 32, no. 1, pp. 42–47, 2012.

[8] A. M. Zbojniewicz, M. E. Maeder, K. H. Emery, and S. R. Salisbury, "Rotator cuff tears in children and adolescents: experience at a large pediatric hospital," *Pediatric Radiology*, vol. 44, no. 6, pp. 729–737, 2014.

[9] X. Li, R. Ma, N. M. Nielsen, L. V. Gulotta, J. S. Dines, and B. D. Owens, "Management of shoulder instability in the skeletally immature patient," *The Journal of the American Academy of Orthopaedic Surgeons*, vol. 21, no. 9, pp. 529–537, 2013.

[10] A. V. Mohana-Borges, C. B. Chung, and D. Resnick, "Superior labral anteroposterior tear: classification and diagnosis on MRI and MR arthrography," *American Journal of Roentgenology*, vol. 181, no. 6, pp. 1449–1462, 2003.

[11] K. Ogawa, W. Inokuchi, and N. Matsumura, "Physeal injuries of the coracoid process are closely associated with sports activities: a systematic review," *Orthopaedic Journal of Sports Medicine*, vol. 8, no. 12, 2020.

[12] C. Cooper, E. M. Dennison, H. G. Leufkens, N. Bishop, and T. P. van Staa, "Epidemiology of childhood fractures in Britain: a study using the general practice research database," *Journal of Bone and Mineral Research*, vol. 19, no. 12, pp. 1976–1981, 2004.

[13] K. Ogawa, A. Yoshida, M. Takahashi, and M. Ui, "Fractures of the coracoid process," *Journal of Bone and Joint Surgery. British Volume*, vol. 79-B, no. 1, pp. 17–19, 1997.

[14] G. W. V. Cross, P. Reilly, and M. Khanna, "Salter-Harris type 1 coracoid process fracture in a rugby playing adolescent," *BJR Case Reports*, vol. 4, no. 3, 2018.

[15] A. I. Froimson, "Fracture of the coracoid process of the scapula," *The Journal of Bone and Joint Surgery. American Volume*, vol. 60, no. 5, pp. 710-711, 1978.

[16] R. P. Goldberg and B. Vicks, "Oblique angled view for coracoid fractures," *Skeletal Radiology*, vol. 9, no. 3, pp. 195–197, 1983.

[17] J. J. Protass, F. V. Stampfli, and J. C. Osmer, "Coracoid process fracture diagnosis in acromioclavicular separation," *Radiology*, vol. 116, no. 1, pp. 61–64, 1975.

[18] D. P. Shi, S. C. Zhu, Y. Li, and J. Zheng, "Epiphyseal and physeal injury: comparison of conventional radiography and magnetic resonance imaging," *Clinical Imaging*, vol. 33, no. 5, pp. 379–383, 2009.

[19] E. F. Alaia, Z. S. Rosenberg, I. Rossi et al., "Growth plate injury at the base of the coracoid: MRI features," *Skeletal Radiology*, vol. 46, no. 11, pp. 1507–1512, 2017.

[20] I. Anwar, D. Amiras, M. Khanna, and M. Walker, "Physes around the shoulder girdle: normal development and injury patterns," *Clinical Radiology*, vol. 71, no. 7, pp. 702–709, 2016.

[21] T. Mondori, Y. Nakagawa, S. Kurata et al., "New system for the classification of epiphyseal separation of the coracoid process: evaluation of nine cases and review of the literature," *Advances in Orthopedics*, vol. 2020, Article ID 9749515, 9 pages, 2020.

[22] T. Mwaturura and R. Bourne, "An unusual cause of shoulder pain: undisplaced Salter-Harris type I fracture of the coracoid process," *American Journal of Orthopedics*, vol. 38, no. 6, pp. E101–E103, 2009.

[23] I. Taga, M. Yoneda, and K. Ono, "Epiphyseal separation of the coracoid process associated with acromioclavicular Sprain," *Clinical Orthopaedics and Related Research*, vol. 207, pp. 138–141, 1986.

[24] A. K. Holst, J. V. Christiansen, and A. K. Holst, "Epiphyseal separation of the coracoid process without acromioclavicular dislocation," *Skeletal Radiology*, vol. 27, no. 8, pp. 461-462, 1998.

[25] P. G. van Doesburg, S. El Saddy, T. D. Alta, A. van Noort, and C. J. van Bergen, "Treatment of coracoid process fractures: a systematic review," *Archives of Orthopaedic and Trauma Surgery*, vol. 141, no. 7, pp. 1091–1100, 2021.

[26] J. W. Galvin, J. Kang, R. Ma, and X. Li, "Fractures of the coracoid process: evaluation, management, and outcomes," *The Journal of the American Academy of Orthopaedic Surgeons*, vol. 28, no. 16, pp. e706–e715, 2020.

[27] D. M. Knapik, S. H. Patel, R. J. Wetzel, and J. E. Voos, "Prevalence and management of coracoid fracture sustained during sporting activities and time to return to sport: a systematic review," *The American Journal of Sports Medicine*, vol. 46, no. 3, pp. 753–758, 2018.

[28] M. DiPaola and P. Marchetto, "Coracoid process fracture with acromioclavicular joint separation in an American football player: a case report and literature review," *American Journal of Orthopedics*, vol. 38, no. 1, pp. 37–39, 2009.

[29] V. Pedersen, W. C. Prall, B. Ockert, and F. Haasters, "Non-operative treatment of a fracture to the coracoid process with acromioclavicular dislocation in an adolescent," *Orthopedic Reviews*, vol. 6, no. 3, pp. 103–106, 2014.

[30] A. R. Chitre, H. M. Divecha, M. Hakimi, and H. A. Marynissen, "Traumatic isolated coracoid fractures in the adolescent," *Case Reports in Orthopedics*, vol. 2012, Article ID 371627, 4 pages, 2012.

[31] K. Thomas, V. Y. Ng, and J. Bishop, "Nonoperative management of a sagittal coracoid fracture with a concomitant acromioclavicular joint separation," *International Journal of Shoulder Surgery*, vol. 4, no. 2, pp. 44–47, 2010.

# 6

# Hook Plate Technique for Bony Mallet Thumb

**Fumihiro Mukasa**,[1,2] **Yoshimasa Tomita**,[1] **Hideyuki Hirasawa**,[1] **and Kazuo Kaneko**[2]

[1]*Department of Orthopedic Surgery, Tokyo Rosai Hospital, 4-13-21, Omori-minami, Ota-ku, Tokyo 143-0013, Japan*
[2]*Department of Orthopedic Surgery, Juntendo University School of Medicine, 3-1-3, Hongo, Bunkyo-ku, Tokyo 113-8431, Japan*

Correspondence should be addressed to Fumihiro Mukasa; fumihiro_m1009@yahoo.co.jp

Academic Editor: Elke R. Ahlmann

Bony mallet is a common sport injury, but bony mallet thumb is rarely encountered. We performed open reduction and fixation of bony mallet thumb using a hook plate procedure on a 27-year-old man under general anesthesia. The patient began working one day after surgery. Six months postoperatively, the patient had excellent dexterity according to Crawford's evaluation criteria and no difficulties at work or playing softball. Tension band fixation, compression pins, and the extension block technique are commonly used to manage bony mallet. Despite the anatomical reduction, rigid fixation, and early resumption of motion skills offered by the hook plate technique, to our knowledge, no previous reports of its application to bony mallet thumb were found. In this case, the hook plate technique was chosen and made an early return to work possible and brought about a successful result.

## 1. Introduction

Mallet finger is a common sport injury, but bony mallet thumb is rarely encountered because the thumb is shorter than the other fingers and the extensor pollicis longus (EPL) is thicker than the other extensors [1]. It is reported that bony mallet thumb has been managed by tension band fixation, compression fixation pins, or the extension block technique [2–4]. The anatomical reduction, rigid fixation, early resumption of motion activity, and early return to the work offered by the hook plate technique for bony mallet finger have not previously been reported in bony mallet thumb injuries, so far as we know. This is the first report that the hook plate technique was applied to the bony mallet thumb.

## 2. Case Report

The patient was a 27-year-old man who sprained his right thumb while playing softball, resulting in tenderness and swelling around the interphalangeal (IP) joint. He was a software engineer, and his dominant hand was the right hand. Physical examination revealed complete loss of active extension and also that passive extension and active flexion of the IP joint were full. The IP joint was stable against radial and ulnar stress. The images of plain radiography and computed tomography showed an avulsion fracture of one-third to half of its articular surface at the base of the distal phalanx (Figure 1). Using the hook plate technique, open reduction was performed under general anesthesia 19 days after the injury (Figure 2). An incision was made along the crease on the dorsal side of the IP joint. The fracture was reduced and fixed using a hook plate adapted from a 1.5 mm micro module (KLS Martin, Germany, Figure 3(a)). One of the holes was cut, and one-third of its circumference was removed. The ends of the crescent arc were bent approximately 100° by pliers to form two sharp pointed hooks (Figure 3(b)). Two small longitudinal incisions were made at the EPL. The hook plate was slid under the nail matrix, the hooks were inserted through the slips, and the bone fragment was gripped. The screw was inserted into the plate hole to add compression to the fragment. The articular congruency and stability of the fragment in the direction of passive flexion were checked, and the wound was closed.

The splint was maintained for 1 week before motion of the IP joint was allowed, and the patient returned to work 1 day after surgery. Bone union was achieved and the plate

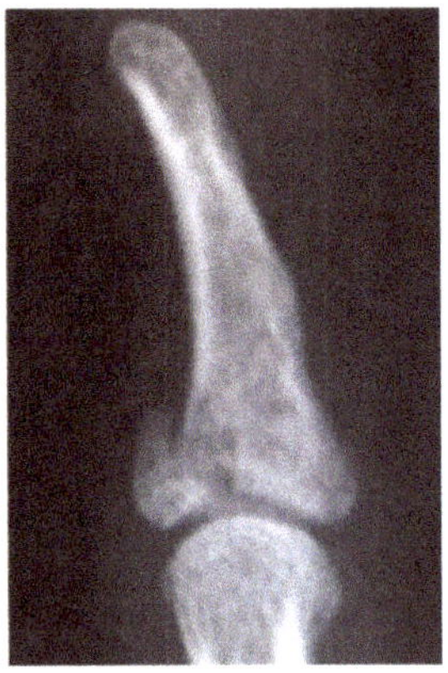

FIGURE 1: Lateral radiograph at the injury site.

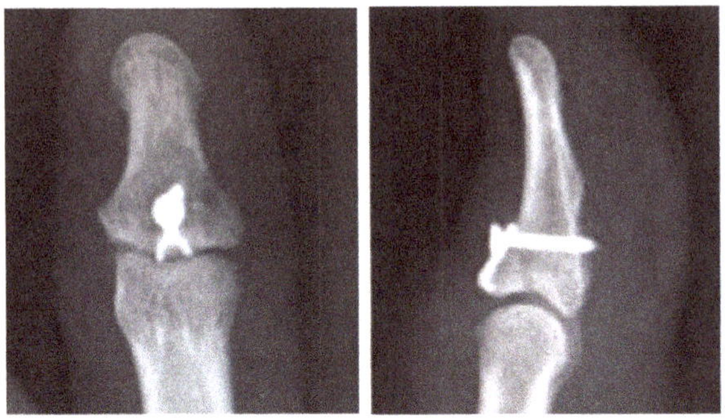

FIGURE 2: The radiograph images after reduction and fixation.

was removed 3 months after the procedure (Figure 4). At the last follow-up of 6 months after surgery, the active range of motion at the IP joint was 80 degrees of flexion and 8 degrees of extension. The range of motion on the contralateral side was 85 degrees of flexion and 10 degrees of extension (Figures 5(a) and 5(b)). The patient had a transverse line nail deformity (Figure 6) that gradually improved. According to Crawford's evaluation criteria [5], the result was excellent. The patient experienced no injury-related difficulties both at work and while playing softball.

## 3. Discussion

Bony mallet thumb is a very rare injury, only one in 160 mallet fractures according to Wehbe and Schneider [6]. The thumb is protected because it is shorter than the other fingers and the EPL is thicker than those of other fingers [1]. Bony mallet thumb requires more precise reduction and more rigid fixation than the other bony mallet fingers because the thumb's terminal tendon is short, approximately 4 mm [7], and the range of extension at the IP joint is larger than those of the other DIP joints. Therefore, extension lag can easily result from deformity of the IP joint surface.

The surgical options for bony mallet thumb include tension band fixation, compression fixation pins, and the extension block technique [2–4]. Teoh and Lee and Theivendran et al. have described the use of the hook plate technique for bony mallet finger, but not bony mallet thumb, to obtain anatomical reduction and stable fixation with early mobilization

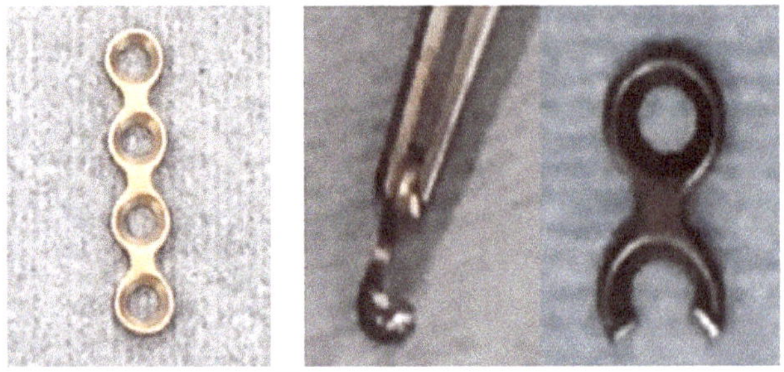

(a) (b)

FIGURE 3: The 1.5 mm mini plate before (a) and after the plate was modified by cutting the hole and bending the ends of crescent arc (b).

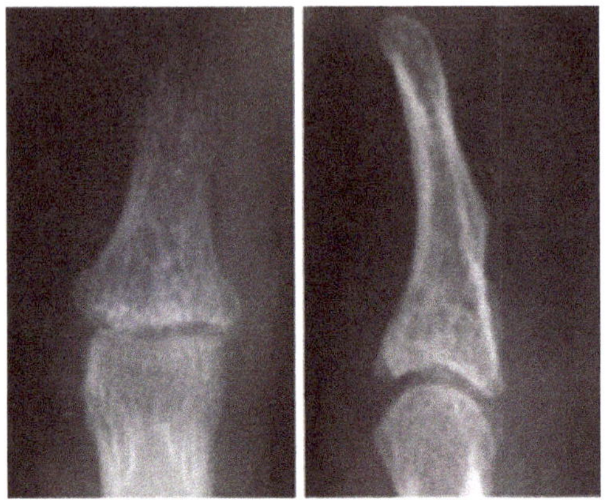

FIGURE 4: Follow-up radiographs showing the healed fracture.

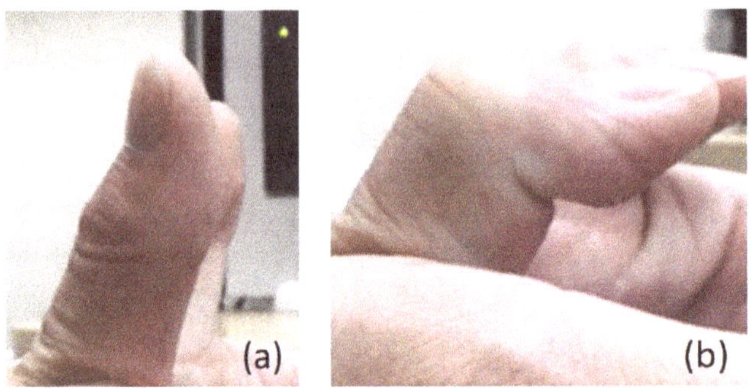


(a) (b)

FIGURE 5: Active range of motion of the IP joint of 8° of extension (a) and 90° of flexion (b).

[8, 9]. In this patient, the hook plate technique was used to repair bony mallet thumb and achieve satisfactory anatomical reduction and rigid fixation without requiring percutaneous pins, which allowed early resumption of motion activity. He was a software engineer and was able to resume work which required the use of a computer keyboard. The extension block technique (Ishiguro's method) and its modifications are very good options for the bony mallet finger, because they were reported to be easier than open reduction and obtain successful results [10]. But the extension block technique cannot allow early mobilization and requires meticulous percutaneous pin care. So, if the extension block technique had been used, he would not have resumed work

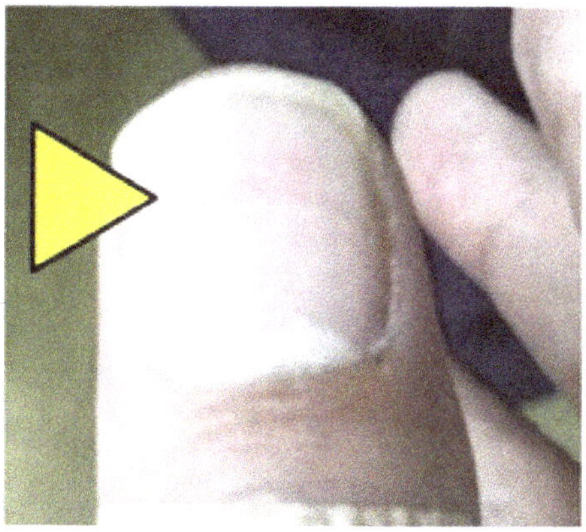

FIGURE 6: Transverse line deformity of the nail that gradually disappeared.

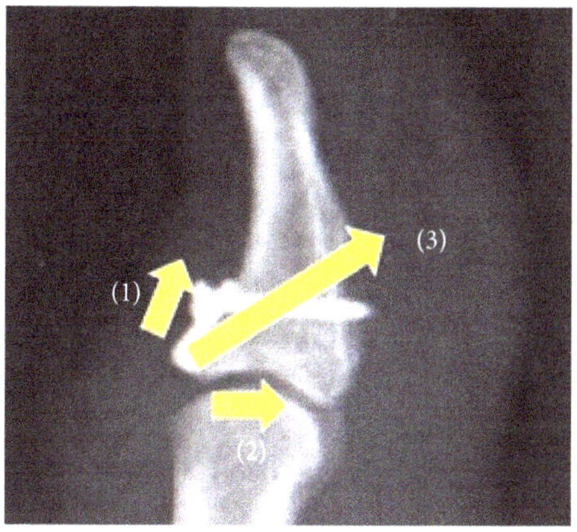


FIGURE 7: The mechanism of compression force generation involved. (1) Force in the distal direction produced by the hook. (2) Force in the horizontal direction produced by the screw and plate. (3) Compression force is applied to the fragment.

so early. When considering early resumption of work, the hook plate technique seems to be a good indication.

The hook plate technique has advantages that include control and anatomical reduction of even large dorsal fragments and can be used to manage thin or avulsion fractures. It can also apply compression and stability to the fragment. The hook produces the force in the distal direction (Figure 7 (1)), the screw and the plate produce the force in the horizontal direction (Figure 7 (2)), and they are combined to be a compression force applied to the fragment (Figure 7 (3)). The hook plate technique permits early resumption of joint motion and does not require meticulous percutaneous pin care [8]. The reported postoperative complications of the hook plate technique include articular cartilage damage, nail deformities, extensor tendon lesions, and skin irritation [8]. Damage of the articular cartilage of the middle phalanx head may result from inadequate length or shape of the hook. In this patient, the hook was placed into the distal fragment through the EPL and articular cartilage damage did not occur. Nail deformities can occur following damage of the nail matrix by the screw or the plate, but the deformity that occurred in this patient did not occur when the plate was located. The deformity may have happened at the time of injury. The nail matrix is located close to the bony insertion of the terminal extensor tendon. The distance from the terminal extensor tendon insertion to the proximal edge of the germinal nail matrix is approximately 1.2 mm [11]. If the hook plate rests on the nail bed, damage of the germinal nail matrix will produce nail deformity. As the hook plate was placed under the nail matrix, the chance of nail deformity was minimized.

Teoh and Lee reported stable fixation and early mobilization with the use of the hook plate technique in mallet finger [8]. However, to the best of our knowledge, no previous cases have reported the use of the hook plate technique for bony mallet thumb. According to this case experience, the hook plate technique can be recommended as an option for the treatment of bony mallet thumb. Further follow-up is needed to assess the long-term benefits of this technique for managing mallet thumb, including the incidence of osteoarthritis. In conclusion, although not a minimally invasive surgery, the hook plate technique offers good anatomical reduction and rigid fixation. It allows early resumption of motion and provides satisfactory results in a patient with bony mallet thumb. And it is considered that when the early return to work is required, the hook plate technique seems to be a good indication.

## References


[1] T. Yamada, Y. Kino, Y. Hattori et al., “Treatment of closed mallet thumb,” *Rinsho Seikei Geka*, vol. 27, pp. 1311–1314, 1992.

[2] R. Bischoff, U. Buechler, R. De Roche, and J. Jupiter, “Clinical results of tension band fixation of avulsion fractures of the hand,” *The Journal of Hand Surgery*, vol. 19, no. 6, pp. 1019–1026, 1994.

[3] K. Yamanaka and T. Sasaki, “Treatment of mallet fractures using compression fixation pins,” *Journal of Hand Surgery*, vol. 24, no. 3, pp. 358–360, 1999.

[4] R. Nishimura, S. Matsuura, T. Miyawaki, and M. Uchida, “Bony mallet thumb,” *Hand Surgery*, vol. 18, no. 01, pp. 107–109, 2013.

[5] G. P. Crawford, “The molded polythene splint for mallet finger deformities,” *The Journal of Hand Surgery*, vol. 9, no. 2, pp. 231–237, 1984.

[6] M. A. Wehbe and L. H. Schneider, “Mallet fractures,” *The Journal of Bone and Joint Surgery. American Volume*, vol. 66, no. 5, pp. 658–669, 1984.

[7] A. B. Dagum and J. L. Mahoney, “Effect of wrist position on extensor mechanism after disruption separation,” *The Journal of Hand Surgery*, vol. 19, no. 4, pp. 584–589, 1994.

[8] L. C. Teoh and J. Y. L. Lee, “Mallet fractures: a novel approach to internal fixation using a hook plate,” *Journal of Hand Surgery (European Volume)*, vol. 32, no. 1, pp. 24–30, 2007.

[9] K. Theivendran, A. Mahon, and V. Rajaratnam, "A novel hook plate fixation technique for the treatment of mallet fractures," *Annals of Plastic Surgery*, vol. 58, no. 1, pp. 112–115, 2007.

[10] A. Darder-Prats, E. Fernandez-Garcia, R. Fernandez-Gabarda, and A. Darder-Garcia, "Treatment of mallet finger fractures by the extension-block K-wire technique," *Journal of Hand Surgery*, vol. 23, no. 6, pp. 802–805, 1998.

[11] C. Shum, R. J. Bruno, S. Ristic, M. P. Rosenwasser, and R. J. Strauch, "Examination of the anatomic relationship of the proximal germinal nail matrix to the extensor tendon insertion," *The Journal of Hand Surgery*, vol. 25, no. 6, pp. 1114–1117, 2000.

7

# Prosthetic Joint Infection of a Revision Knee Arthroplasty with *Candida parapsilosis*

**Martine Christine Keuning,[1] Aziz Al Moujahid,[2] and Wierd Pieter Zijlstra[1]**

[1]*Department of Orthopaedic Surgery, Medical Center Leeuwarden, Leeuwarden, Netherlands*
[2]*Center for Infectious Diseases Friesland, Izore, Leeuwarden, Netherlands*

Correspondence should be addressed to Martine Christine Keuning; m.c.keuning@isala.nl

Academic Editor: Dimitrios S. Karataglis

We report a case of an infected total knee arthroplasty with *Candida parapsilosis*. The patient was successfully treated with a two-stage exchange arthroplasty, local antifungal treatment, and systemic antifungal treatment. This specific combination therapy to treat *C. parapsilosis* joint infection has not been previously reported.

## 1. Introduction

Prosthetic joint infections (PJIs) continue to pose challenges in total joint arthroplasty. Although PJIs are a dreaded complication and a common cause of revision surgery, treatment guidelines have made gram-positive or gram-negative PJIs controllable. A rare PJI, though increasing in prevalence, is a fungal infection. Fungal PJI represents 1% of all PJIs [1–3].

If fungal pathogens are isolated from periprosthetic tissue or joint aspirations, it can be considered a fungal PJI. Isolating the infecting organism can be a challenge with fungi, and repeated joint aspiration may be needed [4]. Management of fungal PJI, surgical as well as therapeutic, is considered more challenging due to the higher risk of persistent infection [5]. Current literature advises a two-stage exchange arthroplasty, combined with local and systemic antifungal therapy to manage fungal PJI [3–7].

Systemic as well as local antifungals can be used in medical treatment of the fungal PJI. Most frequent agents for a systemic treatment are fluconazole and amphotericin B given either orally or intravenously [4, 5]. Local antifungal agent administration can be applied by implanting an impregnated cement spacer, by placing intra-articular powder, or by daily intra-articular lavage. From these three, spacers loaded with antifungal drugs have mainly been reported [4].

PJIs with fungi are referred to as difficult to treat, and treatment has not yet been well described [1, 3, 5, 7]. Relatively few case reports and literary reviews have been published assessing a fungal PJI, mostly following different treatment regimens. Due to its rarity, no standard guidelines exist for the diagnosis and treatment of these infections. Recent proceedings of the International Consensus Meeting on Periprosthetic Joint Infection, though based on limited level of evidence, did establish recommendations regarding fungal PJI [4].

Our case describes a case of an infected total knee arthroplasty with *Candida parapsilosis*. The patient was successfully treated with a two-stage exchange arthroplasty, local antifungal treatment, and unique systemic antifungal treatment.

## 2. Case Report

A 72-year-old woman, diagnosed with rheumatoid arthritis and psoriasis, received a right total knee arthroplasty (TKA) in August 2009 for primary arthrosis with complaints of a large Baker's cyst. The procedure and follow-up went uneventfully. In May 2016, the patient returned with large swelling in the right knee cavity. A white cell scan showed signs of a prosthetic joint infection of the TKA. A DAIR (debridement, antibiotics, and implant retention) was performed on June 10 (2016) and because of persistent wound

Table 1: *Candida parapsilosis* antibiogram.

| Antifungal agent | MIC (mg/l) | EUCAST guidelines | | Interpretation |
|---|---|---|---|---|
| | | Susceptible | Resistant | |
| Amphotericin B | **0.125** | **1** | **1** | Susceptible |
| Anidulafungin | **0.5** | **0.002** | **4** | Susceptible |
| Caspofungin | **1** | Note 1 | Note 1 | |
| Fluconazole | **2** | **2** | **4** | Susceptible |
| Micafungin | **0.25** | **0.002** | **2** | Susceptible |
| Voriconazole | **0.063** | **0.125** | **0.25** | Susceptible |

Note 1: EUCAST breakpoints have not yet been established for caspofungin, due to significant interlaboratory variation in MIC ranges for caspofungin.

leakage again on June 27. All cultures remained sterile. No clinical improvement was followed, and therefore, the TKA was removed on July 14 (2016) and a cement spacer was placed. These cultures showed *Staphylococcus aureus* and *Staphylococcus epidermidis*, for which antibiotic treatment was started. The therapeutic regimen consisted of flucloxacillin 1200 mg daily intravenously combined with rifampicin 450 mg twice daily for 2 weeks, followed by moxifloxacin 400 mg once daily combined with rifampicin 450 mg twice daily for 6 weeks.

In February 2017, the right TKA was reimplanted (Scorpio NRG, posterior stabilized), whilst vancomycine was given. The perioperative cultures remained negative, and the vancomycine was stopped after 2 weeks and replaced with linezolid for 4 weeks. Patient follow-up in the months after the reimplantation was good, and there were no signs of infection, until January 2018, when she returned with swelling and pain in the right knee. On admission, laboratory studies revealed the following: C-reactive protein (CRP) (16 mg/ml) and erythrocyte sedimentation rate (ESR) (67 mm/h). X-ray of the knee showed a total knee prosthesis with no signs of loosening or osteolysis. A white cell scan was done which was inconclusive. A preoperative diagnostic arthrocentesis was performed. The drained synovial fluid was sent to the clinical microbiological laboratory for culture. By day 3 of incubation, the culture showed yeast using BBL CHROMagar Candida Medium (Becton Dickinson). The yeast was identified as *Candida parapsilosis* by using MALDI-TOF-MS (matrix-assisted laser desorption ionization/time-of-flight mass spectrometry). A diagnosis of chronic infection of total knee arthroplasty with *C. parapsilosis* was established. After which, the decision to undertake a two-stage revision procedure was made. The *C. parapsilosis* isolate showed susceptibility to voriconazole (minimum inhibitory concentration (MIC), 0.063 $\mu$g/ml), amphotericin B (MIC, 0.125 $\mu$g/ml), 5-fluorocytosine (MIC, 0.125 $\mu$g/ml), fluconazole (MIC, 2 $\mu$g/ml), micafungin (MIC, 0.25 $\mu$g/ml), anidulafungin (MIC, 1 $\mu$g/ml), and caspofungin (MIC, 1 $\mu$g/ml) (Table 1). An antifungal susceptibility test was performed according to the European Committee on Antimicrobial Susceptibility Testing (EUCAST) criteria. Minimal inhibitory concentrations (MICs) were established by using a microdilution-based method, and the MICs were interpreted according to the EUCAST breakpoint (Table 1).

On March 8, 2018, the TKA was extracted. After the joint had been accessed via the preexisting incision, the patient underwent rigorous debridement of infected and devitalized tissues. The total knee arthroplasty components were removed. Once debridement was performed, the joint was extensively irrigated using iodine and 6 l of saline solution. After preparation of the joint cavity, an amphotericin B-impregnated spacer was inserted. During this procedure, 8 separate intraoperative tissue samples from various anatomical sites were collected and sent for culture. After 3 days of incubation, all eight intraoperative cultures showed *C. parapsilosis*. Blood cultures remained negative. Postoperatively, combination antifungal therapy was started. The patient was treated with intravenous voriconazole (with a loading dose of 6 mg/kg twice daily on the first day, followed by a maintenance dose of 4 mg/kg twice daily) and micafungin 200 mg once daily. Intravenous combination antifungal treatment was maintained for 4 weeks before switching to oral voriconazole monotherapy 300 mg twice daily for additional 4 weeks. Two weeks after taking the medication, the patient experienced a moderate alteration of liver enzyme levels, which was attributed to the use of micafungin. Therefore, the dose of micafungin was reduced from 200 mg to 100 mg once daily for 5 days until the enzyme levels returned to normal.

On May 18, 2018, the TKA was reimplanted. Two weeks before reimplantation, voriconazole was discontinued in order to obtain reliable tissue samples for culture. During this surgical procedure, the spacer was removed and a new semi-constrained prosthesis with a stemmed tibial component (Triathlon Total Stabilizer) was implanted. Augmentation was used for the femur (5 medial and 10 lateral) and tibia (10 medial). Also, several tissue samples were obtained preoperatively and sent for culture. Postoperatively, the patient received cefuroxime empirically and 2 weeks of combination therapy of intravenous voriconazole (with a loading dose of 6 mg/kg twice daily on the first day for 2 doses, followed by a maintenance dose of 4 mg/kg twice daily) and micafungin 200 mg once daily. After two weeks of incubation, culture of intraoperative specimen during reimplantation yielded one colony of *C. parapsilosis* in one out of seven samples with the same antibiogram as described previously; therefore, the intravenous regimen was followed up by 2 weeks of voriconazole 300 mg twice daily. Since bacterial cultures remained negative, cefuroxime was discontinued after 7 days.

Since reimplantation, the patient has been doing well and there have been no more complaints of pain and dysfunction of the knee. She reports no functional impairment. The last follow-up was June 2019. Lab results then showed CRP of 4 mg/ml, BSE of 56 mm/h (which can be related to rheumatoid arthritis), and white blood cell count of $9.7 \times 10^9$.

## 3. Discussion

The treatment of fungal prosthetic joint infections remains a diagnostic and therapeutic challenge. A fungal PJI is difficult to eradicate, partly because of the considerable diagnostic delay for weeks to months due to the indolent clinical presentation. Repeated removal and reimplantation of the prosthetic joint may be necessary, sometimes resulting in a permanent removal of the prosthetic joint. Chance of failure (persistent infection) after surgical and antifungal treatment is 15-23% [5, 6, 8]. These infections often occur in immunocompromised patients (our patient has a medical history of rheumatoid arthritis) and patients who underwent previous surgeries of the affected joint (which also applies to our patient) [4–6].

We therefore considered this PJI difficult to treat. Following standard PJI guidelines and current literature on fungal PJIs [4, 5], the patient was therefore treated with a two-stage exchange arthroplasty. This treatment regimen involved removal of the implant, a rigorous surgical debridement, placement of a spacer supplemented with antifungals mixed with the bone cement, and a new combination of systemic antifungal therapy. We believe that this combination made reimplantation of the TKA thus far successful.

Due to the lack of clinical trials and the paucity of reported cases, the optimal treatment strategy for patients with fungal PJI remains a topic of discussion. The therapeutic approach is mainly based on reported experience and anecdotal evidence. Biofilm formation is considered a virulence factor of *C. parapsilosis* in PJI. To eradicate these infections, prolonged antifungal treatment with an antifungal agent that displays good biofilm activity is required. Micafungin is an example with these properties against *Candida* species.

Recent evaluation studies of susceptibility of *Candida* biofilms showed that the echinocandins, particularly micafungin, had the highest antifungal activities [9]. The use of systemic amphotericin B to treat osteomyelitis is not recommended [10]. Voriconazole achieves adequately high therapeutic concentrations in bone tissue, and micafungin is active against slow-growing organisms and biofilms. Given the mentioned pharmacokinetics and pharmacodynamics and the low MIC value of voriconazole, the combination of voriconazole and micafungin was considered an ideal therapeutic option to manage this infection.

To the best of our knowledge, this combination therapy to treat *C. parapsilosis* joint infection has not been previously reported and makes this case report unique.

## 4. Conclusion

Based on the positive therapeutic result of this case of PJI with *Candida parapsilosis*, we would advise a two-stage exchange arthroplasty combined with local antifungals mixed in bone cement and the combination of systemic voriconazole and micafungin as a new treatment option.

## Consent

The patient described in this case report gave her informed consent for the inclusion in this publication.

## Acknowledgments

We appreciate the advice provided by Prof. Dr. P.E. Verweij of Radboud University.

## References

[1] R. O. Darouiche, R. J. Hamill, D. M. Musher, E. J. Young, and R. L. Harris, "Periprosthetic candidal infections following arthroplasty," *Clinical Infectious Diseases*, vol. 11, no. 1, pp. 89–96, 1989.

[2] S. Kurtz, K. Ong, E. Lau, F. Mowat, and M. Halpern, "Projections of primary and revision hip and knee arthroplasty in the United States from 2005 to 2030," *The Journal of Bone and Joint Surgery. American Volume*, vol. 89, no. 4, pp. 780–785, 2007.

[3] B. Schoof, O. Jakobs, S. Schmidl et al., "Fungal periprosthetic joint infection of the hip: a systematic review," *Orthopedic Reviews*, vol. 7, no. 1, 2015.

[4] K. Belden, L. Cao, J. Chen et al., "Hip and knee section, fungal Periprosthetic joint infection, diagnosis and treatment: proceedings of international consensus on orthopedic infections," *The Journal of Arthroplasty*, vol. 34, no. 2S, pp. S387–S391, 2019.

[5] J. Nace, A. Siddiqi, C. T. Talmo, and A. F. Chen, "Diagnosis and management of fungal periprosthetic joint infections," *The Journal of the American Academy of Orthopaedic Surgeons*, vol. 27, no. 18, pp. e804–e818, 2019.

[6] J. W. P. Kuiper, M. P. J. van den Bekerom, J. van der Stappen, P. A. Nolte, and S. Colen, "2-stage revision recommended for treatment of fungal hip and knee prosthetic joint infections: An analysis of 164 patients, 156 from the literature and 8 own cases," *Acta Orthopaedica*, vol. 84, no. 6, pp. 517–523, 2013.

[7] O. Jakobs, B. Schoof, T. O. Klatte et al., "Fungal periprosthetic joint infection in total knee arthroplasty: a systematic review," *Orthopedic Reviews*, vol. 7, no. 1, 2015.

[8] F. Cobo, J. Rodríguez-Granger, A. Sampedro, L. Aliaga-Martínez, and J. M. Navarro-Marí, "*Candida* prosthetic joint infection. A review of treatment methods," *Journal of Bone and Joint Infection*, vol. 2, no. 2, pp. 114–121, 2017.

[9] M. Seidler, S. Salvenmoser, and F. M. Muller, "In vitro effects of micafungin against *Candida* biofilms on polystyrene and central venous catheter sections," *International Journal of Antimicrobial Agents*, vol. 28, no. 6, pp. 568–573, 2006.

[10] I. Stratov, T. M. Korman, and P. D. R. Johnson, "Management of *Aspergillus* osteomyelitis: report of failure of liposomal amphotericin B and response to voriconazole in an immunocompetent host and literature review," *European Journal of Clinical Microbiology and Infectious Diseases*, vol. 22, no. 5, pp. 277–283, 2003.

8

# Lisfranc Sprain with Second Metatarsal Base Adaptive Stress Response in High-Level Athletes: Case Series and Novel Perspective on a Distinct Entity of Chronic Low-Energy Lisfranc Injury

**WanYin Lim,[1,2] Jonathan Heysen,[1] James Ilic,[3] Ben Beamond,[2,4] and Steven Zadow[1,5]**

[1]*Dr Jones and Partners Medical Imaging, 226 Greenhill Road, Eastwood, South Australia 5063, Australia*
[2]*Radiology Department, Royal Adelaide Hospital, 1 Port Rd, South Australia 5000, Australia*
[3]*Wakefield Sports and Exercise Medicine Clinic, Calvary Adelaide Hospital, South Australia, Australia*
[4]*Wakefield Orthopaedic Clinic, Calvary Adelaide Hospital, South Australia, Australia*
[5]*Flinders Medical Centre, South Australia, Australia*

Correspondence should be addressed to WanYin Lim; ynyn146@gmail.com

Academic Editor: Johannes Mayr

Lisfranc injury is increasingly being recognised in the high-performance athletic cohort, particularly in contact sports. In this cohort, there is a pattern of low-energy Lisfranc injury which combines magnetic resonance findings of both ligamentous sprain and adaptive bone stress response that infers a longer timeframe of stress than the duration of symptoms would suggest. This has not been previously described, and the authors believe that this is an unrecognized subset of midfoot sprain in the context of sustained stress to the midfoot. This retrospective case report describes MRI findings of three index cases of this entity in professional athletes presenting with acute foot pain. Two responded with conservative management whilst the third ultimately required surgery. All athletes were eventually able to return to play.

## 1. Introduction

Foot injury accounts for 16% of all sports-related injuries of which low-energy Lisfranc injury is uncommon but increasingly being diagnosed, presumably from the increased awareness of this condition and the increased use of magnetic resonance imaging (MRI) in imaging of foot pain [1–5]. In contact sports such as soccer and American football where running, jumping, and twisting of the foot in plantarflexion are common, the Lisfranc injury incidence can be as high as 1.9-4% per year [5–7]. This pattern of injury is quoted to have a misdiagnosis rate of up to 39% at first presentation, although the actual prevalence or rate of underdiagnosis is unknown, with significant long-term consequences which include career-ending morbidity [7].

In elite international athletes that we have imaged in the acute setting, we have noticed a pattern of Lisfranc injury that has not been previously described, which includes a mixed picture of acute Lisfranc sprain and chronic adaptive response of the Lisfranc bone unit. It has also come to the authors' attention that there is a relative paucity in radiology literature on Lisfranc ligamentous injury in athletes with low-energy Lisfranc injuries.

This manuscript showcases three high-level athletes with Lisfranc ligament injury demonstrating chronic stress response in the metatarsal bases. It provides a hypothesis for the imaging findings.

## 2. Case Presentation

This is a retrospective study from January 2019 to June 2020. Three international athletes who presented to the radiology clinic for investigation of acute-onset foot pain were identified. All the studies were reported by dedicated musculoskeletal radiologists with combined experience of 45 years.

*2.1. Case 1.* A 19-year-old international-level male soccer player presents with a two-week history of midfoot pain, worse with running. This occurred during an overseas match. There was no single traumatic event recalled. There was no other medical comorbidity. Routine panel of metabolic and blood screen including calcium and vitamin-D level was normal at the start of the season.

The MRI showed localized marrow oedema signal centered at the base of the second metatarsal with suspicion of an avulsion fracture at the footprint of the plantar Lisfranc ligament (Figure 1(a)). The cortex of the metatarsal base was thickened, with intracortical fluid-hyperintense signal present, consistent with chronic stress response. The Lisfranc ligament was thickened and returns intermediate signal with surrounding soft tissue oedema, compatible with a grade II sprain or partial tear (Figures 1(b) and 1(c)).

The undisplaced avulsion fracture was confirmed on computed tomography (CT) (Figures 1(d) and 1(e)).

He was treated conservatively with protected weight-bearing for 6 weeks with good outcome and was able to return to baseline shortly after.

*2.2. Case 2.* An 18-year-old male Australian footballer presents with sudden onset midfoot pain, exacerbated by running and jumping.

The MRI demonstrated localized marrow oedema signal at the plantar margin of the second metatarsal base (Figure 2(a)). This involved both the interosseous and plantar Lisfranc footprints. There was periligamentous oedema without a ligamentous fiber disruption or elongation, consistent with grade I sprain (Figure 2(a)).

There was second metatarsal cortical thickening centered around the ligamentous attachments (Figure 2(b)). This was also treated conservatively, with return to play after 3 months.

*2.3. Case 3.* A 29-year-old female elite soccer player presents with nonspecific, 1-day history of foot pain during an international soccer tournament. She was unable to complete warmup. There was no history of trauma recalled. There is no significant past medical history apart from mild asthma.

On assessment, she had an antalgic gait.

On imaging, there was periligamentous oedema surrounding the otherwise-intact plantar Lisfranc ligament (Figure 3). Plantar cortical thickening was indicative of adaptive response. Intracortical fluid hyperintensity was also present, suggesting progression to a higher-grade stress response and impending fracture.

Patient had to be taken out of the soccer tournament. Following a 3-month period of failed conservative management, this was surgically managed as a nonhealing stress fracture with drilling and plate fixation of the second metatarsal base. She responded well to treatment and was able to return to game at prior baseline level.

## 3. Discussion

The Lisfranc ligamentous complex confers stability to the tarsometatarsal (TMT) articulation by providing structural support to the transverse arch of the mid- and forefoot. The first intermetatarsal space is held by the dorsal, interosseous, and plantar ligaments extending from the medial cuneiform to the base of the second metatarsal. These three ligaments constitute the Lisfranc proper [4, 8]. The interosseous ligament connects the medial cuneiform to the base of the second metatarsal whilst the plantar Lisfranc ligament connects the medial cuneiform to the base of second and third metatarsals. These two are considered the strongest ligaments in the Lisfranc ligamentous complex and are the primary stabilizer to the medial and middle column of the midfoot [4, 8]. This arrangement allows the foot to perform as a lever arm that propels the foot forward during the gait cycle [9].

Injuries to this Lisfranc complex can be differentiated into high-impact or low-impact trauma. The low-impact trauma, also coined midfoot sprain, constitutes up to a third of Lisfranc injuries and will be the main focus of this manuscript [10]. These are usually a result of indirect forces applied to the foot when the foot is in certain fixed positions. The most common mechanism of injury is when the forefoot is abducted and plantarflexed in a fixed position, such as in the context of sudden rotational change in the direction that occurs during tackling. This results in the weight of the body being placed on the tarsometatarsal joints, resulting in ligamentous failure. More commonly, in sports requiring cleated shoe wear, the mechanism for the injury is from rigidly planted forefoot in a plantarflexed position, resulting in force being transmitted along the metatarsals longitudinally and resulting in compressive forces being applied to the TMT joints and Lisfranc ligament [1, 4]. An example of this is a person or weight falling onto the heel of a plantar-flexed foot of another player who is on the ground [4].

There is a three-stage classification system for low-energy Lisfranc injury or midfoot sprains coined by Nunley and Vertullo [11]. This classification is based on weight-bearing radiographs, measuring the degree of diastasis between the medial cuneiform and the base of the second metatarsus, with increased widening indicating higher-grade injuries [11, 12]. They hypothesized that the dorsal ligament, being the weakest, is the most commonly injured component, followed by injury of the interosseous Lisfranc ligament and then the plantar, as more substantial forces are applied. This classification usually implies an acute injury and does not include MRI findings [13]. Proximal variant patterns of instability have also been described, with transmission of force extending proximally through the intercuneiform joints and exiting via the navicular-

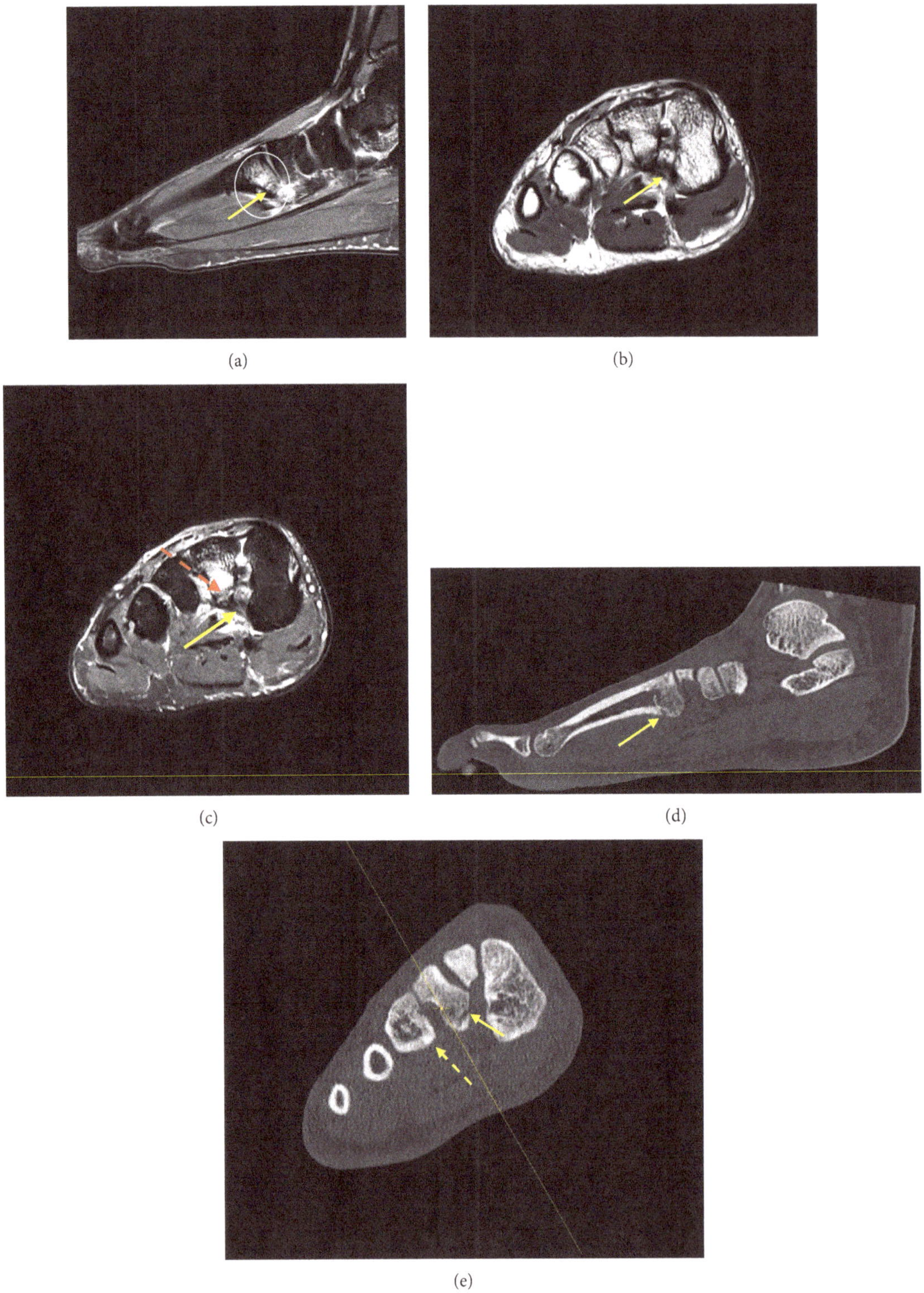

Figure 1: (a) Sagittal proton-density-weighted, fat-suppressed sequence (PDFS) at the level of the second metatarsal. There is localized marrow oedema signal centered at the base of the second metatarsal plantar margin (circled), with adjacent soft tissue oedema. The inferior cortex is thickened, with presence of intracortical high signal consistent with osteitis (arrow). Periosteal oedema present. The intracortical signal traversing the base of the second metatarsal is suspicious for an undisplaced fracture. Axial sequences at the level of the second metatarsal base in proton density (PD) (b) and PDFS (c) show thickening of the plantar Lisfranc ligament (arrow) which returns intermediate signal but is otherwise intact, consistent with grade II sprain or partial tear. Undisplaced fracture at the metatarsal base as shown (dashed arrow). Sagittal (d) and axial (e) CT at the similar level demonstrates the avulsion fracture at the base of the second metatarsal at the site of the plantar Lisfranc ligament insertion (arrow). There is also cortical thickening of the border of the third metatarsal base at the site of plantar Lisfranc attachment (dashed arrow).

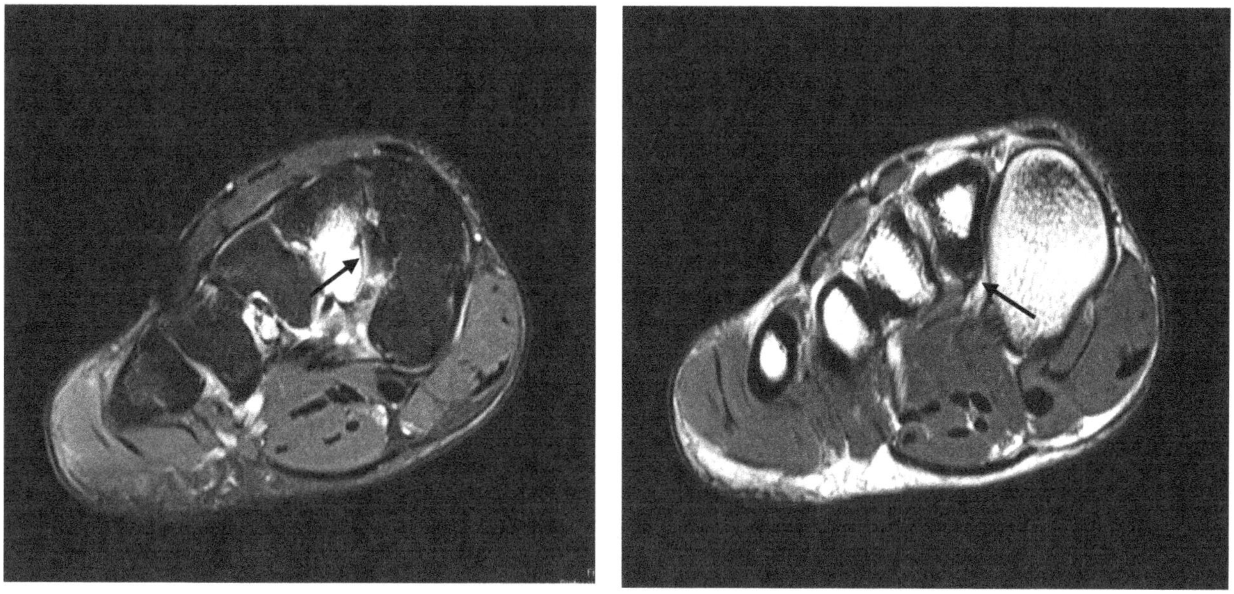

(a) (b)

FIGURE 2: (a, b) An 18-year-old footballer with second metatarsal tenderness worse on running and jumping. Axial PDFS (a) shows localized marrow oedema signal at the plantar margin of the base of the second metatarsal involving both interosseous (arrow) and plantar Lisfranc footprints (dash). Minor Lisfranc proper periligamentous oedema without a discrete tear or elongation identified, consistent with grade I sprain. Axial PD (b) clearly demonstrates the cortical thickening at the second metatarsal base (arrow).

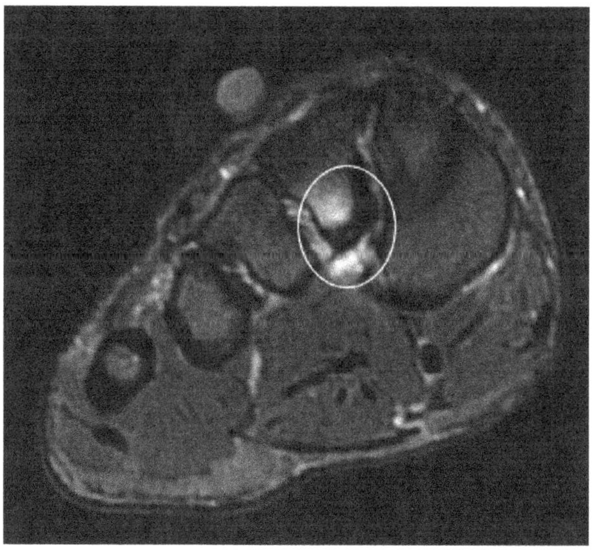

FIGURE 3: A 29-year-old soccer player with progressive midfoot pain. Axial PDFS at the plantar Lisfranc attachment to the second metatarsal base. There is oedema signal associated with the plantar Lisfranc ligament. There is also plantar cortical thickening with intracortical fluid signal (circled).

cuneiform articulation [7, 14]. Whilst traditional teaching dictates that the dorsal ligament often gets injured first, the plantar component is reported to be more commonly injured in athletes [3, 15]. Our case reports reaffirm the observation.

When normal bone is subjected to abnormal or repetitive stress, it undergoes physiologic, adaptive changes with new bone deposition at the sites of the stress [16]. If the stress is sufficient enough to exceed the adaptive response, the bone weakens and becomes increasingly susceptible to injury and fatigue fracture ensues [17, 18]. MRI is superior to other imaging modalities in diagnosis, grading, and hence prognosticating bone stress injuries. On MRI, bone stress injuries often begin with periosteal oedema. This can progress to marrow oedema signal and, if untreated, cortical oedema and stress fracture [18]. Cortical thickening can be observed as part of the remodeling process. There are reports of stress fractures at the base of second metatarsals in high-level athletes which matches our cohort [19] although in the available literature, the Lisfranc ligaments were not specifically assessed.

We also note that stress fractures reported in ballet dancers characteristically occur at the base of the second metatarsals [19]. Whilst acknowledging that Lisfranc ligamentous injury is uncommon in ballet dancers given the en pointe position which imparts compressive rather than shearing force across the TMT joints [9, 20], there is paucity of literature on MRI correlate of ballet dancers with second metatarsal base fractures and Lisfranc ligaments in this cohort of patients. This would be an important area of research because the imaging of these second metatarsal base fractures described in literature are quite similar to our cases, involving the plantar Lisfranc footprints at metatarsal bases [9]. One may assume that chronic Lisfranc sprain could occur in ballet dancers if the technique is poor.

There is one case report in the English literature describing Lisfranc ligamentous injury in a low-energy context in the presence of bone stress reaction, as indicated by cortical reaction and thickening. However, this occurred spontaneously and did not occur in the context of a sports injury.

The patient had a background of autoimmune condition (systemic lupus erythematosus and antiphospholipid syndrome) and osteoporosis. The presentation was also delayed, potentially confounding the imaging findings. Also, an MRI was not performed and Lisfranc ligamentous injury was only inferred based on the fracture which delineated the footprint of the Lisfranc ligament [10].

In our cases, the initial imaging was performed in a relatively short timeframe since the onset of symptoms, showing changes of bone stress response with Lisfranc ligamentous sprain. Extrapolating the available data on athletes and ballet dancers, it is expected that the Lisfranc ligament in this subset of high-performing athletes has to withstand a substantial amount of stress over a prolonged period of time, enough for bony adaptive response at the footprint of the Lisfranc ligaments with cortical remodeling and thickening. The symptoms may only manifest when this adaptive response fails, such as in the context of impending stress fracture. The authors would like to raise chronic stress response as a subset of low-energy injury to the Lisfranc ligament. This hypothesis will have to be further explored with prospective studies, potentially with longitudinal surveillance of these athletes.

Complications of untreated Lisfranc injuries include persistent pain, flattening of the longitudinal arch, and accelerated osteoarthritis in the midfoot. This injury is associated with significant morbidity with up to 18% of affected athletes being unable to return to baseline sports after injury [4]. The treatment goal is aimed at stable and painless midfoot and, hopefully, returning to play [3]. Early treatment and rest can prevent the progression to fracture and associated complication. Most patients can be treated nonoperatively with non-weight-bearing status or protected weight-bearing with boot or cast for 6 weeks, prior to progressive weight-bearing as tolerated [18]. This was the case in two of our athletes. The third athlete did not improve with conservative management and ultimately required internal fixation of the stress fracture, with good response thereafter.

In conclusion, low-energy injuries of the Lisfranc articulation, or midfoot sprain, are increasingly being recognised as a common sports injury, particularly in high-level athletes, with potential long-term morbidity. We present three cases in which the presentation and duration of symptoms of the high-level athletes do not fit with the degree of bone remodeling observed on MRI, suggesting sustained period of stress to the Lisfranc ligament in sporting activities. We speculate that there is a subset of chronic, repetitive, low-energy Lisfranc stress which can manifest as bone adaptive response and ligamentous sprain.

## References

[1] K. J. McHale, B. G. Vopat, B. R. Beaulieu-Jones et al., "Epidemiology and outcomes of Lisfranc injuries identified at the National Football League Scouting Combine," *The American Journal of Sports Medicine*, vol. 45, 8 pages, 2017.

[2] A. H. Stodle, K. H. Hvaal, M. Enger, H. Brogger, J. E. Madsen, and H. E. Ellingsen, "Lisfranc injuries: incidence, mechanisms of injury and predictors of instability," *Foot and Ankle Surgery*, vol. 26, no. 5, pp. 535–540, 2020.

[3] H. Mulcahy, "Lisfranc injury: current concepts," *Radiologic Clinics of North America*, vol. 56, no. 6, pp. 859–876, 2018.

[4] N. A. Siddiqui, M. S. Galizia, E. Almusa, and I. M. Omar, "Evaluation of the tarsometatarsal joint using conventional radiography, CT, and MR imaging," *Radiographics*, vol. 34, no. 2, pp. 514–531, 2014.

[5] M. S. Myerson and R. A. Cerrato, "Current management of tarsometatarsal injuries in the athlete," *The Journal of Bone and Joint Surgery*, vol. 90, no. 11, pp. 2522–2533, 2008.

[6] S. A. Meyer, J. J. Callaghan, J. P. Albright, E. T. Crowley, and J. W. Powell, "Midfoot sprains in collegiate football players," *The American Journal of Sports Medicine*, vol. 22, no. 3, pp. 392–401, 1994.

[7] D. A. Porter, A. F. Barnes, A. Rund, and M. T. Walrod, "Injury pattern in ligamentous Lisfranc injuries in competitive athletes," *Foot & Ankle International*, vol. 40, no. 2, pp. 185–194, 2019.

[8] J. Crim, "MR imaging evaluation of subtle Lisfranc injuries: the midfoot sprain," *Magnetic Resonance Imaging Clinics of North America*, vol. 16, no. 1, pp. 19–27, 2008.

[9] P. Kriz, J. Rafferty, P. Evangelista, S. Van Valkenburg, and C. DiGiovanni, "Stress fracture of the second metatarsal and sprain of lisfranc joint in a pre-professional ballet dancer," *Journal of Dance Medicine & Science*, vol. 19, no. 2, pp. 80–85, 2015.

[10] B. J. O'Neill, L. A. Sweeney, P. J. Moroney, and K. J. Mulhall, "Atypical stress-avulsion fracture of the Lisfranc joint complex," *Foot & Ankle Specialist*, vol. 7, no. 2, pp. 155–158, 2014.

[11] J. A. Nunley and C. J. Vertullo, "Classification, investigation, and management of midfoot sprains: Lisfranc injuries in the athlete," *The American Journal of Sports Medicine*, vol. 30, no. 6, pp. 871–878, 2002.

[12] E. A. Desmond and L. B. Chou, "Current concepts review: Lisfranc injuries," *Foot & Ankle International*, vol. 27, no. 8, pp. 653–660, 2006.

[13] B. Rhim and J. C. Hunt, "Lisfranc injury and Jones fracture in sports," *Clinics in Podiatric Medicine and Surgery*, vol. 28, no. 1, pp. 69–86, 2011.

[14] J. S. Lewis Jr. and R. B. Anderson, "Lisfranc injuries in the athlete," *Foot & Ankle International*, vol. 37, no. 12, pp. 1374–1380, 2016.

[15] K. Kitsukawa, T. Hirano, H. Niki, N. Tachizawa, Y. Nakajima, and K. Hirata, "MR imaging evaluation of the Lisfranc ligament in cadaveric feet and patients with acute to chronic Lisfranc injury," *Foot & Ankle International*, vol. 36, no. 12, pp. 1483–1492, 2015.

[16] J. M. Hughes, K. L. Popp, R. Yanovich, M. L. Bouxsein, and R. W. Matheny Jr., "The role of adaptive bone formation in the etiology of stress fracture," *Experimental Biology and Medicine*, vol. 242, no. 9, pp. 897–906, 2017.

[17] A. Finestone, C. Milgrom, O. Wolf, K. Petrov, R. Evans, and D. Moran, "Epidemiology of metatarsal stress fractures versus tibial and femoral stress fractures during elite training," *Foot & Ankle International*, vol. 32, no. 1, pp. 16–20, 2011.

[18] A. Nattiv, G. Kennedy, M. T. Barrack, A. Abdelkerim, M. A. Goolsby, J. C. Arends et al., "Correlation of MRI grading of bone stress injuries with clinical risk factors and return to play: a 5-year prospective study in collegiate track and field athletes," *The American Journal of Sports Medicine*, vol. 41, no. 8, pp. 1930–1941, 2013.

[19] B. Chuckpaiwong, C. Cook, and J. A. Nunley, "Stress fractures of the second metatarsal base occur in nondancers," *Clinical Orthopaedics and Related Research®*, vol. 461, pp. 197–202, 2007.

[20] D. A. Gunio, E. Vulcano, and C. L. Benitez, "Dynamic stress MRI of midfoot injuries: measurable morphology and laxity of the sprained Lisfranc ligament during mechanical loading: a case report," *JBJS Case Connect*, vol. 9, no. 3, 2019.

# 9

# Bilateral Femoral Neck Fracture in a Postpartum Woman: Beware of the Risk Factors

**Ismail Sahan,[1] Julie De Deken,[2] and Konstantinos Anagnostakos[1]**

[1]*Zentrum für Orthopädie und Unfallchirurgie, Städtisches Klinikum Saarbrücken, Saarbrücken, Germany*
[2]*Klinik für Allgemein-, Viszeral-, Thorax- und Kinderchirurgie, Städtisches Klinikum Saarbrücken, Saarbrücken, Germany*

Correspondence should be addressed to Konstantinos Anagnostakos; k.anagnostakos@web.de

Academic Editor: Christian W. Müller

Bilateral femoral neck fractures pose a rare injury. Literature data describe this entity in association with epileptic seizures, renal osteodystrophy, electric shock, pregnancy-associated transient osteoporosis, and hypocalcemic seizure. In the present work, we report on a rare case of a 28-year-old woman who suffered from such an injury 3 days postpartum. The patient had two predisposing factors (epilepsy history, transient osteoporosis) that were neglected as possible risk factors by the treating physicians. Awareness of the factors might have prevented the emergence of this injury.

## 1. Introduction

Simultaneous bilateral femoral neck fractures are an extremely rare injury. Literature data are scarce about this topic. Single articles have been published, reporting on a possible association with various disorders, such as epileptic seizure [1–3], electric shock injury [4], hypocalcemic seizure [5], and transient osteoporosis during pregnancy [6–8]. Depending on the age of the patient and the type of fracture, either bilateral internal fixation or bilateral total hip arthroplasty have been performed to manage this injury [1–8].

In the present work, we would like to report on an unusual case of a 28-year-old female patient that suffered from bilateral femoral neck fractures three days postpartum.

## 2. Case Report

A 28-year-old woman (1.65 m, 85 kg, BMI 31.2) was referred to our department five days postpartum with a bilateral femoral neck fracture.

During the last two months before the delivery of her first child (begin with the sixth month of gestation), she had complained about increasing weakness and pain in both hips and thighs. In the last two weeks of her pregnancy (begin of the 35$^{th}$ week of gestation), she had to walk on crutches, as she was unable to bear her full weight due to the severe pain in her hips. During this time she took paracetamol daily. Her treating gynaecologist did not initiate any clarification of the symptoms by radiologic imaging methods in this period. Considering her severe pain, it was decided to deliver the child per elective caesarean section (37$^{th}$ +4 week of gestation). Three days postpartum, after being released from the hospital, she had an epileptic seizure and fell. She was admitted to a neurological department of another hospital. During her two-day stay in this department, the woman complained of severe pains in both hips. X-rays and a computer tomography (CT) of the pelvis were performed, revealing bilateral femoral neck fractures. Following this diagnosis, the patient was referred to our department for further treatment.

Regarding her past medical history, she had childhood migraine and epilepsy. She suffered from her first epileptic seizure at the age of 15. She was treated with valproate over 11 years and remained seizure-free during that time. Her treating neurologist stopped the medication two years prior to her pregnancy. The patient did not have any other comorbidities. Particularly, she did not report on any past history of fractures, irregular menstruation, or family history of osteoporosis.

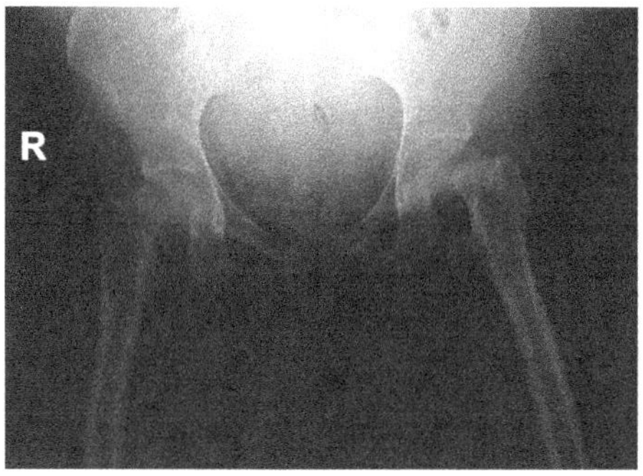


Figure 1: Preoperative anterior-posterior radiographs of the pelvis demonstrating the displaced bilateral femoral neck fractures.

At presentation in our department, the clinical examination showed massively reduced hip movement on both sides because of severe pain. Serum laboratory examination was normal.

Based on the age of the patient, the limited bone quality, the age of the fractures, and their displacement (Figures 1 and 2), it was decided to perform a bilateral hip joint replacement with the use of short-stemmed prostheses (Figure 3). There were no intra- or postoperative complications. Both femoral heads were sent for further histopathological examination. The results of both femoral heads revealed fracture areas with hemorrhagia, proliferation of fibroblasts in the marrow cavities, and formation of focal woven bone as a sign of the bone remodelling, being indicative for a TOH. Postoperatively, the patient was mobilized on crutches under full weight bearing of the operated extremities. After consultation with our Department of Neurology, the patient restarted her valproate medication. Due to this medication, the patient was advised not to breastfeed her child. Since the TOH is regarded to be a self-limiting disorder, no specific osteoporotic treatment was applied. The further course was uneventful, and the patient was dismissed after two weeks.

At 1-year follow-up, the patient is free of any complaints and has no limitation in the range of motion of both hips (extension/flexion 0°-0°-100°, abduction 50°).

## 3. Discussion

As aforementioned, various predisposing factors have been identified at the site of bilateral femoral neck fractures in young patients [1–9]. Knowledge about these factors and their associated diagnosis and treatment might help preventing the emergence of bilateral femoral neck fractures in some cases.

The interpretation of the history of our patient is more important than the treatment itself in the present work. The patient had complaints over both hips and thighs during the past two months of her pregnancy, a symptom that is very typical for the presence of transient osteoporosis [10, 11]. Transient osteoporosis of the hips (TOH) in pregnancy is an uncommon disease, mostly affecting primipara and women in their third trimester of the pregnancy [12]. Unfortunately, no imaging methods such as magnetic resonance imaging (MRI) were used to clarify these symptoms.

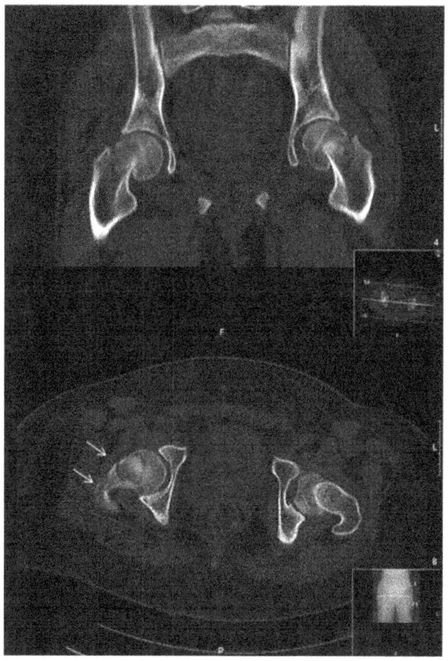

Figure 2: Computed tomography images (coronal and axial plane) confirmed not only the bilateral displacement of the femoral heads but also the presence of a 3-part fracture of the right side (arrows), which helped us to decide for bilateral total hip replacement than internal fixation.

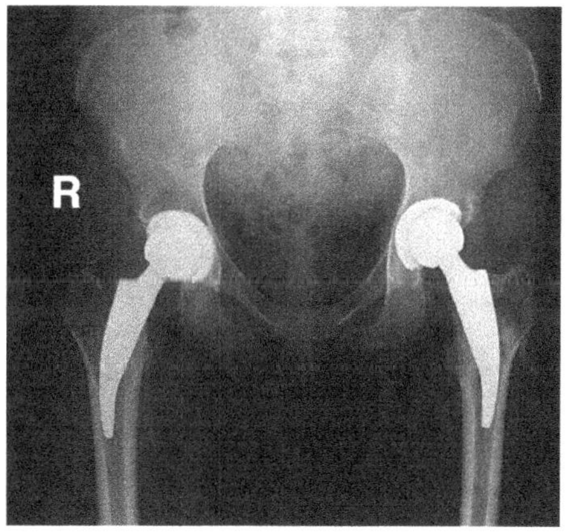


Figure 3: The patient was treated with bilateral implantation of a short-stemmed total hip arthroplasty (Tritanium® cup, Fa. Stryker, Duisburg, Germany; Metha® stem, Fa. Aesculap, Tuttlingen, Germany).

The histopathological examination of both femoral heads confirmed this diagnosis. The deposition of thin seams of woven bone in the marrow spaces and the focal mild fibroblast proliferation, as shown in our case, have been also described in other histopathological studies about TOH [13, 14]. From a retrospective point of view, should a MRI have occurred to an earlier time point, the diagnosis of TOH might have been made, and the associated treatment might have been initiated, hence preventing the further weakness of the bone. The second predisposing factor was her positive history regarding epilepsy. Since the birth of child represents additional stress, it might have been advisable to reevaluate her neurological status and restart her antiepileptic medication in order to prevent any seizure before, during, or after the birth of the child.

The presence of two predisposing factors led in our case to the occurrence of the bilateral femoral neck fracture. It could be assumed that the transient osteoporosis enabled the occurrence of this fracture, and the epileptic seizure was the direct cause for that.

Both conservative and operative treatments have been reported in the literature in the management of transient osteoporosis of the hip. Common themes include restriction of weight-bearing activities and analgesia [11]. TOH associated with femoral neck fracture has to be surgically treated. In the absence of avascular necrosis of the femoral head, young patients with a recent fracture can be treated with a closed or open reduction and internal refixation using cannulated screws or a sliding hip screw [11, 15, 16]. Otherwise, hip joint replacement with a total or hemiarthroplasty is necessary [6].

Based on the age of our patient and the type and age of the fracture, we decided to carry out a bilateral total hip arthroplasty. Due to the young age of the patient, short-stemmed prostheses were implanted. This enabled the patient to a quick and pain-free mobilization.

Proximal femur fractures associated with TOH in pregnancy have been reported in several studies [6, 7, 11, 15–19]. However, our literature search showed no reports of femoral neck fracture associated with TOH in patients with epilepsy. To the best of our knowledge, this report represents the first published case where both entities are represented.

A possible differential diagnosis to TOH that has to be born in mind is the pregnancy-associated osteoporosis (PAO). Although the exact etiology is not completely understood, it is assumed that PAO might be the result of a calcium dysregulation during the last trimester based on insufficient maternal intake of calcium and increased resorption due to the rapid mineralization of the fetal skeleton during this time [20]. Typical predisposing factors for PAO involve anorexia nervosa, a long-term low body weight, and a positive family history of osteoporosis [7]. Measurements of the bone mineral density and of the serum vitamin D level are helpful in confirming this diagnosis [7]. The lumbar spine is frequently affected by PAO resulting to vertebral fractures, whereas involvement of the hip joints is regarded to be rare [7, 20].

Although the bone mineral density and of the serum vitamin D level were not determined in our case, we represent the opinion that our patient was rather affected by TOH than PAO. The patient did not have any of the aforementioned predisposing factors, and she did not have any complaints of the lumbar spine but solely of the hip joints. The PAO cannot be surely excluded, but the TOH appears to be the most probable explanation in the present case.

In conclusion, in pregnant women with hip complaints during the last trimester, a MRI should be performed for exclusion of TOH. Should a pregnant have a positive history of epilepsy, the possibly higher risk of a seizure during or after birth should be acknowledged, and consultation with a neurologist is recommended. The presence of both risk factors might be associated with the emergence of bilateral femoral neck fractures, as shown in the present case. Accurate diagnosis and timely initiation of treatment might prevent further complications during or after birth.

## References


[1] T. Cagırmaz, C. Yapici, M. M. Orak, and O. Guler, "Bilateral femoral neck fractures after an epileptic attack: a case report," *International Journal of Surgery Case Reports*, vol. 6, pp. 107–110, 2015.

[2] M. Grimaldi, H. Vouaillat, J. Tonetti, and P. Merloz, "Simultaneous bilateral femoral neck fractures secondary to epileptic seizures: treatment by bilateral total hip arthroplasty," *Orthopaedics & Traumatology, Surgery & Research*, vol. 95, no. 7, pp. 555–557, 2009.

[3] E. Vanderhooft and M. Swiontkowski, "Bilateral femoral neck fractures following a grand mal seizure," *Annals of Emergency Medicine*, vol. 24, no. 6, pp. 1188–1191, 1994.

[4] M. A. Shaheen and N. A. Sabet, "Bilateral simultaneous fracture of the femoral neck following electrical shock," *Injury*, vol. 16, no. 1, pp. 13-14, 1984.

[5] S. Gür, H. Yilmaz, S. Tüzüner, A. T. Aydin, and G. Süleymanlar, "Fractures due to hypocalcemic convulsion," *International Orthopaedics*, vol. 23, no. 5, pp. 308-309, 1999.

[6] M. J. Emami, H. R. Abdollahpour, A. R. Kazemi, and A. R. Vosoughi, "Bilateral subcapital femoral neck fractures secondary to transient osteoporosis during pregnancy: a case report," *Journal of Orthopaedic Surgery*, vol. 20, no. 2, pp. 260–262, 2012.

[7] K. Kasahara, N. Kita, T. Kawasaki, S. Morisaki, H. Yomo, and T. Murakami, "Bilateral femoral neck fractures resulting from pregnancy-associated osteoporosis showed bone marrow edema on magnetic resonance imaging," *The Journal of Obstetrics and Gynaecology Research*, vol. 43, no. 6, pp. 1067–1070, 2017.

[8] R. Madhok and J. A. Rand, "Ten-year follow-up study of missed, simultaneous, bilateral femoral-neck fractures treated by bipolar arthroplasties in a patient with chronic renal failure," *Clinical Orthopaedics and Related Research*, vol. 291, pp. 185–187, 1993.

[9] M. W. Smith, P. S. Marcus, and L. D. Wurtz, "Orthopedic issues in pregnancy," *Obstetrical & Gynecological Survey*, vol. 63, no. 2, pp. 103–111, 2008.

[10] P. Hadji, J. Boekhoff, M. Hahn, L. Hellmeyer, O. Hars, and I. Kyvernitakis, "Pregnancy-associated transient osteoporosis of the hip: results of a case-control study," *Archives of Osteoporosis*, vol. 12, no. 1, 2017.

[11] S. Lidder, K. Lang, H.-J. Lee, S. Masterson, and R. Kankate, "Bilateral hip fractures associated with transient osteoporosis of pregnancy," *Journal of the Royal Army Medical Corps*, vol. 157, no. 2, pp. 176–178, 2011.

[12] P. Pallavi, S. Padma, and D. Vanitha Anna Selvi, "Transient osteoporosis of hip and lumbar spine in pregnancy," *The Journal of Obstetrics and Gynecology of India*, vol. 62, no. S1, pp. 8-9, 2012, Suppl. 1.

[13] H. PLENK, S. HOFMANN, J. ESCHBERGER et al., "Histomorphology and Bone Morphometry of the Bone Marrow Edema Syndrome of the Hip," *Clinical Orthopaedics and Related Research*, vol. 334, pp. 73–84, 1997.

[14] E. F. McCarthy, "The pathology of transient regional osteoporosis," *The Iowa Orthopaedic Journal*, vol. 18, pp. 35–42, 1998.

[15] C. A. Willis-Owen, J. S. Daurka, A. Chen, and A. Lewis, "Bilateral femoral neck fractures due to transient osteoporosis of pregnancy: a case report," *Cases Journal*, vol. 1, no. 1, 2008.

[16] S. K. Fokter and V. Vengust, "Displaced subcapital fracture of the hip in transient osteoporosis of pregnancy: a case report," *International Orthopaedics*, vol. 21, no. 3, pp. 201–203, 1997.

[17] C. Bircher, K. Afors, and M. Bircher, "Transient osteoporosis of the hip in pregnancy resulting in bilateral fracture of the neck of the femur," *International Journal of Gynecology & Obstetrics*, vol. 116, no. 2, pp. 176-177, 2012.

[18] M. C. Moran, "Iatrogenic Femoral Neck Fracture in Transient Osteoporosis of the Hip," *Clinical Orthopaedics and Related Research*, vol. &NA;, no. 316, pp. 207–210, 1995.

[19] M. L. Wood, C. M. Larson, and L. E. Dahners, "Late presentation of a displaced subcapital fracture of the hip in transient osteoporosis of pregnancy," *Journal of Orthopaedic Trauma*, vol. 17, no. 8, pp. 582–584, 2003.

[20] C. S. Kovacs and S. H. Ralston, "Presentation and management of osteoporosis presenting in association with pregnancy or lactation," *Osteoporosis International*, vol. 26, no. 9, pp. 2223–2241, 2015.

# 10

# Atypical Presentation of Atraumatic Spinal Subdural Hematoma Associated with Warfarin: A Case Report and Review of the Literature

**Abdul Rehman Arain**[1], **Muhammad Moral**[1], **Saadia Shams**[2], **Khusboo Desai**[1] **and Khunwar Kalsa**[1]

[1]*Department of Orthopedics, Albany Medical College, 1267 Washington Ave Suite 202, Albany, NY 12206, USA*
[2]*Rawalpindi Medical College, Pakistan*

Correspondence should be addressed to Abdul Rehman Arain; mrbonelover@gmail.com

Academic Editor: Eyal Itshayek

Nontraumatic spinal subdural hematomas secondary to anticoagulants are remarkably rare. A case of spontaneous, atraumatic subdural hematoma involving the thoracic region in an 80-year-old woman on warfarin is reported. The patient presented with gross motor and sensory loss, delayed onset of incontinence, and no other symptoms. An MRI suggested an epidural hematoma concentrated around the T4-T9 levels. She was taken emergently to the OR approximately 30 hours after the initial onset of symptoms for a T3-T11 laminectomy. No epidural hematoma was noted. However, discoloration and bulging of the thecal sac were noted, and the dura was incised longitudinally from T2 to T10 revealing an expansive jelly-like blood clot which was evacuated. Postoperatively, the patient had regained 1/2 sensory function in the bilateral lower extremities. At the 2-week mark, the patient was still incontinent and showed 2/2 sensory and 2/5 motor functions in select muscle groups in her bilateral lower extremities. Completely nontraumatic, spontaneous subdural hematomas of the spine are very rare, and early surgical decompression within 24 hours from symptom onset may allow neurological recovery. Large extensive laminectomies up to 10 thoracic levels have been shown to be safe and effective in a few cases, including our case.

## 1. Introduction

Spontaneous epidural hematomas of the spine are a rare entity; they are reported in the literature with approximately 600 reported cases [1, 2]. Spontaneous spinal subdural hematomas (SSDH) are extremely rare with only a few cases reported in the literature. Patients usually present with acute low back pain or radicular pain, followed by rapid neurological deterioration.

Emergent surgical decompression is the standard of care for both epidural and subdural hematomas.

Most reported cases of SSDH involve patients on anticoagulants with precipitating events prior to presentation such as a sudden cough, recent lumbar punctures, and a recent increase in physical activities, AV malformation, and neoplasms [1, 3, 4]. To our knowledge, this is the 5$^{th}$ reported case of SSDH involving warfarin [5, 6] and the only case completely absent of accompanying symptoms such as back pain, headache, nausea, and vomiting.

## 2. Case Presentation

We report on an 80-year-old Caucasian woman on warfarin for atrial fibrillation who sustained a spontaneous, atraumatic, spinal subdural hematoma in the thoracic region. The patient awoke in the morning to use the bathroom. Approximately 1 hr after returning to her bed, she was unable to move bilateral lower extremities and was incontinent. She reported no back pain, headache, nausea, vomiting, or any constitutional symptoms. She was

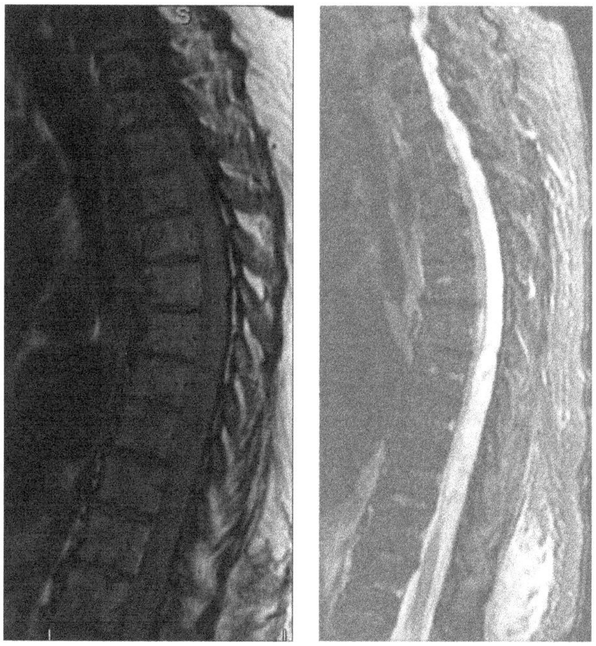

(a) Sagittal T1 (b) Sagittal STIR

FIGURE 1: Sagittal T1 (a) and STIR (b) images of the thoracolumbar spine. A large hyperintense signal from the proximal thoracic to the lumbar spine can be seen on the STIR image.

transferred to an outside hospital and underwent an MRI, which as read by an attending senior radiologist who suggested an epidural hematoma concentrated around the T4-T9 levels (Figures 1(a) and 1(b)). She was reversed for an INR of 3.6 and then transferred to Albany Medical Center for further management. On examination, the patient was comfortable without any pain. She had a loss of bowel and bladder function and had no sensory or motor function below T5. The patient was seen by a fellowship-trained orthopaedic spine surgeon, and her spinal cord injury was classified as a T5 ASIA impairment scale A.

She was taken emergently to the OR approximately 30 hours after the initial onset of symptoms. After a T3-T11 laminectomy, the spinal cord was fully visible, but no epidural hematoma was noted. However, discoloration and bulging of the thecal sac were noted, and the dura was incised longitudinally from T2 to T10 revealing an expansive jelly-like blood clot. The hematoma was evacuated, and the dura closed with a 4′0-NUROLON.

Postoperatively, the patient had regained 1/2 sensory function in the bilateral lower extremities. At the 2-week mark, the patient was still incontinent, showed 2/2 sensory and 2/5 motor functions in select muscle groups in her bilateral lower extremities. The patient's spinal cord injury was classified as an L2 ASIA impairment scale C. An MRI demonstrated a multilevel decompressive thoracolumbar laminectomy (Figures 2(a) and 2(b)), and the patient was discharged to a rehabilitation facility. At the two-month follow-up period, the patient had transitioned to a long-term nursing care facility and her neurological status remained unchanged.

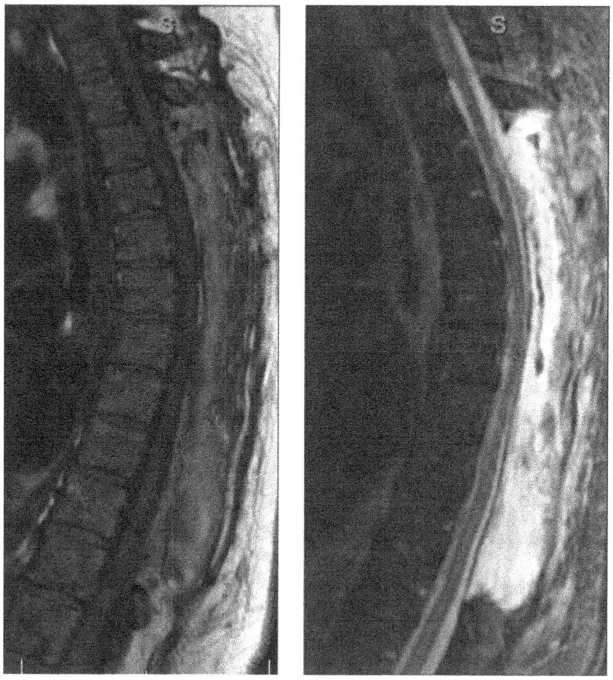

(a) Sagittal T1 (b) Sagittal STIR

FIGURE 2: Sagittal T1 (a) and STIR (b) postoperative MRI images of the thoracolumbar spine showing a large multilevel thoracolumbar laminectomy. Postoperative fluid collections are demonstrated on the STIR image.

## 3. Discussion

The true pathophysiology of spontaneous subdural hematomas is limited to two theories. Minor trauma, or increased intra-abdominal/thoracic pressure, may be associated with the rupture of valveless radiculomedullary veins in the subarachnoid space [7]. Alternatively, similar mechanisms may damage the few thin, delicate extra-arachnoidal vessels located on the inner dural surface, which then break through the arachnoid into the subarachnoid space leading to subdural hematomas [8, 9].

The classic clinical presentation of anticoagulant-associated spontaneous subdural hematoma is severe back pain, neck pain, or radicular pain, often preceding neurological demise [10]. Signs of increased intracranial pressure such as headache, nausea, and giddiness is also frequently reported during this prodromal phase [11]. In all reported cases, neurological symptoms of cord compression were rapidly progressive, and within a few hours of initial symptom onset, most patients had a complete loss of bowel and bladder function. In contrast to previously reported cases, our patient had no pain or prodromal symptoms. The patient's neurological symptoms included incontinence with complete loss of motor and sensory functions, which were all sudden and not progressive. Therefore, clinicians should be aware that even in the absence of classic prodromal symptoms, a spinal hemorrhage should be on the list of differentials for any patient on anticoagulants presenting with rapid neurological compromise.

Although MRI findings in spinal hematomas can vary based on the clot, age, and oxygenation, it remains the gold standard for diagnosis. Within the first 24 h after symptom onset, the hematoma shows isointensity on T1WI and hyperintensity on T2WI. After 24 h, it appears as a high signal on T1WI and as a low signal on T2WI. On sagittal images, subdural hematomas appear clumped and loculated with concave delineation. In contrast, epidural hematomas usually have a convex shape. However, the differentiation of epidural and subdural hematomas with an MRI is challenging. Similar to our case, Badge and Chan describe a case in which an initial MRI showing an epidural hematoma was realized to be a subdural hematoma intraoperatively [11]. In both cases, the decision to incise the dura, evacuate the hematoma, and repair the dura was made intraoperatively. It is difficult to assess if these unexpected intraoperative obstacles had any negative effects on the overall outcome for both patients. Due to the possible conflict between preoperative imaging and intraoperative findings, it is reasonable that any surgeon attempting to evacuate an epidural hematoma be prepared with appropriate tools and surgical backup, if needed, to perform intradural work in case a subdural hematoma is encountered.

Acute surgical decompression and discontinuation of anticoagulants is the standard of care in any patient on anticoagulants who is suspected of having a subdural hematoma [12–15]. Studies involving subdural and epidural hematomas of various etiologies suggest optimum results when surgical decompression occurs within 24 hours from the onset of symptoms [13, 16]. Large multilevel laminectomies for spinal hematoma management have shown to be safe and effective based on the limited literature available. Our case, a 9-level thoracic laminectomy is the second largest laminectomy reported for treating a spontaneous subdural hematoma. Visocchi et al. describe a 10-level thoracic laminectomy for a subdural hematoma occurring a few weeks after a lumbar puncture in a patient who improved from an ASIA impairment scale A to an ASIA impairment scale D at the 36 mo mark [16].

In our case, surgical management was delayed secondary to workup at an outside hospital. The patient's benign symptomatology, with a complete lack of pain and discomfort, may have thwarted an immediate transfer to a level 1 trauma center. The patient was transferred after an MRI showed a spinal hematoma. Upon arrival at our institution, the patient had to be triaged through the emergency department, with multiple teams evaluating the patient prior to the spine surgery team, which further delayed surgical management. We believe streamlined transfers from outside hospitals with adequate communication between the transferring team and surgical team assuming care of the patient would be invaluable in optimizing time-sensitive surgical outcomes, such as those involving spinal hemorrhage.

## 4. Conclusion

Atraumatic subdural hematoma is a rare but devastating entity associated with rapid neurological compromise. MRI is the imaging of choice, but differentiation between an epidural and a subdural hematoma remains a challenge. Although subdural hematomas are not frequently reported in the literature, the actual incidence may be higher as these can be mistaken for epidural hematomas, are often diagnosed intraoperatively, and may go unreported. Therefore, clinicians should be prepared to tackle either entity prior to surgical management of any spinal hemorrhage. Early surgical decompression within 24 hours from symptom onset is ideal for optimum neurological recovery. Large extensive laminectomies up to 10 thoracic levels are safe and effective.

## References


[1] D. Kreppel, G. Antoniadis, and W. Seeling, "Spinal hematoma: a literature survey with meta-analysis of 613 patients," *Neurosurgical review*, vol. 26, no. 1, pp. 1–49, 2003.

[2] C. Tawk, M. el Hajj Moussa, R. Zgheib, and G. Nohra, "Spontaneous epidural hematoma of the spine associated with oral anticoagulants: 3 case studies," *International journal of surgery case reports*, vol. 13, pp. 8–11, 2015.

[3] J. M. Castillo, H. F. Afanador, E. Manjarrez, and X. A. Morales, "Non-traumatic spontaneous spinal subdural hematoma in a patient with non-valvular atrial fibrillation during treatment with rivaroxaban," *The American journal of case reports*, vol. 16, pp. 377–381, 2015.

[4] M. Domenicucci, A. Ramieri, P. Ciappetta, and R. Delfini, "Nontraumatic acute spinal subdural hematoma," *Journal of Neurosurgery: Spine*, vol. 91, no. 1, pp. 65–73, 1999.

[5] X. Morandi, L. Riffaud, E. Chabert, and G. Brassier, "Acute nontraumatic spinal subdural hematomas in three patients," *Spine*, vol. 26, no. 23, pp. E547–E551, 2001.

[6] R. A. Bruce-Brand, G. C. Colleran, J. M. Broderick et al., "Acute nontraumatic spinal intradural hematoma in a patient on warfarin," *The Journal of emergency medicine*, vol. 45, no. 5, pp. 695–697, 2013.

[7] E. C. Kirsch, M. S. Khangure, D. Holthouse, and W. McAuliffe, "Acute spontaneous spinal subdural haematoma: MRI features," *Neuroradiology*, vol. 42, no. 8, pp. 586–590, 2000.

[8] Y. Kakitsubata, S. J. Theodorou, D. J. Theodorou et al., "Spontaneous spinal subarachnoid hemorrhage associated with subdural hematoma at different spinal levels," *Emergency radiology*, vol. 17, no. 1, pp. 69–72, 2010.

[9] S.-D. Kim, J.-O. Park, S.-H. Kim, Y.-H. Lee, D.-J. Lim, and J.-Y. Park, "Spontaneous thoracic spinal subdural hematoma associated with fibromuscular dysplasia," *Journal of Neurosurgery: Spine*, vol. 8, no. 5, pp. 478–481, 2008.

[10] J. L. Tomarken, "Spinal subdural hematoma: a case report and literature review," *The American journal of emergency medicine*, vol. 5, no. 2, pp. 123–125, 1987.

[11] R. Badge and D. Chan, "Spinal subdural haematoma in association with anticoagulant therapy, an unusual presentation: a case report and review of literature," *Cases journal*, vol. 2, no. 1, 2009.

[12] M. W. A. ROSCOE and T. W. BARRINGTON, "Acute spinal subdural hematoma. A case report and review of literature," *Spine*, vol. 9, no. 7, pp. 672–675, 1984.

[13] W. Küker, R. Thiex, S. Friese et al., "Spinal subdural and epidural haematomas: diagnostic and therapeutic aspects in acute and subacute cases," *Acta neurochirurgica*, vol. 142, no. 7, pp. 777–785, 2000.

[14] M. Guthikonda, H. H. Schmidek, L. J. Wallman, and T. M. Snyder, "Spinal subdural hematoma: case report and review of the literature," *Neurosurgery*, vol. 5, no. 5, pp. 614–616, 1979.

[15] H. Jimbo, S. Asamoto, T. Mitsuyama, K. Hatayama, Y. Iwasaki, and Y. Fukui, "Spinal chronic subdural hematoma in association with anticoagulant therapy: a case report and literature review," *Spine*, vol. 31, no. 6, pp. E184–E187, 2006.

[16] M. Visocchi, G. La Rocca, F. Signorelli, R. Roselli, Z. Jun, and A. Spallone, "10 levels thoracic no-intrumented laminectomy for huge spontaneous spinal subdural hematoma removal. Report of the first case and literature review," *International Journal of Surgery Case Reports*, vol. 15, pp. 57–62, 2015.

# 11

# Chromium-Cobalt Intoxication with Intense Systemic Complications following Total Hip Revision after Per-Operative Ceramic Fracture

**Paul Lecoanet, Mathias Blangis, Matthieu Garcia, Yohan Legallois, and Thierry Fabre**

*CHU de Bordeaux, Place Amélie Raba-Léon, 33000 Bordeaux, France*

Correspondence should be addressed to Paul Lecoanet; paul.lecoanet@chu-bordeaux.fr

Academic Editor: Athanassios Papanikolaou

*Introduction.* Heavy metal intoxication after arthroplasty is extremely rare but could be lethal. *Case Report.* We report the case of a 69-year-old woman, who presented intense systemic symptoms of chromium-cobalt intoxication after revision of per-operative fractured ceramic components with metal-on-polyethylene. Systemic toxicity occurred a year after surgery and expressed brutally with mostly central neurological symptoms. Chelation associated with revision surgery allowed rapid regression of all symptoms. *Conclusion.* Revision of fractured ceramic, even per-operatively, should not be done with metal-on-polyethylene components, in order to avoid potentially lethal metal intoxication.

## 1. Introduction

Heavy metal intoxication after arthroplasty is extremely rare, but a few cases are reported in literature [1–4]. These cases of cobalt toxicity generally result in replacing fractured ceramic parts with metal-on-metal (MoM) or metal-on-polyethylene (MOP) implants, creating a third-body wear. Friction between residual parts of the ceramic and cobalt-chromium implants creates metal debris, releasing into synovial fluid and the bloodstream. This causes elevated blood cobalt levels and systemic toxicity [5]. Most frequent symptoms of cobalt toxicity are peripheral neuropathy, hearing and visual loss, cognitive decline, and thyroid and cardiac toxicity [6]. Impairment of neurological basal ganglia and caudate nucleus was never described before. This case's interest lies in the severity of symptoms and the fast recovery after appropriate treatment.

## 2. Case Presentation

We report the case of a 69-year-old woman without significant history, who suffered from chromium-cobalt intoxication following total hip arthroplasty (THA). This patient underwent primary arthroplasty to the left hip in 2013 in another orthopedic department, with ceramic bearing. Postoperative course was uncomplicated until 2016 when she experienced three dislocations. Unipolar revision surgery for instability was performed, with per-operative ceramic acetabular liner fracturing in order to remove it. Dual-mobility cup with metal-on-polyethylene components was then implanted. Less than a year after revision surgery, the patient presented to our hospital with fever, asthenia, tachycardia, weight loss, and left groin pain. First clinical and biological evaluation suggested prosthetic joint infection. Plain radiographs and CT scan showed massive collection around the left prosthesis (Figures 1 and 2). A few days later, the patient reported rapid cognitive decline with behavioral disorders, lack of memory, and brutal hearing and visual loss with worsening of asthenia and weight loss (15 kg in 6 weeks due to decreased oral intake, attributed to dysgeusia with metallic taste). Puncture of the periprosthetic collection was performed, revealing metallosis. Neurological exam with MRI showed heavy metal accumulation in the basal ganglia and caudate nucleus (Figure 3). Ophthalmologic and otologic

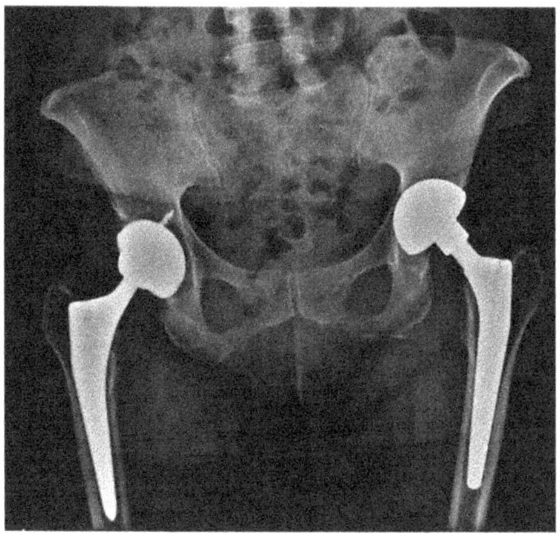

Figure 1: Pelvic A-P view at symptom onset, April 2017. Left periprosthetic collection with hydroaeric levels.

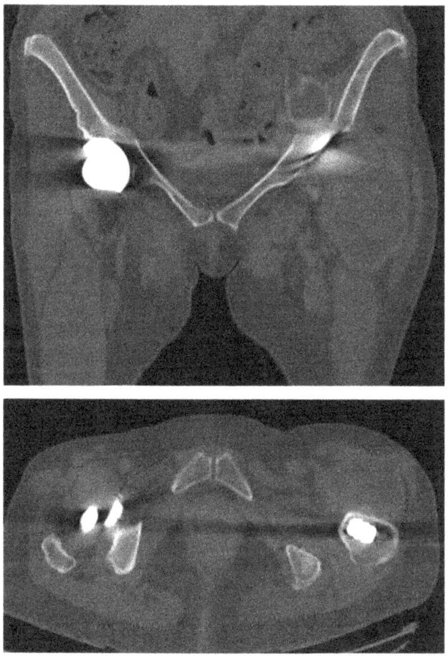

Figure 2: Frontal and axial views of the CT scan showing the important left periprosthetic collection.

examinations confirmed metal damages to the eyes with bilateral papilledema and to the ears with sensorineural hearing loss limited to 55 dB.

Heavy metal blood levels revealed huge concentrations of cobalt 24808 nmol/L (normal: 0.3-9) (i.e., 1461 $\mu$g/L) and chromium 1268 nmol/L (normal: 1-5) (i.e., 65.9 $\mu$g/L). Urinary dosage also revealed explosive levels of cobalt 8234 $\mu$g/g of creatinine (normal < 2) and chromium 151 $\mu$g/L (normal < 1). Regarding these systemic symptoms of metal toxicity, our patient received immediate calcicodisodic EDTA (ethylenediaminetetraacetic acid) and DMSA (dimercaptosuccinic acid) chelation.

One-stage bipolar revision surgery was also performed shortly after, in our institution. Considerable black-liquid collection (around 500 mL, cobalt dosage in liquid > 1 g/L, culture negative for infection) was found around the prosthesis

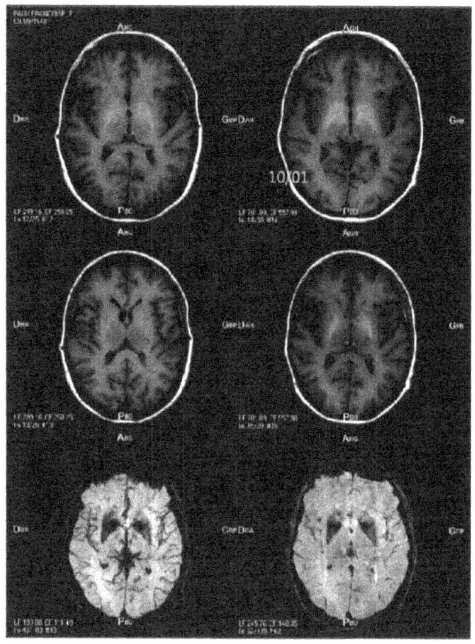

Figure 3: MRI showing the important metal accumulation in the basal ganglia and caudate nucleus with T1 hypersignal and T2 hyposignal.

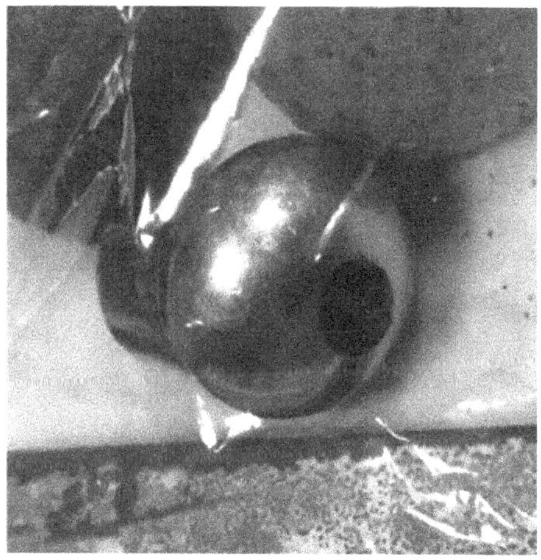

Figure 4: Per-operative aspect of the femoral chromium-cobalt head, flattened with a hole in it. 18 g of metal loss explaining metallosis with systemic repercussions.

with black staining in periprosthetic tissues and gluteal muscles necrosis. Every component was removed and the cobalt-chromium femoral head was severely worn, with a hole in it (Figure 4). Laboratory exam of the head revealed an 18 g of metal loss, explaining heavy metal intoxication. Ceramic particles around polyethylene and chromium-cobalt head were also found, contributing to metal debris formation. We performed a large and exhaustive synovectomy and debridement of the muscles necrosis and were obliged to implant a dual mobility cup in order to maintain stability of this multioperated hip.

All symptoms along with hip pain rapidly improved after treatment. Cognitive functions were progressively restored. Patient regained audition and vision at functional level.

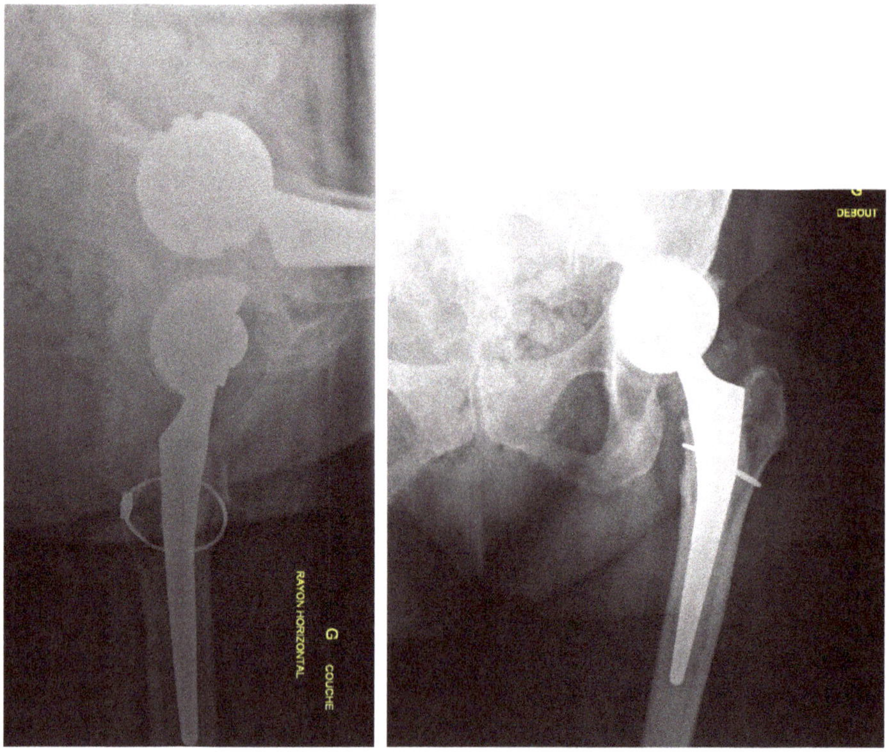


Figure 5: Post revision surgery X-rays at six-month follow-up.

Asthenia, behavioral disorders, and memory loss also disappeared. New MRI examination at 3 months showed reduced T1 hypersignal of the basal ganglia and caudate nucleus. These improvements accompanied a decrease in cobalt and chromium levels. Serum cobalt level went down to 34 and 17 $\mu$g/L at, respectively, 1 and 6 months follow-up. Chromium serum levels were at 50 and 40 $\mu$g/L at 1 and 6 months. Urinary cobalt level was at 483 $\mu$g/g of creatinine and urinary chromium level at 82 $\mu$g/L at 6 months. Standard X-rays at the six-month follow-up showed no radiological complications of the left hip revision (Figure 5). Patient could walk without limping or crutches and the Harris Hip Score was 75/100.

## 3. Discussion

In this case of severe metallosis after revision of fractured ceramic components with MOP, neurological repercussions of chromium-cobalt intoxication were put forward, especially, impairment of the neurological basal ganglia and caudate nucleus, as seen on the MRI, that were never described before in this type of case.

Ceramic failure can be usually seen on head component after a traumatic event. In this case, ceramic shattering occurred per-operatively when removing the acetabular liner.

Onset of metallosis systemic symptoms is normally seen within 2 years after revision surgery, and serum levels of cobalt usually ranges from 10 to 2000 times than the normal values [7]. Our patient presented systemic repercussion of metallosis less than a year after revision surgery, with cobalt levels around 3000 times that the normal values. Heavy metal serum levels will be screened on a regular basis, every year for follow-up, as well as clinical and radiological aspects.

Compared to third-body wear from revision of failed ceramic components, toxicity from failed metal-on-metal THAs has been reported to be significantly lower due to the lower levels of cobalt in the blood [8].

Symptomatic cobalt toxicity after revision of failed ceramic component to MOP is well described in literature [7, 9, 10]. After ceramic fracture (although less common since recent advances in manufacturing new generation ceramics [11]), metal-on-polyethylene with synovectomy is often chosen to limit residual ceramic particles and avoid metallosis. Sharma et al. reported a 10-year survivorship in 5 patients if a complete and thorough synovectomy can be performed [12]. However, totally removing all ceramic particles with extensive synovectomy has been proven to be very difficult [13].

## 4. Conclusion

Revision of failed ceramic arthroplasties, even immediate ceramic fracture occurring per-operatively, needs a large synovectomy for removing all ceramic debris and should be done with new ceramic components instead of metal-on-polyethylene, if stability is obtained, in order to avoid metal toxicity, which could be lethal.

## 5. Clinical Message

Cardiomyopathy, visual and hearing loss, or central neurological symptoms appearing after revision of failed ceramic arthroplasty with MOP implants should incite to look for metallosis, even a few years after revision surgery [7].

## References

[1] M. C. Rizzetti, P. Liberini, G. Zarattini et al., "Loss of sight and sound. Could it be the hip?," *The Lancet*, vol. 373, no. 9668, p. 1052, 2009.

[2] K. Dahms, Y. Sharkova, P. Heitland, S. Pankuweit, and J. R. Schaefer, "Cobalt intoxication diagnosed with the help of Dr House," *The Lancet*, vol. 383, no. 9916, p. 574, 2014.

[3] K. A. Fox, T. M. Phillips, J. H. Yanta, and M. G. Abesamis, "Fatal cobalt toxicity after total hip arthroplasty revision for fractured ceramic components," *Clinical Toxicology*, vol. 54, no. 9, pp. 874–877, 2016.

[4] M. Oldenburg, R. Wegner, and X. Baur, "Severe cobalt intoxication due to prosthesis wear in repeated total hip arthroplasty," *The Journal of Arthroplasty*, vol. 24, no. 5, pp. 825.e15–825.e20, 2009.

[5] D. R. Bijukumar, A. Segu, J. C. M. Souza et al., "Systemic and local toxicity of metal debris released from hip prostheses: a review of experimental approaches," *Nanomedicine: Nanotechnology, Biology and Medicine*, vol. 14, no. 3, pp. 951–963, 2018.

[6] S. M. Bradberry, J. M. Wilkinson, and R. E. Ferner, "Systemic toxicity related to metal hip prostheses," *Clinical Toxicology*, vol. 52, no. 8, pp. 837–847, 2014.

[7] A. Harris, J. Johnson, P. K. Mansuripur, and R. Limbird, "Cobalt toxicity after revision to a metal-on-polyethylene total hip arthroplasty for fracture of ceramic acetabular component," *Arthroplasty Today*, vol. 1, no. 4, pp. 89–91, 2015.

[8] S. S. Tower, "Arthroprosthetic cobaltism associated with metal on metal hip implants," *BMJ*, vol. 344, no. 3, pp. e430–e430, 2012.

[9] R. M. Peters, P. Willemse, P. C. Rijk, M. Hoogendoorn, and W. P. Zijlstra, "Fatal cobalt toxicity after a non-metal-on-metal Total hip arthroplasty," *Case Reports in Orthopedics*, vol. 2017, 5 pages, 2017.

[10] M. Hasegawa, A. Sudo, and A. Uchida, "Cobalt-chromium head wear following revision hip arthroplasty performed after ceramic fracture—a case report," *Acta Orthopaedica*, vol. 77, no. 5, pp. 833–835, 2006.

[11] P. Massin, R. Lopes, B. Masson, and D. Mainard, "Does Biolox® Delta ceramic reduce the rate of component fractures in total hip replacement?," *Orthopaedics & Traumatology: Surgery & Research*, vol. 100, no. 6, pp. S317–S321, 2014.

[12] V. Sharma, A. S. Ranawat, V. J. Rasquinha, J. Weiskopf, H. Howard, and C. S. Ranawat, "Revision total hip arthroplasty for ceramic head fracture," *The Journal of Arthroplasty*, vol. 25, no. 3, pp. 342–347, 2010.

[13] G. Matziolis, C. Perka, and A. Disch, "Massive metallosis after revision of a fractured ceramic head onto a metal head," *Archives of Orthopaedic and Trauma Surgery*, vol. 123, no. 1, pp. 48–50, 2003.

# 12

# Concurrent Primary Repair of a Glenoid Labrum Articular Disruption and a Bankart Lesion in an Adolescent: A Case Report of a Novel Technique

**Avinesh Agarwalla,[1] Richard N. Puzzitiello,[1] Natalie L. Leong,[2] and Brian Forsythe[1]**

[1]*Midwest Orthopaedics at Rush, Rush University Medical Center, Chicago, IL, USA*
[2]*Department of Orthopaedic Surgery, University of Maryland, College Park, MD, USA*

Correspondence should be addressed to Brian Forsythe; forsythe.research@rushortho.com

Academic Editor: Kiyohisa Ogawa

Glenoid labrum articular disruption (GLAD) lesions are an uncommon concomitant injury associated with labral tears, occurring in 1.5-2.9% of cases. In previous reported cases, the articular lesion is debrided during repair of the labral injury, which may predispose patients to osteoarthritis, a longitudinal complication seen in articular debridement of the hip. We report the case of a 15-year-old healthy adolescent male swimmer who sustained a labral injury with a concomitant GLAD lesion. During operative management, three Polyetheretherketone (PEEK) SutureTaks were placed on the glenoid. #2 FiberWire was used to imbricate capsular tissue, passed beneath the labrum, and was then subsequently advanced through the fibrous rim of the displaced cartilage flap/GLAD lesion at the site of each suture anchor. This construct restored tension to the anterior band of the inferior glenohumeral ligament, recreated the anteroinferior labral bumper, and effectively reduced the cartilage flap/GLAD lesion to the anterior inferior glenoid. By six months postoperatively, the patient demonstrated near-normal function with full range of motion and evidence of a stable construct on MRI. Unlike previously described cases, this is the first report of a hybrid technique that simultaneously performed a primary repair of both labral and articular injuries without the use of additional implants for the articular lesion. Primary repair of the labral and articular lesions should provide longitudinal benefit to the patient by reducing the risk of developing glenohumeral osteoarthritis.

## 1. Introduction

Anterior inferior glenolabral injuries occur secondary to anterior shoulder dislocations and are often associated with concomitant injuries such as the Bankart lesion, anterior labral periosteal sleeve avulsions (ALPSA), Perthes lesions, and glenoid labral articular disruption (GLAD) lesions [1]. GLAD lesions are the least common of these concomitant injuries, occurring in 1.5-2.9% of anterior inferior glenolabral injuries. This injury most commonly occurs with forced adduction while the arm is abducted and externally rotated and is often a significant source of anterior shoulder pain in these patients [1–3].

GLAD lesions are characterized by an avulsion of the articular glenoid cartilage that is associated with the inferior glenoid labrum, due to the continuity of the deep fibers of these structures [2, 4]. A high degree of clinical suspicion is needed due to the infrequency of these injuries. Furthermore, GLAD lesions are not readily visualized on standard MRI [5]; thus, higher resolution studies such as magnetic resonance arthrography (MRA) may be needed to detect this injury pattern [1, 3, 5]. Management of GLAD lesions involves arthroscopic debridement or chondroplasty to correct the uneven chondral layer that may be the source of discomfort, in addition to a stabilization procedure for concurrent labral injury [1, 2, 6].

In this case report, we present an adolescent male with a previous history of arthroscopic shoulder surgery who experienced a shoulder dislocation while swimming. The patient was diagnosed with an anterior inferior glenolabral tear with a GLAD defect and underwent primary arthroscopic labral repair with concomitant glenolabral cartilage disruption repair, utilizing a previously unreported single suture anchor construct.

## 2. Case Report

The patient is a 15-year-old competitive male swimmer with a history of bilateral arthroscopic subacromial decompression within the preceding year. The patient continued regular follow-up with the senior author until he reached maximal medical improvement (MMI) from these procedures. One week following this visit, the patient suffered a right shoulder dislocation while swimming, which was self-reduced. He presented to the clinic 3 days following the injury. At this time, he reported mild pain (3/10), and his self-reported functionality was less than 20% of normal.

Upon presentation, the patient was not in acute distress, and there was no obvious deformity of the right shoulder. He reported tenderness to palpation on the bicipital groove and achieved 150 degrees of scaption, 45 degrees of external rotation, and internal rotation to the T10 level. He demonstrated a positive Neer test, Hawkins test, O'Brien's test, and valgus sheer test. He demonstrated a positive anterior load test. He demonstrated a negative posterior load test, belly test, and a lift-off test. An MRI was ordered to evaluate his labrum, which demonstrated a humeral head subluxation with posterior humeral head contusion and Buford complex. Conservative management with physical therapy was recommended at this time.

After six weeks of physical therapy, the patient returned for evaluation and noted moderate pain (4/10), function less than 50% of normal, and instability. He was experiencing serious discomfort using a ladder and experienced an episode of shoulder subluxation. His physical examination findings were largely unchanged from his previous visit but exhibited discomfort with apprehension and anterior load examinations.

Following examination, his previous MRI was again reviewed. While the official report described a Buford complex, the abnormal-appearing labrum was located more inferior than the typical Buford complex—consistent with an anterior labral tear (Figure 1). Given his inability to return to sport activities and MRI results consistent with a labral injury, it was recommended that he undergo arthroscopic anterior labral repair due to his lack of progress from conservative management. The patient and his family elected to proceed with operative management.

During the procedure, the patient was placed in the lateral decubitus position. Standard anterior and posterior portals were established with an accessory anterior superolateral viewing portal. Diagnostic arthroscopy was significant for complete disruption of the labral tissue between the 3 o'clock and 6 o'clock positions (Figures 2(a) and 2(b), respectively). It was also revealed that there was an articular glenoid cartilage lesion measuring 6 mm × 8 mm anteroinferiorly (Figure 3). The posterior and superior labrums were intact, and there was no damage to any rotator cuff tendon or the biceps tendon.

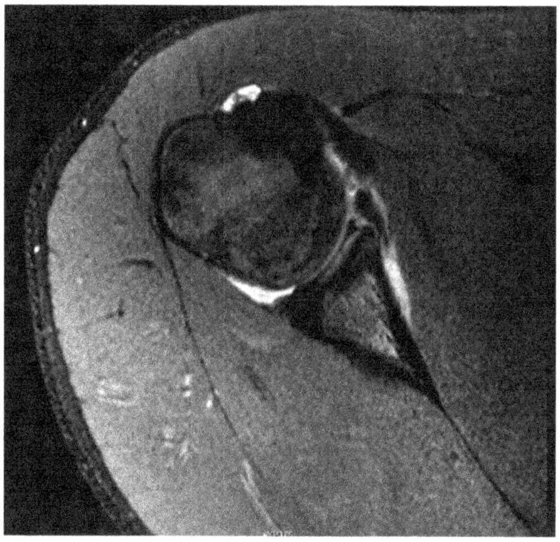

Figure 1: Preoperative MRI that was initially read as a Buford complex, but after failed conservative management, the lesion was reevaluated as an anterior inferior labral tear.

Before the labral repair, the calcified cartilage layer along the anterior-inferior glenoid, beneath the cartilage flap, was gently debrided and removed with an arthroscopic shaver and an arthroscopic curette (Figure 4). An arthroscopic biter and shaver were utilized to trim the fibrillated margins of the cartilage tissue. Three 2.4 mm Polyetheretherketone (PEEK) (Arthrex, Naples, FL) SutureTaks were placed at the 6, 4:30, and 3 o'clock positions on the glenoid. A 25-degree right angle suture lasso (Arthrex, Naples, FL) was used to imbricate several millimeters of capsular tissue. The suture lasso was then passed beneath the labrum at the site of each suture anchor and was then subsequently advanced through the fibrous rim of the displaced cartilage flap/GLAD lesion. The Nitinol wire was used to shuttle #2 FiberWire though the cartilage flap, around the labrum, and through the capsular tissues to establish 3 fixation points (Figures 5(a) and 5(b)). A simple knot configuration was tied with sliding arthroscopic Weston knots followed by three alternating half stitches, repeated 3 times, beginning inferiorly at 6 o'clock, progressing superiorly to 4:30 and 3 o'clock. This construct restored tension to the anterior band of the inferior glenohumeral ligament, recreated the anteroinferior labral bumper, and effectively reduced the cartilage flap/GLAD lesion to the anterior inferior glenoid (Figures 6(a) and 6(b)).

Three months postoperative, the patient reported no pain and 85% of normal function. On physical examination, he achieved 165 degrees of scaption, 65 degrees of external rotation, and internal rotation to the level of T9. At this time, he was instructed to continue physical therapy as per standard institutional protocol.

Five months postoperative, the patient suffered a traumatic fall backwards and landed on his outstretched, extended hand. He felt that his shoulder may have subluxed and noted moderate pain with activity (5/10). On physical examination, he achieved 150 degrees of scaption with discomfort, 45 degrees of external rotation with discomfort,

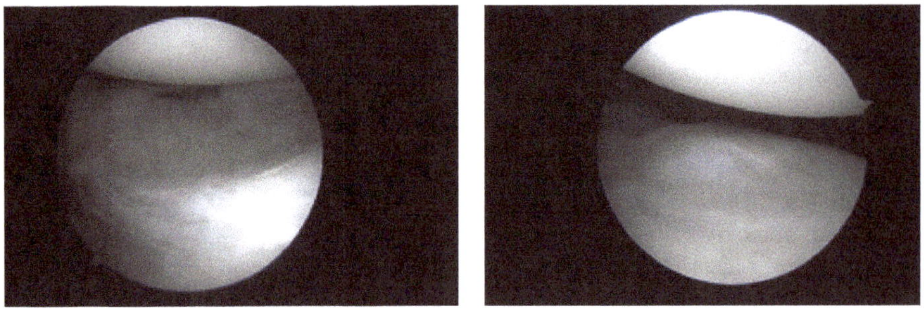

(a) (b)

Figure 2: Anterior inferior labral injury at the 3 o'clock (a) and 6 o'clock (b) positions.

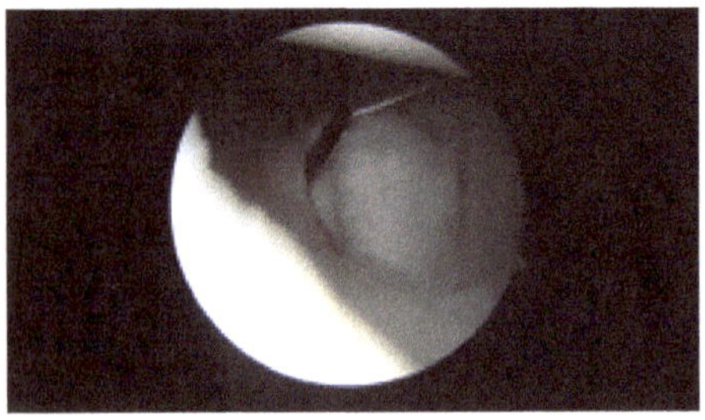

Figure 3: Identification of a 6 mm × 8 mm glenolabral articular defect (GLAD).

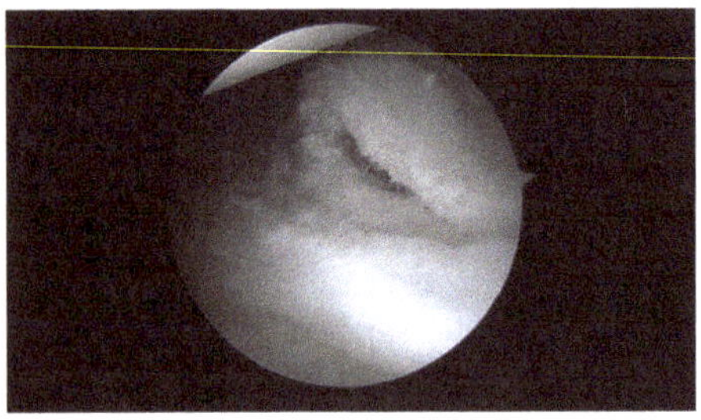

Figure 4: GLAD lesion following arthroscopic debridement of the underlying bony surface.

and internal rotation to the level of T10. He had discomfort with apprehension, which was relieved with relocation, as well as discomfort with anterior load and shift. An MRI was performed which revealed an intact GLAD lesion repair and labral repair (Figures 7(a) and 7(b), respectively). The GLAD lesion repair remained intact. Given the acuity of the injury, it was recommended that he undergo conservative treatment for one month.

The patient was seen one month later at his 6-month postoperative visit and reported no pain and 95% normal function. On physical examination, he achieved 170 degrees of scaption, 50 degrees of external rotation, and internal rotation to the level of T5 without any discomfort. He exhibited no tenderness to palpation and demonstrated a negative Neer test, O'Brien's test, valgus sheer stress, belly press test, anterior load test, and posterior load test. The apprehension test was similarly negative. The patient was instructed to continue with his home exercise regimen.

## 3. Discussion

Management of glenoid labral articular disruption (GLAD) is predicated on creating an even articular surface by debriding chondral tissue and removing loose bodies from the glenohumeral joint space [1, 2, 6]. The course of operative management is often determined by the degree of the articular lesion. If a small lesion is encountered, the unstable articular flap can be debrided, and the labrum can be advanced into the defect; however, if there is diffuse damage, only the articular surface is debrided, and the defect is left unfilled [7]. In this case report, we present an adolescent male who suffered an anterior shoulder dislocation which caused an anterior inferior labral tear with a concomitant GLAD lesion, which were both arthroscopically repaired concurrently with a single suture anchor construct. We believe that our technique is novel and previously unreported.

Traditionally, glenoid labral articular defects are repaired separately to labral lesions. Galano et al. utilized a cartilage fixation device to repair the GLAD lesion followed by labral repair with multiple suture anchors [8]. Additionally, Page and Bhatia reported a technique that utilized multiple suture anchors to first imbricate labral tissue and fasten it to the glenoid bone [9]. During fixation, the labral tissue was overlapped with the chondral edge to provide stability to the articular lesion, while additional anchoring stitches were then implanted to further secure the articular tissue. While primary repair of the GLAD lesion was described, none of these aforementioned techniques utilized a single suture anchor construct to concurrently repair both chondral and labral lesions.

Several studies have shown radiographic and clinical evidences demonstrating that patients receiving knee meniscectomies are at an increased risk of developing osteoarthritis due to loss of cartilage [10–12]. While studies have yet to establish a relationship between articular damage and the development of glenohumeral osteoarthritis, the same principles of increased humeral-to-glenoid contact following cartilage deficit lead to bony lesions within the glenohumeral joint. In older patients with glenohumeral osteoarthritis, surgical management typically includes arthroscopic debridement in mild cases, and in refractory or severe cases, a total shoulder arthroplasty [13, 14]. In younger patients, the treatment algorithm is not as clearly elucidated since radiologic

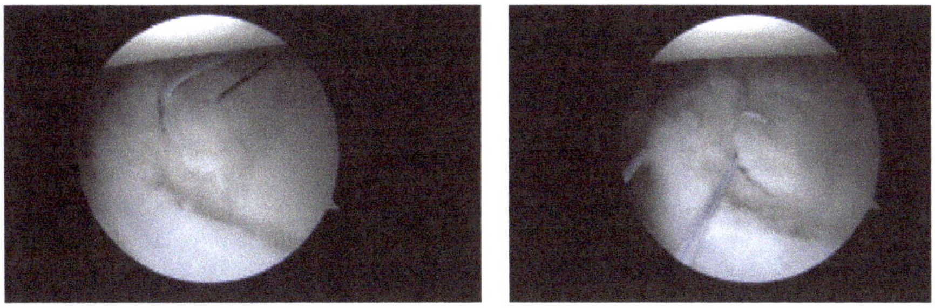

(a) (b)

FIGURE 5: Primary repair of the GLAD lesion. #2 suture is passed through the cartilage (a) with the fixation being incorporated into anchor constructs of the labral repair.

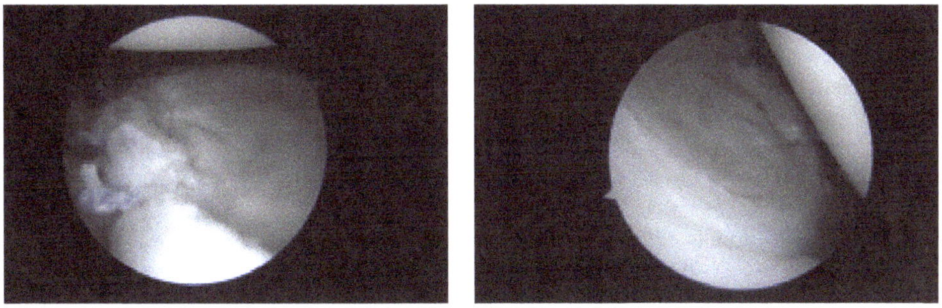

(a) (b)

FIGURE 6: Final repair of the anterior inferior labrum and GLAD lesion.

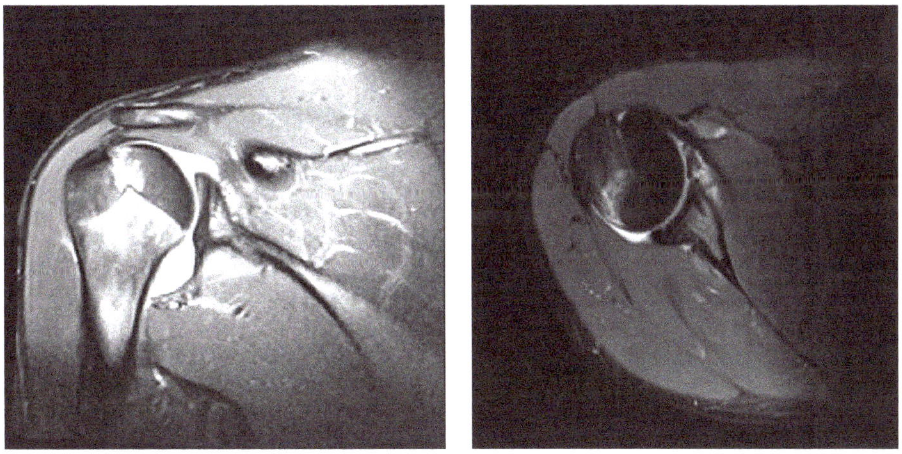

(a) (b)

FIGURE 7: Coronal (a) and axial (b) MRI performed 5 months postoperative due to traumatic injury reveals a Hill-sachs lesion. After nonconservative treatment resulted in improvement, the patient was instructed to follow-up only as needed.

and clinical outcomes following intervention are less favorable than in older patients [15].

Although the complications and outcomes of labral injuries with concomitant articular damage in the shoulder have not been thoroughly determined, within the hip literature, labral tears are frequently associated with articular lesions in the anterior acetabulum [16]. This injury predisposes patients to hip instability and osteoarthritis secondary to the labral defect and articular damage, respectively [17]. Although patients receiving labral repairs have favorable outcomes, those with concomitant cartilage defect are at an increased risk of osteoarthritis due to increased contact pressure of the femoral head on the acetabulum [18, 19]. Due to the analogous anatomy and physiology between the structures of the shoulder and hip joints, labral injuries with concomitant cartilage defect in the shoulder may lead to the development of osteoarthritis over time.

While concomitant injuries and fixation techniques impact the outcomes of shoulder labral repair in adolescents, patients exhibit good to excellent outcomes following arthroscopic repair [20]. The recurrence rate of instability following operative management is higher among the adolescent population than adults (18.7% vs. 25.1%, respectively); however, nearly 82% of adolescent patients return to their preinjury sport [21–23]. Due to the infrequent nature of GLAD lesions, outcomes following this injury have not been reported. Gross et al. performed a systematic review on cartilage restorative and reparative procedures of the glenohumeral joint, and while each injury and corrective procedure reported favorable outcomes, sample heterogeneity and a small sample size prohibited a direct comparison [24].

Management of GLAD lesions has been previously described with the purpose of reducing the uneven chondral surface within the glenohumeral joint in order to reduce pain [1, 2]. However, chondral debridement may predispose to glenohumeral arthritis. In this report, a patient who suffered an anterior inferior labral tear with concomitant GLAD lesion underwent concurrent primary repair of both the GLAD lesion and labral tear, utilizing a single suture anchor construct. Nonabsorbable sutures were used instead of absorbable sutures because they provide a more durable fixation during the healing phase (first four weeks postoperative). The simple stitch configuration is of a low profile; thus, no suture knot crosses the articular surface in this repair construct. If the GLAD lesion was managed with articular debridement, exposure of the underlying glenoid bone may have eventually predisposed to discomfort, instability, pain, and osteoarthritis. Glenohumeral arthritis may evolve to a debilitating disability with effects on quality of life comparable to chronic medical conditions such as chronic heart failure or diabetes [25]. Our approach to concurrent anterior labral and GLAD lesion repair should benefit the patient longitudinally by reducing the risk of developing osteoarthritis.

## References

[1] S. Waldt, A. Burkart, A. B. Imhoff, M. Bruegel, E. J. Rummeny, and K. Woertler, "Anterior shoulder instability: accuracy of MR arthrography in the classification of anteroinferior labroligamentous injuries," *Radiology*, vol. 237, no. 2, pp. 578–583, 2005.

[2] T. J. Neviaser, "The GLAD lesion: another cause of anterior shoulder pain," *Arthroscopy*, vol. 9, no. 1, pp. 22-23, 1993.

[3] G. E. Antonio, J. F. Griffith, A. B. Yu, P. S. H. Yung, K. M. Chan, and A. T. Ahuja, "First-time shoulder dislocation: high prevalence of labral injury and age-related differences revealed by MR arthrography," *Journal of Magnetic Resonance Imaging*, vol. 26, no. 4, pp. 983–991, 2007.

[4] P. Boileau, M. Villalba, J. Y. Hery, F. Balg, P. Ahrens, and L. Neyton, "Risk factors for recurrence of shoulder instability after arthroscopic Bankart repair," *The Journal of Bone & Joint Surgery*, vol. 88, no. 8, pp. 1755–1763, 2006.

[5] R. Pavic, P. Margetic, M. Bensic, and R. L. Brnadic, "Diagnostic value of US, MR and MR arthrography in shoulder instability," *Injury*, vol. 44, Supplement 3, pp. S26–S32, 2013.

[6] R. S. Page, "Managing chondral lesions of the glenohumeral joint," *International Journal of Shoulder Surgery*, vol. 2, no. 4, pp. 77-78, 2008.

[7] F. Elser, S. Braun, C. B. Dewing, and P. J. Millett, "Glenohumeral joint preservation: current options for managing articular cartilage lesions in young, active patients," *Arthroscopy*, vol. 26, no. 5, pp. 685–696, 2010.

[8] G. J. Galano, B. M. Weisenthal, and D. W. Altchek, "Articular shear of the anterior-inferior quadrant of the glenoid: a glenolabral articular disruption lesion variant," *American Journal of Orthopedics*, vol. 42, no. 1, pp. 41–43, 2013.

[9] R. Page and D. N. Bhatia, "Arthroscopic repair of a chondrolabral lesion associated with anterior glenohumeral dislocation," *Knee Surgery, Sports Traumatology, Arthroscopy*, vol. 18, no. 12, pp. 1748–1751, 2010.

[10] M. Englund and L. S. Lohmander, "Risk factors for symptomatic knee osteoarthritis fifteen to twenty-two years after meniscectomy," *Arthritis & Rheumatism*, vol. 50, no. 9, pp. 2811–2819, 2004.

[11] E. M. Roos, H. P. Roos, L. S. Lohmander, C. Ekdahl, and B. D. Beynnon, "Knee Injury and Osteoarthritis Outcome Score (KOOS)—development of a self-administered outcome measure," *Journal of Orthopaedic & Sports Physical Therapy*, vol. 28, no. 2, pp. 88–96, 1998.

[12] R. J. Johnson, D. B. Kettelkamp, W. Clark, and P. Leaverton, "Factors effecting late results after meniscectomy," *The Journal of Bone & Joint Surgery*, vol. 56, no. 4, pp. 719–729, 1974.

[13] D. M. Weinstein, J. S. Bucchieri, R. G. Pollock, E. L. Flatow, and L. U. Bigliani, "Arthroscopic debridement of the shoulder for osteoarthritis," *Arthroscopy*, vol. 16, no. 5, pp. 471–476, 2000.

[14] C. S. Radnay, K. J. Setter, L. Chambers, W. N. Levine, L. U. Bigliani, and C. S. Ahmad, "Total shoulder replacement compared with humeral head replacement for the treatment of primary glenohumeral osteoarthritis: a systematic review," *Journal of Shoulder and Elbow Surgery*, vol. 16, no. 4, pp. 396–402, 2007.

[15] P. J. Denard, M. A. Wirth, and R. M. Orfaly, "Management of glenohumeral arthritis in the young adult," *The Journal of Bone and Joint Surgery-American Volume*, vol. 93, no. 9, pp. 885–892, 2011.

[16] J. C. McCarthy, P. C. Noble, M. R. Schuck, J. Wright, and J. Lee, "The watershed labral lesion: its relationship to early arthritis of the hip," *The Journal of Arthroplasty*, vol. 16, no. 8, Supplement 1, pp. 81–87, 2001.

[17] J. C. McCarthy, P. C. Noble, M. R. Schuck, J. Wright, and J. Lee, "The role of labral lesions to development of early degenerative hip disease," *Clinical Orthopaedics and Related Research*, vol. 393, pp. 25–37, 2001.

[18] M. Beck, M. Kalhor, M. Leunig, and R. Ganz, "Hip morphology influences the pattern of damage to the acetabular cartilage: femoroacetabular impingement as a cause of early osteoarthritis of the hip," *The Journal of Bone and Joint Surgery-British Volume*, vol. 87, no. 7, pp. 1012–1018, 2005.

[19] J. D. Harris, "Hip labral repair: options and outcomes," *Current Reviews in Musculoskeletal Medicine*, vol. 9, no. 4, pp. 361–367, 2016.

[20] A. B. Imhoff, P. Ansah, T. Tischer et al., "Arthroscopic repair of anterior-inferior glenohumeral instability using a portal at the 5:30-o'clock position: analysis of the effects of age, fixation method, and concomitant shoulder injury on surgical

outcomes," *The American Journal of Sports Medicine*, vol. 38, no. 9, pp. 1795–1803, 2010.

[21] G. D. Rose, M. Borroni, and A. Castagna, "The role of arthroscopic capsulo-labral repair in unidirectional post-traumatic shoulder instability in adolescent athletes participating in overhead or contact sports," *Joints*, vol. 1, no. 3, pp. 108–111, 2013.

[22] J. Deitch, C. T. Mehlman, S. L. Foad, A. Obbehat, and M. Mallory, "Traumatic anterior shoulder dislocation in adolescents," *The American Journal of Sports Medicine*, vol. 31, no. 5, pp. 758–763, 2003.

[23] A. D. Mazzocca, F. M. Brown, D. S. Carreira, J. Hayden, and A. A. Romeo, "Arthroscopic anterior shoulder stabilization of collision and contact athletes," *The American Journal of Sports Medicine*, vol. 33, no. 1, pp. 52–60, 2005.

[24] C. E. Gross, P. N. Chalmers, J. Chahal et al., "Operative treatment of chondral defects in the glenohumeral joint," *Arthroscopy*, vol. 28, no. 12, pp. 1889–1901, 2012.

[25] G. M. Gartsman, M. R. Brinker, M. Khan, and M. Karahan, "Self-assessment of general health status in patients with five common shoulder conditions," *Journal of Shoulder and Elbow Surgery*, vol. 7, no. 3, pp. 228–237, 1998.

# 13

# Complete Traumatic Trifocal Failure of the Extensor Mechanism of the Knee: A Case Report and Review of the Literature

**Alexander J. Johnson, Katharine D. Harper, and Christopher Haydel**

*Temple University Hospital Department of Orthopaedics and Sports Medicine, USA*

Correspondence should be addressed to Alexander J. Johnson; ajj8952@gmail.com

Academic Editor: John Nyland

The unique case of a rare 3-level extensor mechanism failure in a 28-year-old male, involving a tibial tubercle avulsion fracture, a patellar tendon avulsion off the tibial tubercle fragment, and a severely comminuted patella fracture, and the surgical technique required to repair such an injury is presented. Focus is spent on the unique repair of a tendon injury when both proximal and distal bony attachments are damaged. Trifocal knee extensor mechanism is a rare clinical entity with minimal literature available—to date, this injury has only been reported in a retrospective review of combat-related injuries in military personnel. It is important to maintain an understanding of knee extensor mechanism anatomy and perform thorough investigation of high-energy knee injuries to ensure adequate treatment of all injuries. The outcome presented in this case shows that positive results after complex extensor mechanism injuries may be achieved, but limited data exists to elucidate optimum treatment. It is essential for surgeons to have firm grasp of techniques used to treat each segment of the extensor mechanism so that they may be combined when a patient presents with complex, multifocal injury.

## 1. Introduction

Traumatic extensor mechanism injuries are common, especially in those under 40 years of age. Most commonly, when the extensor mechanism fails, the failure occurs at a single location along the chain, with patella fractures being more common than other locations. [1] This paper will discuss in detail the unique case of a 3-level extensor mechanism failure and the surgical technique required to repair such an injury. The patient presented had a comminuted patellar fracture, a patellar tendon avulsion off the tibial tubercle, and a tibial tubercle fracture. Focus will be spent on the unique repair of a tendon injury when both proximal and distal bony attachments are damaged.

## 2. Case Details

A 28-year-old male presented to the emergency department after a motor vehicle accident (MVC). The patient had a body mass index (BMI) of 36, no significant past medical history, and no history of smoking. There was a possible history of remote, pediatric "knee surgery," but this history could not be confirmed by the patient. He was driving an 18-wheeler truck in the accident, which had the front end of the cab collapse into the cabin. At time of presentation to the trauma bay, he was initially assessed by the trauma service via Advanced Trauma Life Support (ATLS) standards and was determined to be hemodynamically stable with an isolated orthopaedic injury to his left lower extremity. The left lower extremity had two visible approximately 5 cm wounds over the anterior knee (Figure 1). Initial radiographs showed a tibial tubercle fracture and comminuted patella fracture (Figure 2). Computerized tomography (CT) scan was acquired that showed a vertical fracture line in the coronal plane of the tibial tubercle and comminuted patellar fracture (Figure 3). The patient received 2 g cefazolin in the emergency room for prophylaxis for his open fracture, as well as a tetanus vaccine. He was then emergently brought to the operating room for

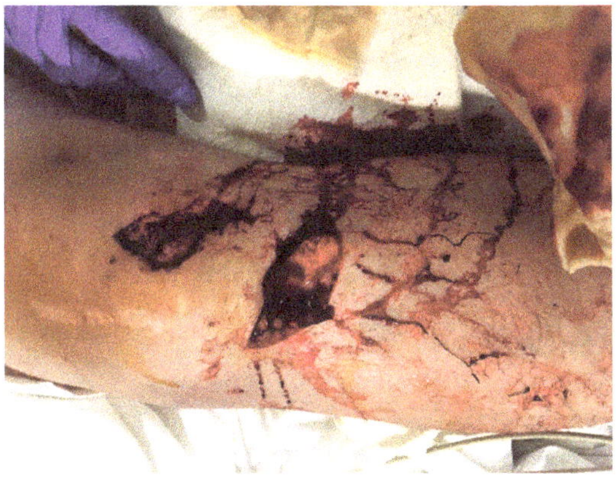

FIGURE 1: Picture demonstrating the wounds sustained in the initial injury, with underlying exposed bone of the fracture site.

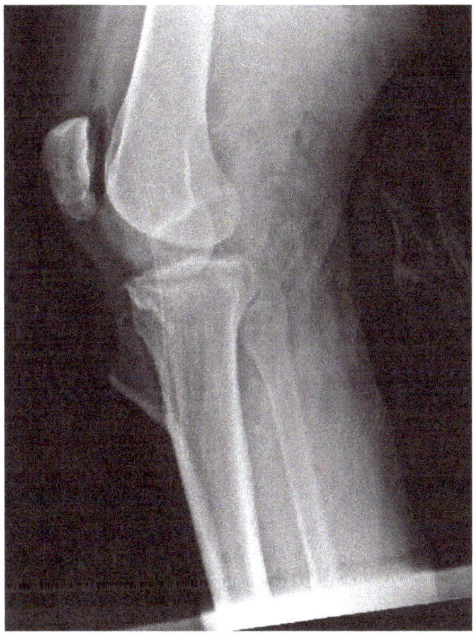

FIGURE 2: Lateral radiograph demonstrating tibial tubercle fracture and comminuted patellar fracture with overlying soft tissue defects.

irrigation and debridement of his open fracture wounds and ORIF for his patella and tibia. In the operating room, the injury was classified as a Gustilo-Anderson Grade II open tibia fracture with associated Gustilo-Anderson Grade II open patella fracture by the operative attending based on the wounds each measuring < 10 cm with evidence of vascular injury and no need for soft tissue coverage procedure.

## 3. Surgical Technique

There were two large wounds, one overlying the anterior tibia (with visualized tubercle fracture) as well as one overlying the patella (Figure 1). The distal-most, transverse wound was extended distally to improve visualization of the underlying fracture. These wounds were initially explored, and the patellar tendon was identified and mobilized from the overlying and underlying tissue. Once the tendon was mobilized, it was discovered to have avulsed from its tibial tubercle insertion. The most distal wound was extended distally along the lateral aspect of the tibial crest for complete visualization of the fracture. The fracture was mobilized and debrided of soft tissue, periosteum, and hematoma. After debridement, initial irrigation of the open wound was performed with 3L NS by low-pressure gravity tubing. Following that, an anatomical reduction was achieved on the fracture fragment and K-wire placement performed for initial fixation. Following that, two Synthes 3.5 mm cortical lag screws (Synthes DePuy; Warsaw, IN) were placed in the proximal and distal aspect of the fracture fragment. Adequate compression was achieved at the fracture site. Screw placement was confirmed under fluoroscopy to be in adequate position (Figure 4).

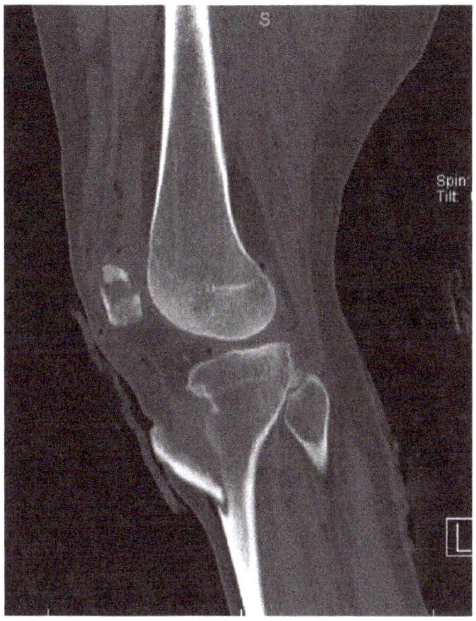


FIGURE 3: CT scan delineating the vertical, coronal plane fracture line of the extra-articular tibial tubercle fracture with overlying soft tissue injury. Also demonstrates a large bony defect in the patella, confirming the comminute nature of the fracture.

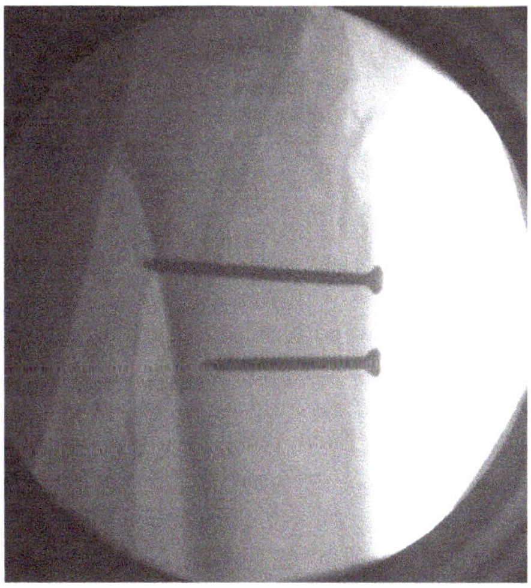

FIGURE 4: Intraoperative fluoroscopic images confirming anatomic reduction of the tibial tubercle fragment with 4.0 cannulated bicortical screws, placed in a lag screw fashion.

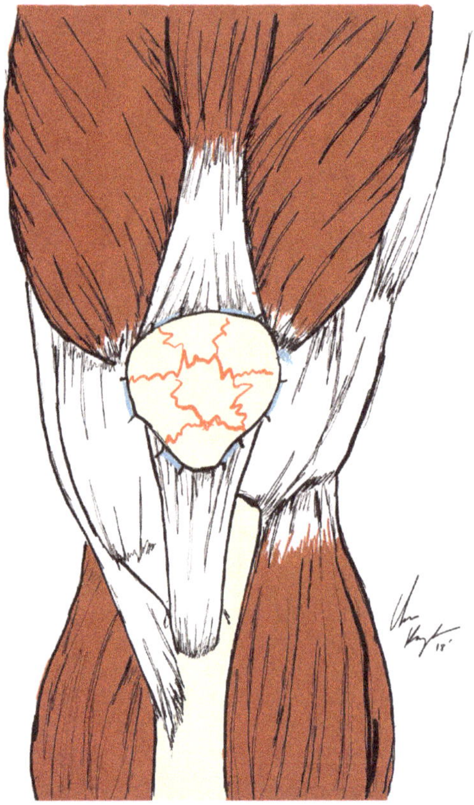

Figure 5: An illustration demonstrating the unique, purse-string technique employed for fixation of the patella fracture with overlying soft tissue deficit.

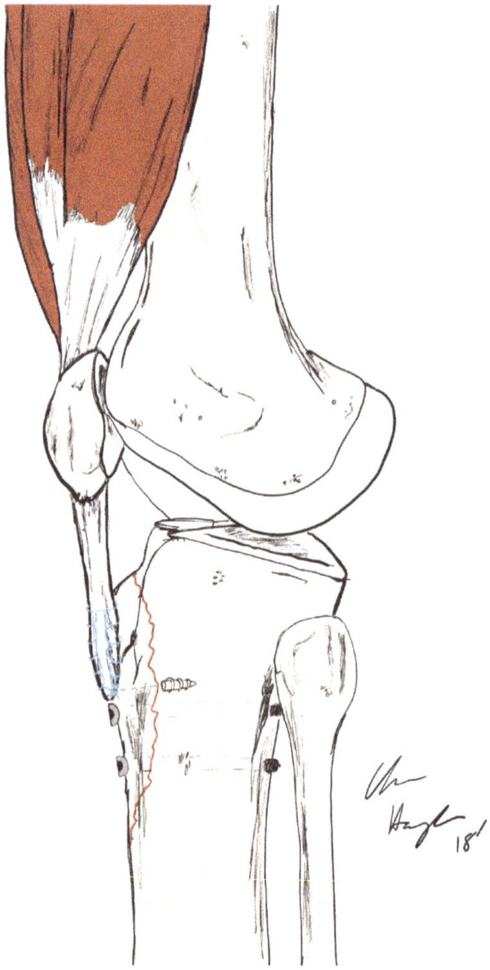

Figure 6: An illustration demonstrating the placement of anchor suture drill holes for fixation of the patellar tendon insertion, bypassing previously fixated fracture site.

Attention was then turned to the patellar fracture. Patellar retinaculum was investigated and determined to be intact, with a comminuted patella fracture underlying with minimal displacement of fragments. A small retinacular window was created to observe the largest fragment, and a point-to-point bone clamp was placed on the medial and lateral aspect of the patella to compress the fracture fragments. Following compression, a #2 fibre wire was placed in a cerclage, purse-string fashion around the patellar retinacular soft tissue and hand tied under tension (Figure 5). Clamp was removed and good compression across comminuted fragments was found with gross alignment maintained. The patella was then irrigated with 3L NS solution, and the retinacular window was closed using #0 vicryl suture in an interrupted fashion.

Finally, the patellar tendon insertion avulsion was addressed. Due to the associated tibial tubercle fracture, this presented a unique challenge in acquiring adequate fixation. Two Arthrex 5.5 mm corkscrew anchor sutures (Arthrex; Naples, FL) were placed at the tibial insertion just medial to and through the previously fixed fracture fragment. The anchors were advanced from anterior to posterior through the fracture fragment and into a stable tibial bone (Figure 6). The anchors were tested manually and found to be well fixed in a stable bone. Attached #2 fibre wire was then stitched through the patellar tendon in a Krakow stitch using a free needle. Two complete distal to proximal then proximal to distal rows of sutures were performed and tied overtop the tendon. The insertion site was then reinforced with #0 vicryl suture. The entire extensor mechanism repair was tested under flexion without evidence of gapping at the tibial tubercle fracture site, patellar fracture site, or patellar tendon repair site (Figure 7).

Following surgery, the patient was hospitalized for 24 hours of antibiotic treatment, compartment monitoring, and pain control. He was discharged with partial weight bearing in a hinged knee brace locked in extension on postoperative day 1. First follow-up visit occurred 10 days after surgery and showed well-healing wounds without evidence of skin necrosis (Figure 8). Final follow-up occurred at 1 year postsurgery; his wounds have healed without issue; he has complete bony union of all fractures, has returned to full activities, and has no complaints at this time. X-rays from final follow-up are shown in Figure 9.

## 4. Discussion

We have described a case of trifocal knee extensor mechanism failure including a tibial tubercle avulsion fracture, a

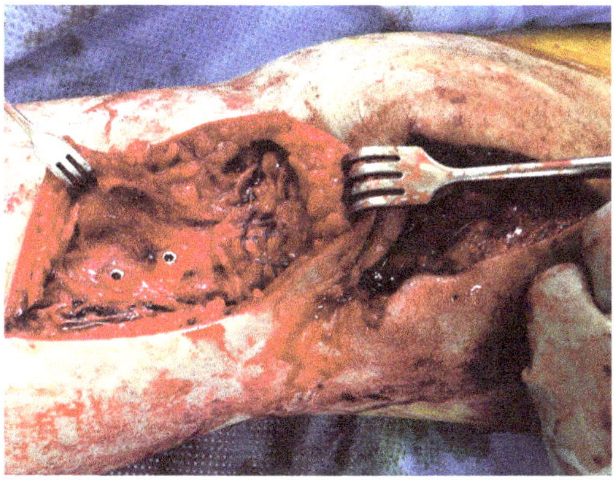

Figure 7: Intraoperative clinical picture showing the completed repair of the tibial tubercle fracture, patellar fracture, and patellar tendon avulsion.

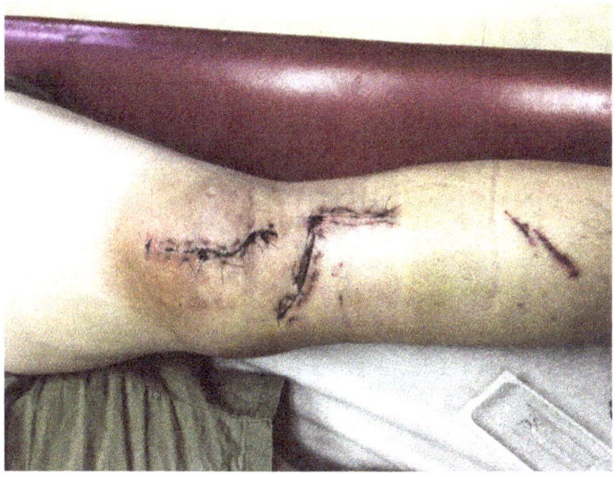

Figure 8: Clinical photograph at first follow-up visit showing well-healing wounds without evidence of skin necrosis, wound breakdown, erythema, or drainage.

patellar tendon avulsion off the tibial tubercle fragment, and a severely comminuted patella fracture. Failure of the knee extensor mechanism in three locations is exceedingly rare with the only identified report in a retrospective review of combat-related injuries in military personnel [1]. In that series, 17 reviewed complex open extensor mechanism injuries were caused by explosive devices in 15 cases and high energy gunshots in 2 cases compared to the current case which involved a restrained tractor trailer driver in a high-speed motor vehicle collision. The authors proposed a novel classification scheme based on the segment of the extensor mechanism that was injured, soft tissue status, and associated distal femur or proximal tibia fracture requiring fixation. According to this classification, the injury in the current case would be labeled a 345A0, an injury combination that was not present in any of the 17 reviewed cases. The series did include 4 cases of trifocal extensor mechanism failure and 1 case of four-level failure.

In adults, patellar tendon avulsions/ruptures are more common in patients with elevated body mass index (BMI), underlying systemic illness, or steroid use [2]. The patient in the current case did have an elevated BMI of 36, but did not clearly possess any other risk factors, although no dedicated workup of systemic illness was performed. Generally, patellar avulsion and tendinous failure of the extensor mechanism occur via force applied across a flexed knee, while comminuted or open patella fractures occur via direct trauma [2]. The injury in the current case is most likely related to a combined mechanism evidenced by the tubercle avulsion fracture and the comminuted patella fracture with overlying open wound. At 10-month follow-up, our patient has minimal pain over the anterior knee, intact extensor mechanism with 5 out of 5 knee extension strength, and range of motion of 0 to 130 degrees at the knee. He was able to return to activities of daily living and employment as a truck driver with frequent requirements to lift heavy objects and has returned to weight training in the gym, reporting focus on squat exercises. The authors consider this patient to have a better than expected outcome given the extent of injury. In one previous outcome study, there was a trend for patients with open patella fractures to have more associated injuries, higher pain scores, lower functional outcome scores, and higher incidence of complications, though this data did not reach statistical significance [3].

In limited case series, patella fractures were open in 7-13% of cases and were treated with antibiotics, incision, and debridement and various forms of fracture fixation with or without internal fixation [3–5]. In the current case, the patient was treated with immediate antibiotics and incision and debridement. The fracture was treated with purse-string closure of the overlying periosteum without internal fixation because the highly comminuted fracture had limited fixation options and high risk of infection existed given large open wound. While the previously cited series reported infection rates between 0 and 10.7% [3–5], there was no evidence of infection in the current case.

Although examples of trifocal extensor mechanism failure are lacking in nonmilitary series, there are a number of reports of bifocal failure. Kang et al. summarized these reports and presented a case of bifocal knee extensor mechanism disruption in an 84-year-old male after a motorcycle accident resulting in an open avulsion fracture of the inferior patellar pole and avulsion fracture of the tibial tubercle [6]. In this case, the patellar avulsion was repaired with three nonabsorbable number 2.0 Ethibond sutures using a vertical wiring technique [7], and the tibial tubercle avulsion was repaired with a 4.0 cannulated screw. The authors also proposed a classification system for double disruptions of the knee extensor mechanism. The injury presented in the current case resembles a type 1 injury under this classification system—avulsion fracture of tibial tubercle with patellar ligament avulsion off the tibial tubercle—with an ipsilateral comminuted patella fracture. In the literature review presented by Kang et al., 14 reported cases of type 1 injuries were identified, all in patients 18 years or younger, further illustrating the rarity of the case presented here in a 28-year-old patient [6].

Though reports of such injuries are limited in adult literature, several repair techniques have been described in pediatric cases of combined tibial tubercle and patella tendon avulsion injuries. Common to most of these reported

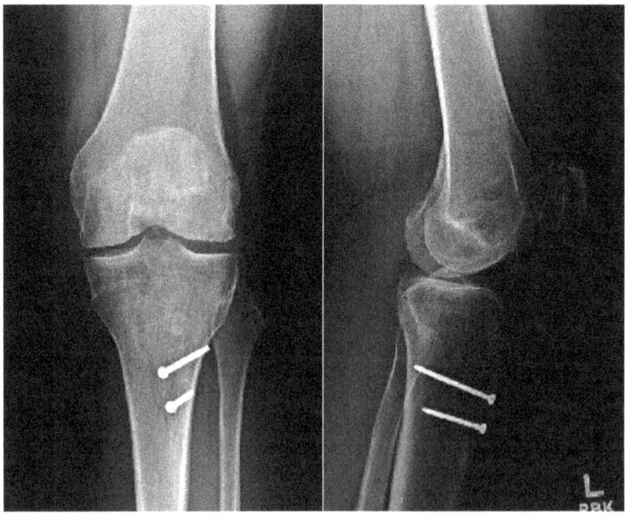


FIGURE 9: AP and lateral radiograph taken at 1-year follow-up showing healed fracture and no evidence of hardware complications.

techniques is open reduction and internal fixation of the tubercle fragment with screw fixation, but K-wire and staple fixation have also been described [6]. Multiple techniques for repairing the patella tendon injury have been described including staple fixation of the patellar tendon to the tibia distal to the tubercle fracture [8], suture fixation of the patellar tendon through transverse transosseous tunnels in the tibia distal to the tubercle fragment [9], and suture repair of the patella tendon to the tibial periosteum distal to the tubercle fracture [10]. Regardless of the method used, the repair of the avulsed tendon is commonly performed with fixation distal to the reduced tibial tubercle fragment, as it was in this case.

## 5. Conclusion

Although the injury described in this case does appear to be extremely rare, it is important to maintain a complete understanding of knee extensor mechanism anatomy and perform thorough investigation of high-energy knee injuries to ensure adequate treatment and improved outcomes in injuries that could be otherwise devastating to future function. The case and technique reviewed in this case demonstrate that acceptable outcomes after complex extensor mechanism injuries are possible, but limited data exists to elucidate optimum treatment. It is essential for surgeons who may encounter similar injuries to have firm grasp of techniques used to treat injury to each segment of the extensor mechanism so that they may be combined accordingly when a patient presents with complex, multifocal injury.

## References


[1] R. C. Andersen, K. W. Wilson, J. A. Bojescul, T. J. Mickel, W. T. Gordon, and B. K. Potter, "Open, combat-related loss, or disruption of the knee extensor mechanism: treatment strategies, classification, and outcomes," *Journal of Orthopaedic Trauma*, vol. 28, no. 11, pp. e250–e257, 2014.

[2] M. R. Garner, E. Gausden, M. B. Berkes, J. T. Nguyen, and D. G. Lorich, "Extensor mechanism injuries of the knee: demographic characteristics and comorbidities from a review of 726 patient records," *The Journal of Bone and Joint Surgery-American Volume*, vol. 97, no. 19, pp. 1592–1596, 2015.

[3] S. Anand, J. C. Hahnel, and P. V. Giannoudis, "Open patellar fractures: high energy injuries with a poor outcome?," *Injury*, vol. 39, no. 4, pp. 480–484, 2008.

[4] M. Torchia and D. Lewallen, "Open fractures of the patella," *Journal of Orthopaedic Trauma*, vol. 10, no. 6, pp. 403–409, 1996.

[5] J. Catalano, W. Iannacone, S. Marczyk et al., "Open fractures of the patella: long-term functional outcome," *The Journal of Trauma: Injury, Infection, and Critical Care*, vol. 39, no. 3, pp. 439–444, 1995.

[6] S. Kang, P. H. Chung, Y. S. Kim, H. M. Lee, and J. P. Kim, "Bifocal disruption of the knee extensor mechanism: a case report and literature review," *Archives of Orthopaedic and Trauma Surgery*, vol. 133, no. 4, pp. 517–521, 2013.

[7] K. H. Yang and Y. S. Byun, "Separate vertical wiring for the fixation of comminuted fractures of the inferior pole of the patella," *The Journal of Bone and Joint Surgery. British volume*, vol. 85-B, no. 8, pp. 1155–1160, 2003.

[8] J.-H. Seo, M.-W. Kim, D.-H. Kim, and S.-S. Seo, "Avulsion fracture of the tibial tuberosity with patellar ligament rupture in an adolescent patient," *Arthroscopy and Orthopedic Sports Medicine*, vol. 2, no. 1, pp. 48–50, 2015.

[9] M. Louis Rizio and M. Kenneth Swan Jr, "Combined avulsion fracture of the tibial tubercle and avulsion of the patellar ligament," *Orthopedics*, vol. 30, no. 7, pp. 571-572, 2007.

[10] U. Frankl, S. A. Wasilewski, and W. L. Healy, "Avulsion fracture of the tibial tubercle with avulsion of the patellar ligament. Report of two cases," *The Journal of Bone & Joint Surgery*, vol. 72, no. 9, pp. 1411–1413, 1990.

# 14

# Electronic Cigarette Burns: A Case Report and Review of Current Literature

**Rachel Michael, Nabil Ebraheim, Jacob Maier, Mina Tanios, and Anthony Kouri**

*University of Toledo Medical Center Department of Orthopaedic Surgery, 3000 Arlington Ave Toledo, OH 43614, USA*

Correspondence should be addressed to Rachel Michael; rachel.michael@utoledo.edu

Academic Editor: Christian W. Müller

Due to the development of electronic cigarettes and their use in our patient population, this article seeks to evaluate the safety and associated morbidity that may result from their use. This article also presents a patient case regarding an explosion of an electronic cigarette battery and the resultant injury and deformity that occurred.

## 1. Introduction

In recent years, Electronic Nicotine Delivery Systems (ENDS), also known as electronic cigarettes (e-cigarettes) have gained increased popularity. While viewed as a healthier alternative to traditional tobacco cigarettes, ENDS present new dangers. In 2016, the National Electronic Injury Surveillance System (NEISS) reported 26 cases of ENDS-related burn injuries that were presented to emergency departments, which translates to a national average of 1007 ENDS-related burn injuries [1]. Corey et al. also report that the majority of these burns (77.3%) were located on the patient's upper trunk/lower leg, which is a result of explosions occurring in the shirt or pant pockets. Numerous case studies have shown that, in addition to the thigh, the genitalia are often injured in these types of explosions [2, 3]. Injuries to the hands and face are also common when the ENDS explodes during use [4, 5]. In addition to burns, maxillofacial fractures have also been documented [6]. Researchers attribute the cause of these explosions to the lithium ion battery that powers the device [7]. This mechanism contributes to the mixed thermal and alkali chemical burns seen in patients [8]. This article focuses on the morbidity-associated burns from ENDS and does not take into account the overall prevalence of burn injuries.

Nicotine-free e-cigarettes appear to be more popular than their nicotine counterparts among the younger generation. One study showed that out of all teenagers that reported using e-cigarettes, 72% used products without nicotine (versus 28% who used products with nicotine) [9]. Ferrari et al. found that there were no immediate adverse effects from nicotine-free e-cigarettes, with respect to fractional concentration of exhaled carbon monoxide and nitric oxide [10]. The use of e-cigarettes has also been shown to mimic cancer. Ring Madsen et al. presented a case that suggests e-cigarettes can induce an inflammatory response similar to responses found in metastatic cancer [11]. Similarly, Fracol et al. found that e-cigarette vapor was cytotoxic to endothelial cells independent of nicotine content [12].

## 2. Case

This case was chosen due to its unique historical presentation and resultant morbidity. A 40-year-old male presented to the emergency department with severe burns on the left posterior thigh that resulted from the spontaneous combustion of an ENDS in his left front pant pocket (Figures 1 and 2). The patient states that the device was turned off while in his pocket. The patient was a nonnicotine e-cigarette user. Due to the nature of his injury, the patient was transported to a nearby hospital burn unit. His injuries were treated with multiple debridements both bedside and in the operating theatre. The patient then underwent a split thickness autograft and additional use of an allograft matrix four days after injury. Following the procedure, the left thigh graft remained

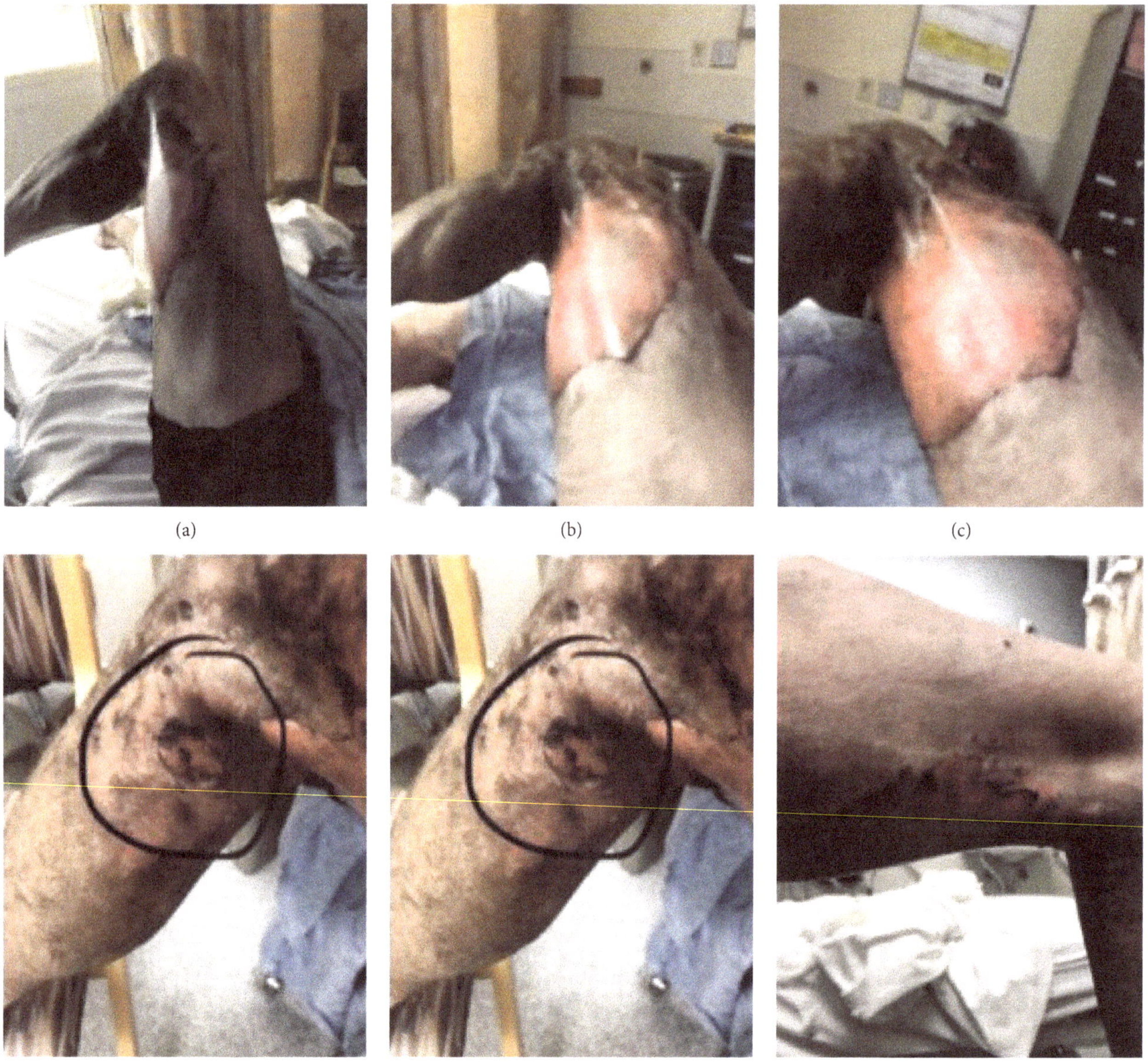

(a) (b) (c)

(d) (e) (f)

Figure 1: Images (a–f) are the presenting burn injuries on the left lower extremity.

viable and had been incorporated fully; however, there was some evidence of graft hypertrophy and signs of contracture around the boundary of the graft.

One month after injury, the patient continued to have intermittent pain, irritation, and numbness over the left posterior thigh burn site and has not returned to a normal gait. The patient states that since his injury, he has noticed a drastic decline in his activities and ability to exercise at the level he did prior to his injury. He also has cosmetic concerns about his burn scars and contractures and thus wears clothes that cover the exposed sites.

Patient examination one month after his injury demonstrated a mildly antalgic gait with external rotation of the left lower extremity with external foot progression compared to the contralateral side. The patient had full tone and motor strength throughout the bilateral lower extremities. There was no cyanosis or edema noted on his examination. Focused examination of the right lower extremity demonstrated a scab over the skin graft harvest site on the anterior thigh (Figure 3). At the donor site on the right thigh, the patient experienced some pain which manifests as tenderness and redness. He was neurovascularly intact distally. Of note, the right lower extremity had quadriceps atrophy compared to the contralateral side (Figure 4).

The left lower extremity demonstrated healing at the skin graft recipient site with mild contraction over the posterior knee and thigh. The graft spanned the posterior aspect of the knee joint and contributed to the loss of terminal extension of the knee joint. There was no surrounding erythema. On the left lower extremity, the quadriceps muscle appears larger due to fascial defects (Figures 4 and 5). Clinically, there was also evidence of iliotibial band tightness compared to the contralateral extremity which may also contribute to the lack of full mobility. Knee range of motion was assessed and was

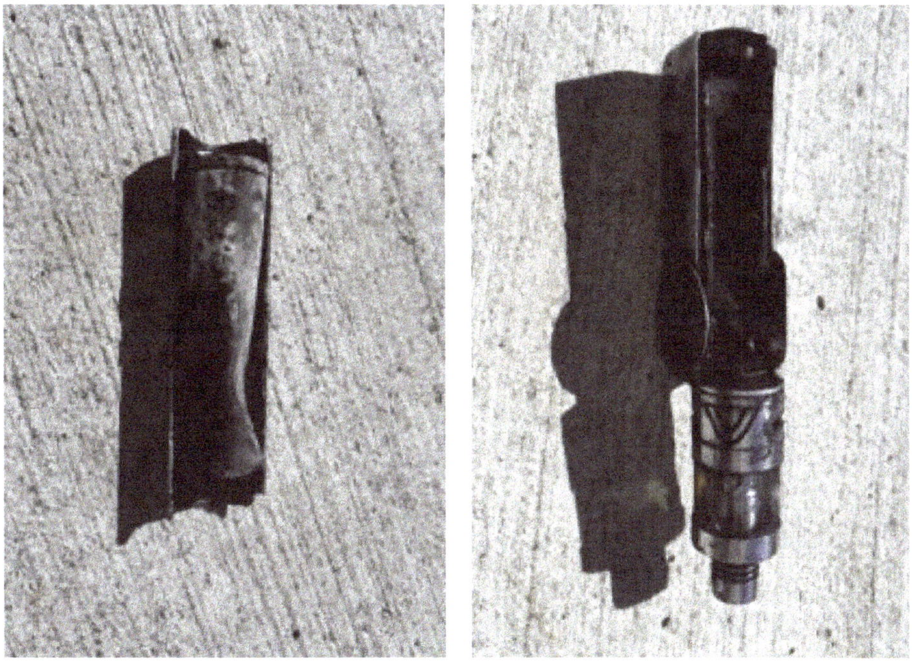

(a) (b)

FIGURE 2: Images (a, b) represent the electronic cigarette after it exploded.

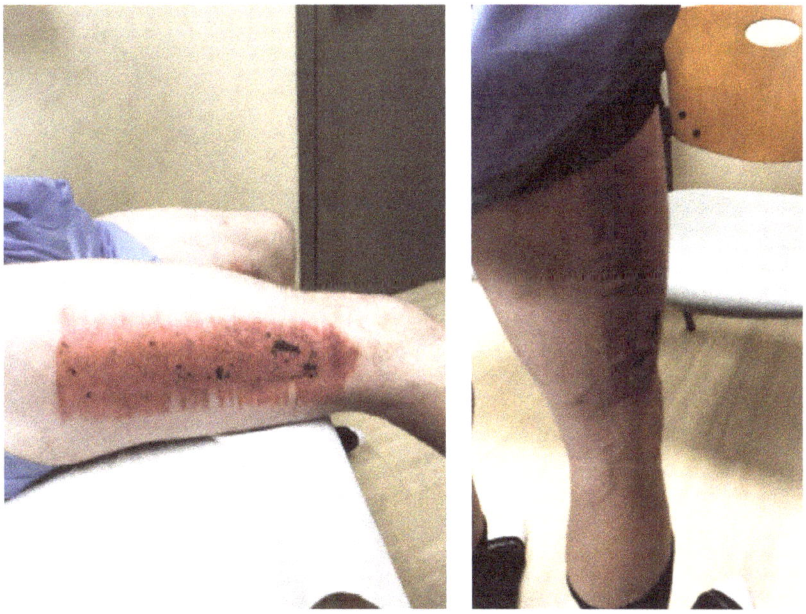

(a) (b)

FIGURE 3: The right thigh site of the split thickness skin graft donor site. The patient is one month after grafting.

15-110 degrees on the left and 5-130 degrees on the right (Table 1). The patient had bilateral hip extension to neutral.

If his symptoms do not respond to conservative measures with physical therapy and scar massage, the patient may require surgical interventions such as revision grafting, iliotibial band release, or possible tendon and skin z-plasties.

The patient also indicated that he is having difficulty coping with his injury. The cosmetic appearance of his graft and donor site is of great emotional concern to the patient. He was recommended for psychological evaluation and treatment to help him cope with the mental trauma associated with his injury.

## 3. Discussion

Cases of severe burns from spontaneous combustion of ENDS are becoming a concern with their increasing popularity as alternatives to traditional cigarette smoking. A large

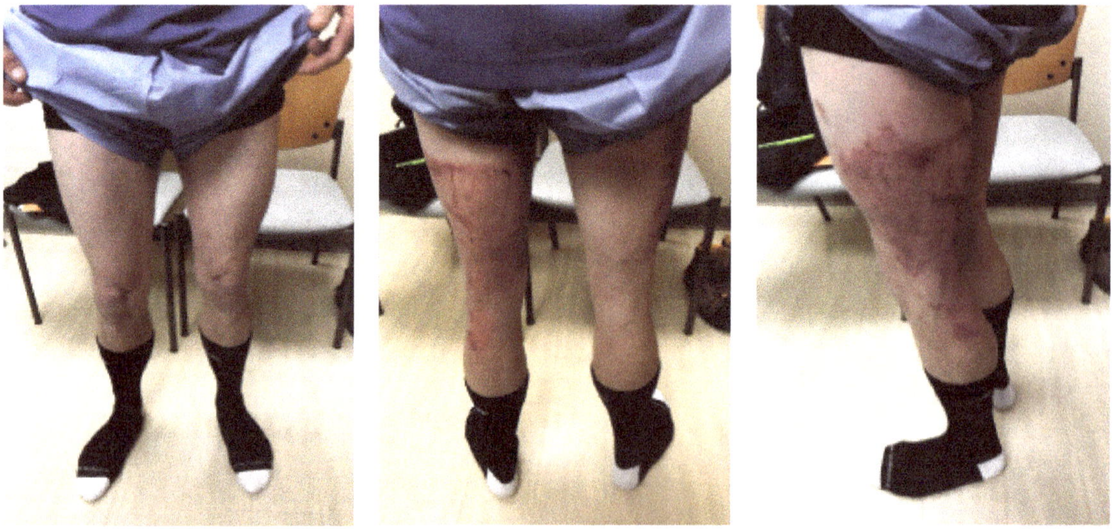

(a) (b) (c)

Figure 4: Anterior, posterior, and lateral gross images of the patient bilateral lower extremities one month after injury. The discrepancy in quadriceps volume can be seen in (a). (b) demonstrates the residual scar from his burns and grafting on the left posterior thigh. (c) is the lateral view of the left lower extremity injury after grafting.

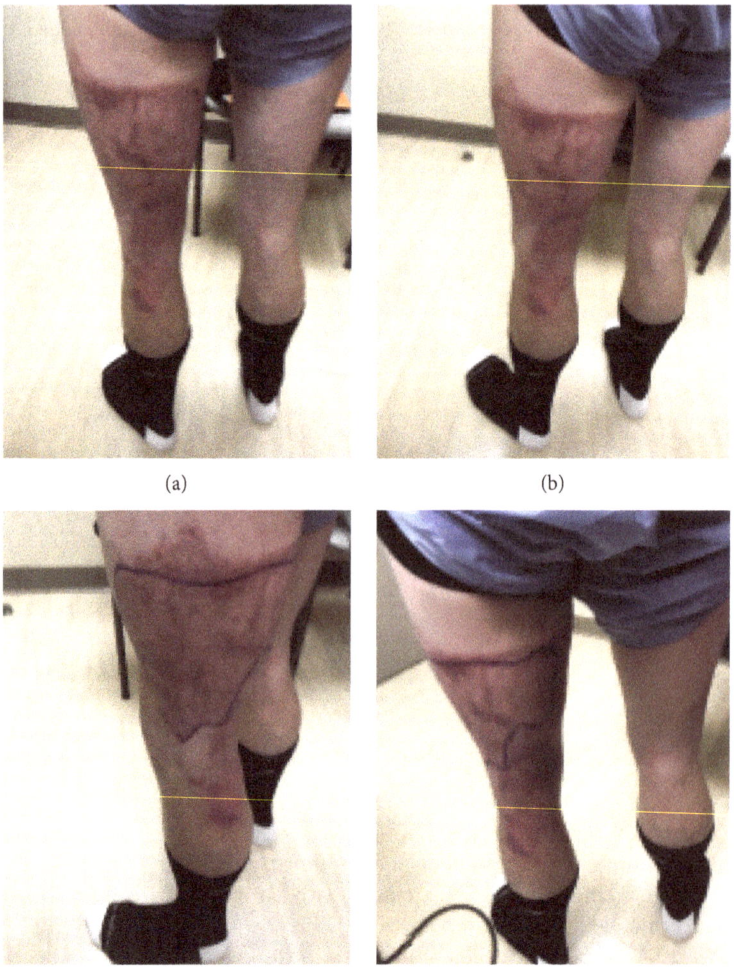

(a) (b)

(c) (d)

Figure 5: Views of the affected left lower extremity one month after injury. (c, d) show the outline of the graft recipient site.

Table 1: Lower extremity range of motion one month after injury.

| | Lower extremity range of motion | |
|---|---|---|
| | Right lower extremity (autograft harvest limb) | Left lower extremity (injured/graft recipient limb) |
| Hip extension | 0° | 0° |
| Hip flexion | 110° | 110° |
| Knee extension | 5° | 15° |
| Knee flexion | 130° | 110° |

percentage of these explosions occur in the pants or shirt pockets which makes the severe burns on the thigh and chest or upper extremity a common presentation. The scar contractures around the knee and hip joints pose a significant functional limitation. The psychiatric effects of the incurred trauma and resultant cosmetic deformity are not well documented in the current literature but present a significant issue for these patients. Our patient struggled with the appearance of burns on his legs, yet many patients have been documented to have prominent burns on their faces and hands. The physiological trauma of this injury cannot be overlooked. It is also postulated that less severe burns may occur with more frequency and are not included in the studies of severe burns requiring surgical treatment. These less severe burns may be treated by family practice or emergency department personnel and are thus not included in the present study population. Further investigation is needed on all burns from ENDS.

It is our intention with this article to demonstrate the dangers of these devices so that the public and our patients may be better informed. The danger of serious burns is related to the combustibility of the lithium battery that powers the devices, which is unique compared to heat burns from traditional tobacco cigarettes. Thus, there needs to be further investigation to compare chemical burns associated with electronic cigarettes versus traditional cigarette burns. We currently recommend against the use of all ENDS, both nicotine-containing and nicotine-free devices, due to the cytotoxicity of the vapors and the potential for device explosion. However, we understand that these devices will continue to be used within our patient population, and thus, it is our recommendation that guidelines for proper storage and care of the devices should be made.

## References


[1] C. G. Corey, J. T. Chang, and B. L. Rostron, "Electronic nicotine delivery system (ENDS) battery-related burns presenting to US emergency departments, 2016," *Injury Epidemiology*, vol. 5, no. 1, p. 4, 2018.

[2] D. Treitl, R. Solomon, D. L. Davare, R. Sanchez, and C. Kiffin, "Full and partial thickness burns from spontaneous combustion of E-cigarette lithium-ion batteries with review of literature," *The Journal of Emergency Medicine*, vol. 53, no. 1, pp. 121–125, 2017.

[3] A. Z. Jiwani, J. F. Williams, J. A. Rizzo, K. K. Chung, B. T. King, and L. C. Cancio, "Thermal injury patterns associated with electronic cigarettes," *International Journal of Burns and Trauma*, vol. 7, no. 1, pp. 1–5, 2017.

[4] D. E. Cason, D. E. Morgan, and J. A. Pietryga, "Injuries from an exploding E-cigarette: a case report," *Annals of Internal Medicine*, vol. 165, no. 9, pp. 678-679, 2016.

[5] R. Harrison and D. Hicklin Jr., "Electronic cigarette explosions involving the oral cavity," *Journal of the American Dental Association*, vol. 147, no. 11, pp. 891–896, 2016.

[6] B. A. Archambeau, S. Young, C. Lee et al., "E-cigarette blast injury: complex facial fractures and pneumocephalus," *The Western Journal of Emergency Medicine*, vol. 17, no. 6, pp. 805–807, 2016.

[7] C. Sheckter, A. Chattopadhyay, J. Paro, and Y. Karanas, "Burns resulting from spontaneous combustion of electronic cigarettes: a case series," *Burns & Trauma*, vol. 4, p. 35, 2016.

[8] K. J. Nicoll, A. M. Rose, M. A. Khan, O. Quaba, and A. G. Lowrie, "Thigh burns from exploding e-cigarette lithium ion batteries: first case series," *Burns*, vol. 42, no. 4, pp. E42–E46, 2016.

[9] H. A. Hamilton, R. Ferrence, A. Boak et al., "Ever use of nicotine and nonnicotine electronic cigarettes among high school students in Ontario, Canada," *Nicotine & Tobacco Research*, vol. 17, no. 10, pp. 1212–1218, 2015.

[10] M. Ferrari, A. Zanasi, E. Nardi et al., "Short-term effects of a nicotine-free e-cigarette compared to a traditional cigarette in smokers and non-smokers," *BMC Pulmonary Medicine*, vol. 15, no. 1, pp. 1–9, 2015.

[11] L. R. Madsen, N. H. V. Krarup, T. K. Bergmann et al., "A Cancer That Went Up in Smoke: Pulmonary Reaction to e-Cigarettes Imitating Metastatic Cancer," *Chest*, vol. 149, no. 3, pp. e65–e67, 2016.

[12] M. Fracol, R. Dorfman, L. Janes et al., "The surgical impact of E-cigarettes: a case report and review of the current literature," *Archives of Plastic Surgery*, vol. 44, no. 6, pp. 477–481, 2017.

# 15

# Recurrent Hematomas following a Revision Total Hip Arthroplasty in Acquired Coagulation Factor XIII Deficiency

**Yoshinori Takashima, Shingo Hashimoto, Tomoyuki Kamenaga, Masanori Tsubosaka, Yuichi Kuroda, Kazuhiro Takeuchi, Koji Takayama, Shinya Hayashi, Ryosuke Kuroda, and Tomoyuki Matsumoto**

*Department of Orthopaedic Surgery, Kobe University Graduate School of Medicine, Kobe, 7-5-1, Kusunoki-cho, Chuo-ku, Kobe 650-0017, Japan*

Correspondence should be addressed to Shingo Hashimoto; shingo1023@theia.ocn.ne.jp

Academic Editor: Mark K. Lyons

Coagulation factor XIII (FXIII) is the final enzyme in the coagulation cascade and plays an important role in catalyzing the intermolecular cross-linking of fibrin polymers. FXIII deficiency is a rare disorder that presents with recurrent soft tissue bleeding. In this case report, we describe a patient with recurrent hematomas, following a revision total hip arthroplasty (THA). A 50-year-old female patient with no past history of bleeding and with a normal perioperative coagulation profile presented with recurrent hip joint hematomas. Her plasma FXIII activity showed a slight decrease (69%). Therefore, the patient was diagnosed with an acquired deficiency and was administered FXIII to correct it. The bleeding did not recur once the FXIII activity had returned to a normal level (76%). At 2 months after the second evacuation procedure, the patient was discharged from the hospital in an ambulatory state. There has been no recurrence of a hematoma since. We managed a rare case of acquired FXIII deficiency, which highlighted that a patient can present with an acquired bleeding disorder despite having a normal coagulation profile. An acquired FXIII deficiency should be suspected in patients with inexplicable, sudden-onset bleeding, as early diagnosis and treatment are important to prevent life-threatening complications.

## 1. Introduction

Coagulation factor XIII (FXIII) exists as a protransglutaminase (FXIII-A2B2) enzyme in the plasma. The enzyme is composed of two catalytic A subunits (FXIII-A2) and two noncatalytic B subunits (FXIII-B2), held together by noncovalent bonds [1, 2]. FXIII is the final enzyme in the coagulation cascade pathway and plays an important role in catalyzing the intermolecular cross-linking of fibrin polymers, thereby stabilizing the fibrin clot [3]. Patients with FXIII deficiency present with symptoms of recurrent soft tissue bleeding and delayed wound healing. To our knowledge, there are few published papers on the management of recurrent hip joint hematoma following a revision total hip arthroplasty (THA), in patients with FXIII deficiency. We report the case of a patient with recurrent postoperative hematomas that led to the diagnosis of this rare bleeding disorder.

## 2. Case Report

A 50-year-old woman underwent a THA of the right hip by the Dall approach, at another hospital, for an idiopathic osteonecrosis of the femoral head. However, she experienced frequent dislocation of the operated joint. She was then referred to our hospital the same year. The patient presented only with right-sided, lateral thigh pain. There was no past history of excessive bleeding following trauma, dental procedures, or surgery. She did not have a family history of excessive bleeding too. Her coagulation profile was within normal limits, with an activated partial thromboplastin time (APTT) of 29.8 s and a prothrombin time international normalized

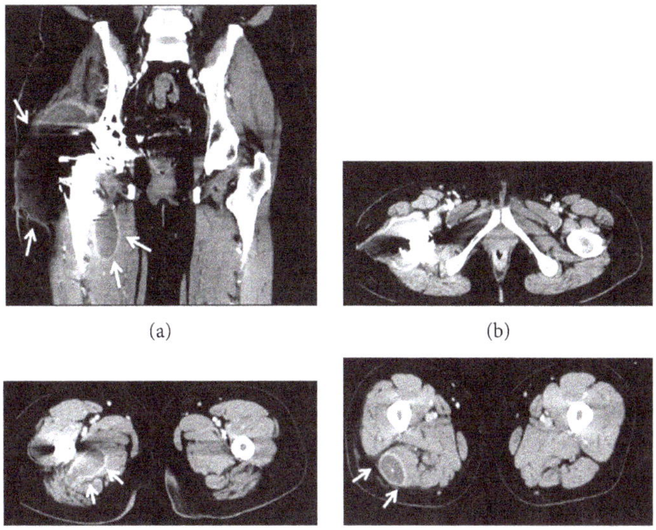

(a) (b) (c) (d)

Figure 1: (a–d) Contrast computerized tomography images of the pelvic cavity at 10 days after the first evacuation procedure. A mass lesion was observed around the right hip joint. Although no active bleeding was observed, a hematoma was visible in this scan (white arrows).

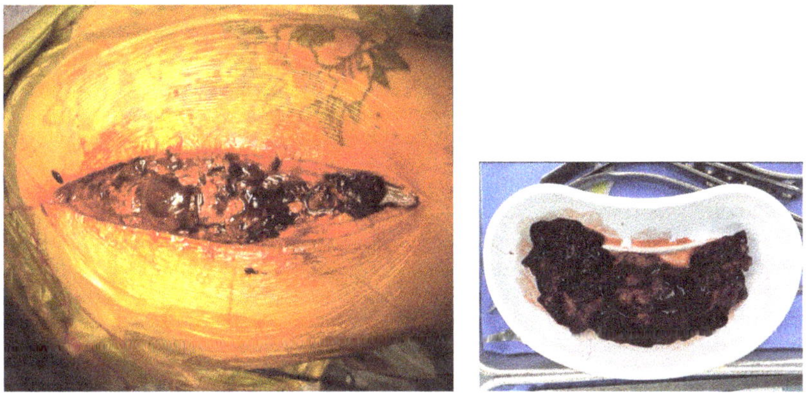

(a) (b)

Figure 2: (a) Intraoperative finding—a large hematoma identified around the right hip. (b) The extracted hematoma, after the second evacuation procedure.

ratio (PT-INR) value of 0.98. A revision THA was performed using constrained liner, and no unexpected bleeding was observed during the operation. However, on postoperative day 21, the patient suddenly experienced acute pain and swelling of the right upper thigh. Her blood tests showed a C-reactive protein level of 495.23 nmol/L, a white blood cell count of $10.9 \times 10^9$/L, and a hemoglobin value of 80 g/L. Her coagulation profile remained normal with APTT and PT-INR values of 28.2 s and 1.11, respectively. We suspected a postoperative infection or a hematoma and performed an emergency operation for an evacuation (of the hematoma), followed by irrigation of the operative site. Apart from a large hematoma identified at the operative site, there was no other significant finding. A tissue culture of the evacuated hematoma tissue did not yield any growth. At 10 days after the evacuation, the surgical wound site was found to be discharging a bloody exudate. A contrast computed tomography (CT) showed a mass lesion extending from the right hip to the proximal femur (Figure 1). The CT imaging and angiography did not reveal any active bleeding. At this time, her blood tests showed a further decrease in hemoglobin to 67 g/L, but her coagulation test results remained within normal limits with an APTT of 26.7 s and a PT-INR of 1.05 and a normal value of the von Willebrand factor. We then assessed the FXIII activity in the plasma, using a Berichrom FXIII kit (Dade Behring, Marburg, Germany) [4], which showed a slight decrease (69%). The patient was therefore diagnosed with an acquired FXIII deficiency, and a third procedure for an evacuation of the hematoma was performed (Figure 2), followed by an administration of human plasma-derived FXIII (Fibrogammin-P®; CSL Behring GmbH, Marburg, Germany) concentrate, at a dose of 1200 U/day for 5 days. After the treatment, the FXIII activity returned to normal levels (76%), and the bleeding did not recur. At 2 months after the second evacuation procedure, the patient was discharged from the hospital in an ambulatory state, mobilized with the aid of a T-cane. There has been no recurrence of a hematoma since.

## 3. Discussion

The most important inference derived from our experience in managing this patient was that an acquired FXIII deficiency should be unfailingly considered in the differential diagnoses when recurrent bleeding after THA is encountered, even when the coagulation profile remains within normal limits. Few studies have reported the complication of a hematoma around an operated hip joint as a result of FXIII deficiency.

The mechanism of FXIII deficiency is unknown and is associated with severe bleeding, spontaneous intracranial hemorrhages, and poor wound healing [2]. In the final step of the coagulation pathway, thrombin activates FXIII, which in turn triggers a cross-linkage of fibrin, a process essential for clot formation. FXIII strengthens fibrin thrombi and protects the fibrin clot from enzymolysis [5]. The resultant blood clot is thus stabilized by FXIII in the coagulation pathways. FXIII also protects against infection by immobilizing and destroying bacteria, in addition to promoting phagocytosis by macrophages [6]. FXIII deficiency is classified as either a congenital or an acquired illness. Hereditary FXIII deficiency is a rare bleeding disorder (incidence of 1 in 5 million) [7]. The major cause is a genetic defect in FXIII. An acquired FXIII deficiency may arise because of specific autoantibodies but may also be consequent to other underlying diseases that result in a decreased synthesis or an increased consumption of FXIII. A decrease in FXIII in adults has been attributed to a variety of causes such as chronic liver disease, leukemia, Henoch-Schönlein purpura, autoimmune diseases, drugs, and trauma [8]. Also, Kanda et al. [9] reported that an infection of the prosthesis subsequent to a revision THA might be one of the risk factors.

Postoperative hematomas tend to occur in patients who have received anticoagulation or hormonal therapy or in those who have thrombocytopenia and hemorrhage. Almost all hematomas spontaneously reduce through internal absorption, but a huge hematoma that may occur following hip surgery can cause nerve palsy, acute thigh pain, and swelling [10, 11]. A hematoma is also a risk factor for a periprosthetic infection [12]. Our patient had no history of risk factors, and her coagulation profile (PT, APTT, platelet count, platelet function assay, and bleeding time) remained within a normal range. However, she developed recurrent hematomas at the operative site, following the revision arthroplasty. Our differential diagnoses for this patient also included other hemorrhagic disorders, such as von Willebrand disease, $\alpha_2$-antiplasmin deficiency, platelet factor 3 deficiency, dysfibrinogenemia, and plasminogen activator inhibitor-1 deficiency [3]. In our case, there was a minor decrease in FXIII activity (69%). However, a FXIII activity level at which hemorrhage may occur is variable and patient-specific [13, 14]. The localized soft tissue damage following the revision THA and the minor FXIII deficiency may have acted additively to affect the bleeding. In addition to that, after 5 days of supplementation, the FXIII activity returned only to 76%. This almost unchanged FXIII activity after the treatment is a strong indicator that a relevant consumption of FXIII has been taking place.

As the presence of a FXIII inhibitor could not be demonstrated conclusively in our patient, we considered her deficiency to have been caused by an increased consumption process. When an autoimmune inhibitor of FXIII is not detected in the plasma, the administration of FXIII concentrate is an effective treatment [15]. If FXIII is not available at hand, fresh frozen plasma administration is also acceptable. Conversely, if a FXIII inhibitor is detected in the plasma, additional immunosuppressive therapy using adrenocorticosteroids, cyclophosphamide, plasma exchange therapy, adsorptive therapy, or high-dose immunoglobulins would be required for an effective outcome [3, 15]. In our patient, the FXIII replenishment was remarkably effective. Additional therapy was not needed, and the patient made steady progress to recovery.

## 4. Conclusion

We managed a rare case of FXIII deficiency and conclude that a patient presenting with an acquired bleeding disorder can have a normal coagulation profile. An acquired FXIII deficiency should be a part of the differential diagnoses when sudden bleeding tendency is observed, especially in a postoperative patient. An early diagnosis and treatment are imperative in preventing the life-threatening complications of an acquired FXIII deficiency.

## References


[1] F. Duckert, E. Jung, and D. H. Shmerling, "A hitherto undescribed congenital haemorrhagic diathesis probably due to fibrin stabilizing factor deficiency," *Thrombosis and Haemostasis*, vol. 5, no. 1, pp. 179–186, 1960.

[2] L. Hsieh and D. Nugent, "Factor XIII deficiency," *Haemophilia*, vol. 14, no. 6, pp. 1190–1200, 2008.

[3] T. F. Gregory and B. Cooper, "Case report of an acquired factor XIII inhibitor: diagnosis and management," *Baylor University Medical Center Proceedings*, vol. 19, no. 3, pp. 221–223, 2006.

[4] K. Fickenscher, A. Aab, and W. Stuber, "A photometric assay for blood coagulation factor XIII," *Thrombosis and Haemostasis*, vol. 65, no. 5, pp. 535–540, 1991.

[5] A. Ichinose, "Physiopathology and regulation of factor XIII," *Thrombosis and Haemostasis*, vol. 86, no. 1, pp. 57–65, 2001.

[6] A. Ichinose, "Factor XIII is a key molecule at the intersection of coagulation and fibrinolysis as well as inflammation and infection control," *International Journal of Hematology*, vol. 95, no. 4, pp. 362–370, 2012.

[7] P. Eshghi, S. B. Mahjour, M. Naderi, J. Dehbozorgian, and M. Karimi, "Long-term prophylaxis in patients with factor

XIII deficiency complicated by intracranial haemorrhage in Iran," *Haemophilia*, vol. 16, no. 2, pp. 383–385, 2010.

[8] A. Dorgalaleh and J. Rashidpanah, "Blood coagulation factor XIII and factor XIII deficiency," *Blood Reviews*, vol. 30, no. 6, pp. 461–475, 2016.

[9] A. Kanda, K. Kaneko, O. Obayashi, and A. Mogami, "The massive bleeding after the operation of hip joint surgery with the acquired haemorrhagic coagulation factor XIII(13) deficiency: two case reports," *Case Reports in Orthopedics*, vol. 2013, Article ID 473014, 5 pages, 2013.

[10] E. P. Su, "Retraction: Post-operative neuropathy after total hip arthroplasty," *The bone & Joint Journal*, vol. 99-B, no. 1, Supplement A, pp. 46–49, 2017.

[11] Y. H. Kim, S. H. Cho, and R. S. Kim, "Drainage versus non-drainage in simultaneous bilateral total hip arthroplasties," *The Journal of Arthroplasty*, vol. 13, no. 2, pp. 156–161, 1998.

[12] J. Parvizi, L. K. Kahl, and C. Dalsey, "Aggressive anticoagulation after TJA: an evaluation of the ACCP guidelines for thromboprophylaxis," *Journal of Long-Term Effects of Medical Implants*, vol. 17, no. 4, pp. 359–365, 2007.

[13] R. Gerlach, A. Raabe, M. Zimmermann, A. Siegemund, and V. Seifert, "Factor XIII deficiency and postoperative hemorrhage after neurosurgical procedures," *Surgical Neurology*, vol. 54, no. 3, pp. 260–266, 2000, discussion 64-65.

[14] W. F. Korte, "F. XIII in perioperative coagulation management," *Best Practice & Research Clinical Anaesthesiology*, vol. 24, no. 1, pp. 85–93, 2010.

[15] A. Ichinose, "Hemorrhagic acquired factor XIII (13) deficiency and acquired hemorrhaphilia 13 revisited," *Seminars in Thrombosis and Hemostasis*, vol. 37, no. 04, pp. 382–388, 2011.

16

# Seizures Causing Simultaneous Bilateral Neck of Femur Fractures

**Dane Gary Maimin**[1] **and Livan Meneses-Turino**[2]

[1]*Madadeni Hospital, Newcastle, South Africa*
[2]*HOD Orthopaedics Northdale Hospital, Pietermaritzburg, South Africa*

Correspondence should be addressed to Dane Gary Maimin; danemaimin@gmail.com

Academic Editor: Paul E. Di Cesare

Neck of femur fractures are a ubiquitous injury seen by orthopaedic surgeons. In the elderly, these fractures usually occur after a low energy fall, and are invariably unilateral injuries. Bilateral neck of femur fractures have been reported in patients with metabolic bone disease, after electroconvulsive therapy, and in association with stress fractures. The otherwise healthy index patient in this case report presented most unusually, with simultaneous, bilateral neck of femur fractures that were sustained during a seizure.

## 1. Introduction

Hip fractures are a common occurrence throughout the world, with the United States alone seeing over 340,000 hip fractures per year [1] with incidences increasing dramatically with age, as bone density decreases and likelihood of falls increases. Between ages 60 and 85 years, the risk of fracture doubles for every 5- to 6-year increase in age [2]. The mechanism of injury is more commonly low energy trauma as this age group has higher rates of osteoporosis as well as osteomalacia, myeloma, renal osteodystrophy, and other metabolic and neoplastic bone diseases. The incidence of neck of femur fractures is highest in European caucasian populations. Denmark, Sweden, and Norway have incidences of 574, 563, and 539 per 100,000, respectively [3]. There is limited data regarding the incidence in South Africa and other African populations; however, several studies concur that the incidence in black African populations is among the lowest in the world [3, 4].

The vast majority of hip fractures occur unilaterally. Bilateral injuries occur very rarely but have been reported in patients with metabolic diseases, after electroconvulsive therapy, and due to stress fractures [4]. This report is interesting and uncommon as the patient presented with simultaneous, bilateral hip fractures sustained during a generalised tonic clonic seizure.

## 2. Case Report

The patient is a 69-year-old gentleman, who is HIV positive. His viral load is undetectable and his CD4 count is 417 cells/mm$^3$. For six years he has been on first line antiretroviral therapy in compliance with the South African Department of Health guidelines i.e. a fixed-dose combination pill taken daily, containing tenofovir, emtricitabine, and efavirenz [5]. He has no history of seizures or other comorbidities. He is an independent and active member of the community. He does not smoke or abuse alcohol.

He first presented to his local clinic with a history of seizure-like activity beginning approximately one week prior. Subsequent to the onset of seizures, the patient had been unable to walk and was experiencing pain in both his hips. There was no history of trauma otherwise. At his clinic, he had a witnessed generalised tonic-clonic seizure which was aborted with a benzodiazepine. He was then referred to Madadeni Provincial Hospital.

On presentation, the patient was noted to be drowsy but rousable, and cooperative. His vitals were normal. Orthopaedic examination showed bilaterally externally rotated lower limbs, with tenderness in the groin and pain on movement of his hips. He had no neurological deficit with a normal vascular exam. There were no signs of trauma or open wounds. Pelvic radiographs showed bilateral Garden 4 subcapital neck of femur fractures (Figure 1).

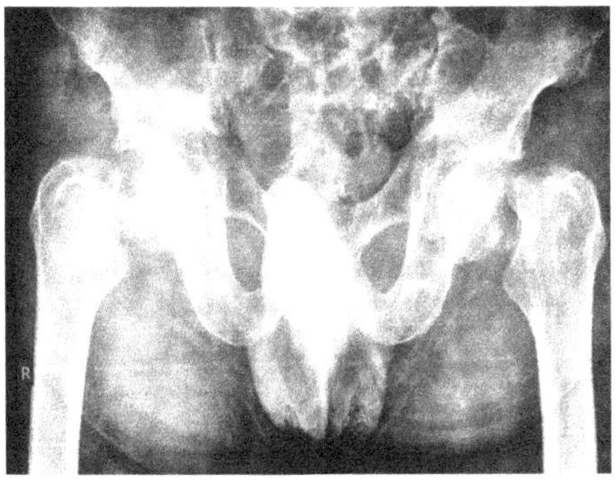

Figure 1

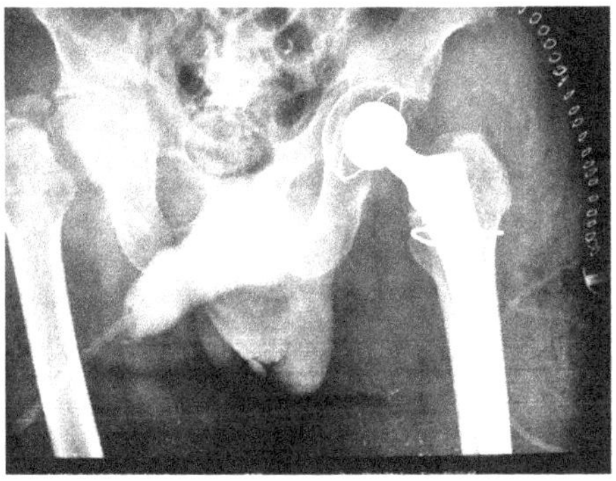

Figure 2

He was admitted for comanagement by internal medicine and orthopaedics. His medical workup revealed an electrolyte abnormality of severe hyponatraemia (115 mmol/L), and, as his other blood tests were normal and CT brain showing only age-related atrophy, the hyponatremia was attributed as the cause of the seizures. The hyponatremia was corrected and he had no further seizures in the ward.

He was kept in bilateral skin traction during his medical optimisation. Staged, bilateral total hip arthroplasties was ultimately performed. Due to lack of theatre time and a high patient load at Madadeni Hospital, the patient waited almost two weeks for his first surgery (Figure 2) and another month before his second surgery (Figure 3). The patient was assessed as a Dorr B, had good intraoperative bone quality and both arthroplasties were thus uncemented. During the first (left) arthroplasty, there were concerns of fracture extension into the intertrochanteric region, and a cabling system was used to reinforce the stem insertion. For both surgeries, a Mathys RM Pressfit cup, with symarec head and a Zimmer Avenir stem, was used. Several bone biopsies were also taken during the first surgery to exclude a pathological fracture. All biopsies were normal.

Postoperatively, the patient was kept on DVT prophylaxis and began in-bed hip and knee range of motion exercises on day two after surgery. The patient was mobilising with the assistance of a physiotherapist and a walking frame within a week of his second surgery and was discharged home with no postoperative complications.

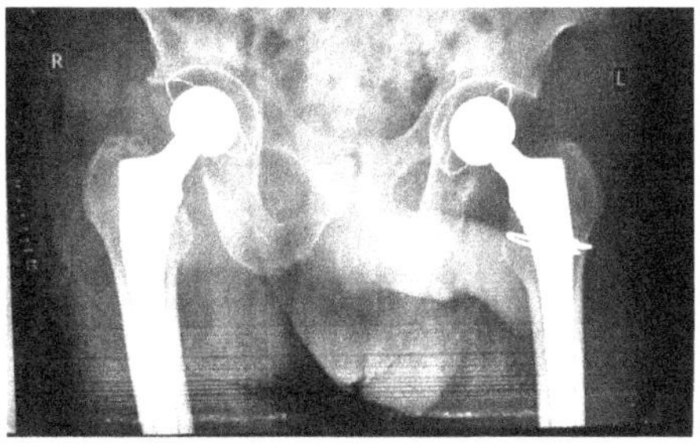

Figure 3

## 3. Discussion

The strong muscle contractions during seizures are known to cause fractures and/or dislocations with an incidence of 1.1% following a convulsion [6]. However, there were very few reported cases of bilateral hip fractures sustained during seizure [4, 6–11]. Those that do occur tend to have an underlying metabolic bone disease such as osteomalacia or decreased bone density as a result of chronic antiepileptic treatment.

Patients presenting with seizures may have several potential reasons for a decreased level of consciousness and further more may need to be sedated and or ventilated as part of their treatment. As such, musculoskeletal injuries, including neck of femur fractures which have very subtle clinical signs, may initially be missed [7]. Any patient presenting with seizures requires a thorough musculoskeletal examination to prevent complications such as avascular necrosis, osteoarthritis, nonunion, functional disability, and legal consequences [10]. This is especially relevant in intracapsular neck of femur fractures in younger patients.

## 4. Conclusion

Musculoskeletal complications postseizures are rare but easily missed. All physicians treating patients with seizures should maintain a high index of suspicion to avoid missing injuries and incurring the complications that may follow.

## Disclosure

The authors confirm that the case report submitted is original and does not transgress plagiarism policies of the journal.

## References

[1] C. A. Brauer, M. Coca-Perraillon, D. M. Cutler, and A. B. Rosen, "Incidence and mortality of hip fractures in the United States," *Journal of the American Medical Association*, vol. 302, no. 14, pp. 1573–1579, 2009.

[2] S. H. Kim, J. P. Meehan, T. Blumenfeld, and R. M. Szabo, "Hip fractures in the United States: 2008 nationwide emergency

department sample," *Arthritis Care & Research*, vol. 64, no. 5, pp. 751–757, 2012.

[3] J. A. Kanis, A. Odén, E. V. McCloskey et al., "A systematic review of hip fracture incidence and probability of fracture worldwide," *Osteoporosis International*, vol. 23, no. 9, pp. 2239–2256, 2012.

[4] F. Paruk, G. Matthews, and B. Cassim, "Osteoporotic hip fractures in black South Africans: a regional study," *Archives of Osteoporosis*, vol. 12, no. 1, p. 107, 2017.

[5] G. Meintjies, M. A. Moorhouse, S. Carmona et al., "Adult antiretroviral therapy guidelines 2017," *Southern African Journal of HIV Medicine*, vol. 18, no. 1, p. 24, 2017.

[6] T. Cagırmaz, C. Yapici, M. M. Orak, and O. Guler, "Bilateral femoral neck fractures after an epileptic attack: a case report," *International Journal of Surgery Case Reports.*, vol. 6, pp. 107–110, 2015.

[7] H. M. Shah, A. Grover, D. Gadi, and K. Sudarshan, "Bilateral neck femur fracture following a generalized seizure- a rare case report," *The Archives of Bone and Joint Surgery*, vol. 2, no. 4, pp. 255–257, 2014.

[8] S. Joshy, "Bilateral femoral neck fracture following convulsions: pitfalls in early diagnosis and management," *The Internet Journal of Orthopedic Surgery*, vol. 2, no. 1, 2004.

[9] H. D. W. Powell, "Simultaneous bilateral fractures of the neck of the femur," *The Journal of Bone and Joint Surgery. British volume*, vol. 42-B, no. 2, pp. 236–252, 1960.

[10] M. Grimaldi, H. Vouaillat, J. Tonetti, and P. Merloz, "Simultaneous bilateral femoral neck fractures secondary to epileptic seizures: treatment by bilateral total hip arthroplasty," *Orthopaedics & Traumatology, Surgery & Research*, vol. 95, no. 7, pp. 555–557, 2009.

[11] R. Ribacoba-Montero and J. Salas-Puig, "Simultaneous bilateral fractures of the hip following a grand mal seizure. An unusual complication," *Seizure*, vol. 6, no. 5, pp. 403-404, 1997.

# 17

# Scaphoid Waist Nonunion in an 8-Year-Old: A Rare Occurrence

**T. M. Gause II, T. E. Moran, J. B. Carr, and D. N. Deal**

*Department of Orthopedic Surgery, University of Virginia Health System, Charlottesville, VA, USA*

Correspondence should be addressed to T. M. Gause II; trentgause@gmail.com

Academic Editor: Mark K. Lyons

*Case.* Historically, the most common pattern of pediatric scaphoid injury described is at the distal pole, which has a high rate of success with nonoperative management. Injury patterns have evolved as children are more commonly presenting with adult-type fracture patterns. We present the case of a scaphoid waist fracture in an 8-year-old male that resulted in nonunion and required surgical fixation. *Conclusion.* This case highlights the trend of adult pattern scaphoid fractures in the pediatric population and the utility of magnetic resonance imaging in patients who do not have complete carpal bone ossification at the time of initial radiographic evaluation.

## 1. Introduction

Scaphoid fractures are the most prevalent carpal bone fracture in the pediatric population, accounting for 3% of pediatric hand and wrist fractures [1]. The most common age for a pediatric scaphoid fracture is 15 years old, with the earliest documented case reported in a 5-year-old male [2]. Scaphoid fractures are difficult to identify in the pediatric population due to incomplete ossification of the scaphoid at the time of radiographic evaluation. Endochondral ossification of the scaphoid starts at approximately 4 years in females and 5 years in males and is completed roughly by 13 and 15 years, respectively [3].

While nonunion is a well-known complication in the management of adult scaphoid fractures, it is rare in the pediatric population with a reported incidence of 0.8% following closed treatment with immobilization [4]. Several unique characteristics of pediatric scaphoid fractures help prevent nonunion and avascular necrosis (AVN). First, the injury often described is a chondral injury as opposed to a pure bony injury due to the process of endochondral ossification. Second, the traditionally described fracture pattern in skeletally immature patients is a distal pole fracture, which preserves the dominant blood supply. Lastly, these distal pole fractures are usually minimally displaced, allowing for closed management.

Despite the classic description, adult injury patterns are occurring in the pediatric population with increased frequency [5, 6]. This is likely due to increasing sports-related activity and higher energy injuries in children, which subject the scaphoid to stresses similar to adults.

We present the case of an 8-year-old male who sustained a scaphoid waist fracture that was not identified until three years after the initial injury due to lack of ossification on radiographs. The importance of this case is threefold: (1) it is the second youngest case of a pediatric scaphoid waist fracture ever reported, (2) it demonstrates the need to recognize adult pattern scaphoid fractures in children, and (3) it advocates for consideration of advanced imaging in pediatric patients with persistent wrist pain following an injury and in the setting of negative radiographs. Consent was obtained from the patient's parents regarding this case being summarized and submitted for publication.

## 2. Case Report

An 8-year-old male with no significant past medical, surgical, or social history initially presented to an emergency department in October 2013 with a chief complaint of right, radial-sided wrist pain after a fall on his right arm while playing soccer. No fracture was seen on radiographs, and he was placed in a removable splint for comfort and discharged. The

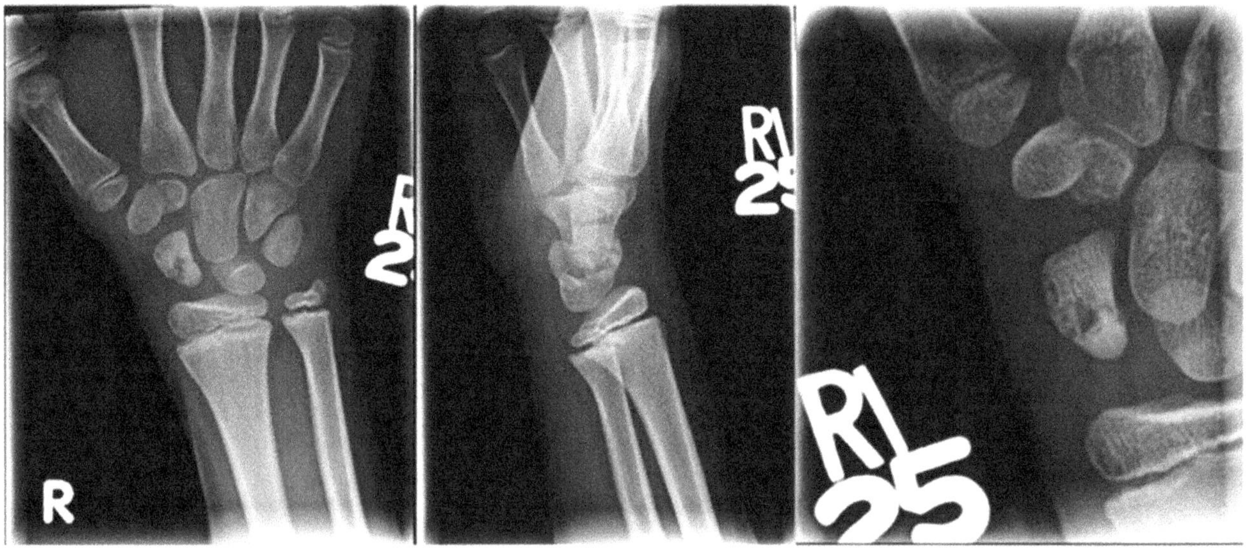


Figure 1: AP and lateral radiographs from November 2016 (approximately 3 years and 1 month from the initial injury) demonstrating a nondisplaced scaphoid waist fracture and a subtle osteosclerotic appearance within the proximal pole. There is also a relative sclerotic appearance of the scaphoid relative to the other carpal bones—a constellation of findings concerning for osteonecrosis [26].

patient was scheduled for follow-up but would not present to an orthopaedic clinic until three years post injury, at age 11. At age 11, when the patient was seen at an outside orthopaedic clinic, he reported continued wrist pain from his initial injury three years prior. He described dull pain in his right wrist with intermittent swelling after several minor falls while playing soccer. Radiographs did not reveal a fracture or other pathology, and the patient was again diagnosed with a wrist sprain and given a brace for comfort. He was compliant with the brace, but 8 months later, he again returned to his pediatrician with continued pain. Interval radiographs revealed a right-sided, displaced scaphoid waist fracture (Figure 1). He was referred to our clinic for further management. He was noted to have tenderness located at the anatomic snuffbox but full range of motion. A magnetic resonance imaging (MRI) scan was ordered to further evaluate for AVN and osseous bridging given the chronicity of his symptoms, and he was placed in a thumb spica wrist brace. His MRI demonstrated the scaphoid waist nonunion with concerns for AVN (Figure 2). At this point, the patient and parents elected to undergo surgical fixation of his nonunion. Due to the concern for AVN on MRI, utilization of a vascularized bone graft was considered. However, it was felt that given the young age of the patient, drilling of the bone would be sufficient to stimulate bone growth and avoid the more aggressive procedure.

The patient underwent surgery at 11 years and 3 months of age. Open reduction and internal fixation was performed using a dorsal approach centered over the scapholunate interval, using 14 and 16 mm headless compression screws to achieve fixation. The patient was placed in a thumb spica splint and discharged home the same day. Two weeks later, he presented to clinic with resolution of pain and intact hardware on imaging (Figure 3). He was transitioned to a thumb spica short arm cast. Six weeks postoperatively, he was placed in a removable thumb spica brace for one month. The patient returned to full activity by 4 months postoperatively. One year postoperatively, the patient remained asymptomatic and maintained a full physical activity level without difficulty or pain.

## 3. Discussion

Diagnosing pediatric scaphoid fractures can be difficult, especially before the scaphoid is fully ossified. Previous approaches to managing scaphoid injuries in children were stratified by age, with the assumption that the progressive ossification of the scaphoid predisposes to discrete fractures [7]. Historically, the most common injury was thought to be a distal pole fracture [8–12]. However, recent literature suggests an increasing number of adult injury patterns in children [5, 7]. Stanciu and Dumont reported on a series of 21 patients (mean age of 13 years) who sustained scaphoid fractures. 12 of these patients (57%) sustained scaphoid waist fractures.

The majority of pediatric scaphoid fractures are treated with closed management [4, 10]. Christodoulou and Colton reported successful closed management in 63 of 64 patients aged 8 to 14 years [13]. Surgical treatment is usually reserved for patients who demonstrate nonunion or initial displacement of a waist or proximal pole fracture. The most common method of surgical fixation is screw fixation with or without bone grafting, which has yielded good functional outcomes with regard to range of motion and absence of pain, as well as fusion rates approaching 100% [4, 14–19]. Mintzer et al. reported on 13 scaphoid fractures managed operatively, in which 12 resulted in successful union and 1 requiring revision fixation [17]. Complications following both nonsurgical and surgical treatment are rare with nonunion being the most commonly reported for both treatment modalities [14]. In the setting of failed closed management, surgical treatment

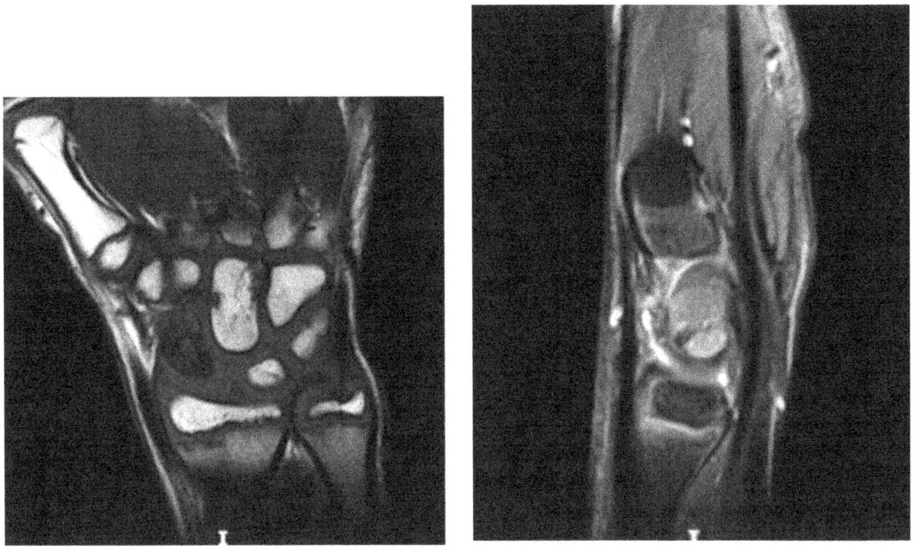


FIGURE 2: (a) Coronal T1-weighted magnetic resonance (MR) image of the right wrist showing diffuse loss of signal throughout the scaphoid bone that is concerning for osteonecrosis; (b) sagittal fat-suppressed PD-w MR image of the right wrist. The presence of a fracture line is indicative of nonunion.

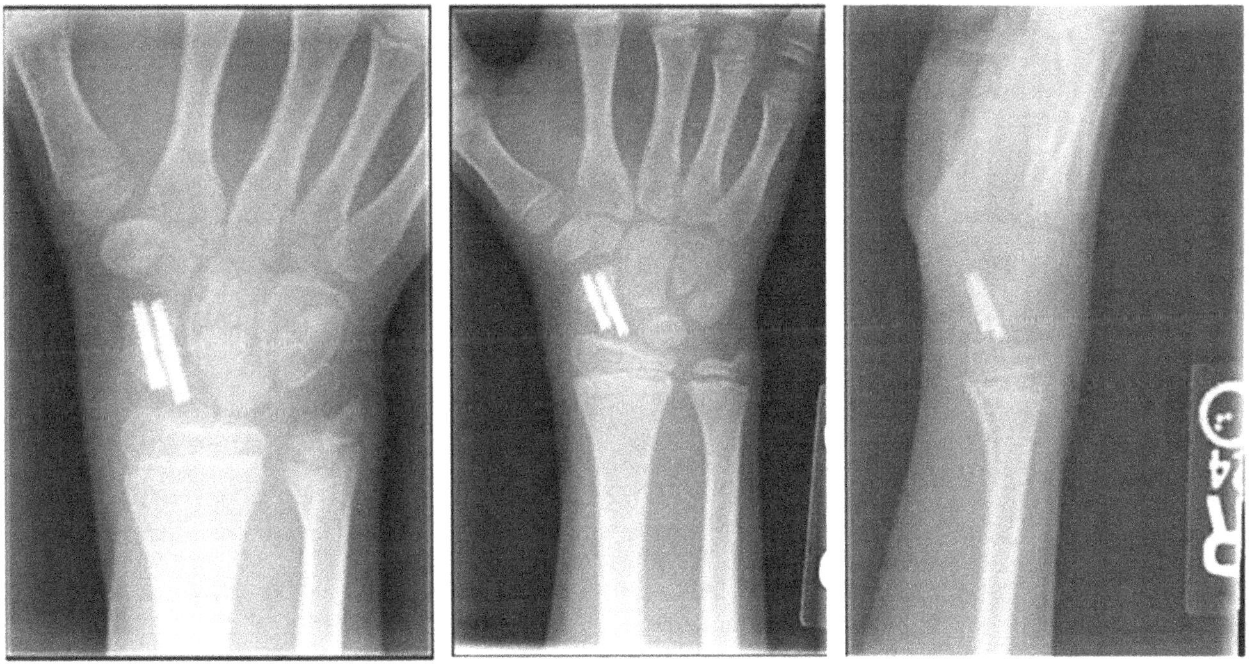

FIGURE 3: AP and lateral radiographs taken two weeks postsurgical fixation using two Arthrex micro screws.

is the treatment of choice with excellent outcomes even in the setting of nonunion [19, 20].

The current case report highlights that pediatric patients with wrist pain and negative radiographic imaging should be closely monitored in the acute setting. We recommend that pediatric patients who sustain an injury to the wrist without radiographic evidence of fracture should require close follow-up with consideration of advanced imaging if symptoms do not improve as expected. If wrist pain does not resolve within 6 weeks, it is reasonable to consider advanced imaging modalities such as ultrasound or MRI. MRI is not user dependent and can readily diagnose a scaphoid fracture regardless of the ossification stage. MRI scans can be positive in as little as two days after the injury, and the reported negative predictive value is close to 100%, which may eliminate the need for additional follow-up imaging in the setting of a negative scan [21–25].

Lastly, our study presents an adult type scaphoid waist fracture in an eight-year-old patient, which advocates for greater suspicion for a potentially missed scaphoid fracture in pediatric patients with persistent wrist pain. Furthermore, this case report demonstrates the need for appropriate immobilization in instances of pediatric scaphoid fracture, as it is rare for a scaphoid fracture in a young patient to demonstrate nonunion with proper immobilization. Appropriate immobilization may have been facilitated by the earlier use of advanced imaging for diagnosis of scaphoid fracture in this patient, as scaphoid pathology is difficult to reliably demonstrate radiographically prior to skeletal maturity due to lack of ossification.

## 4. Conclusion

Scaphoid fractures are exceedingly rare within the first decade, particularly in children eight years old and younger. More recent literature shows an increased frequency in identification of adult pattern scaphoid fractures in the pediatric population. Anatomic location of pediatric scaphoid fractures is important since fractures of the scaphoid waist are more susceptible to nonunion and may require prolonged immobilization to achieve union or surgical fixation if there is initial fracture displacement. In patients who are not skeletally mature enough to reliably show scaphoid fractures on radiographs, the use of advanced imaging can aid in identifying scaphoid pathology in cases of unresolved wrist pain and more adequately guide management. In cases of scaphoid nonunion, optimal treatment is controversial, but surgical fixation may be considered and can deliver favorable outcomes. Finally, this case demonstrates that a high index of suspicion for scaphoid fracture must be maintained when treating a pediatric patient with wrist pain and incomplete scaphoid ossification.

## References

[1] B. Ting, A. Sesko Bauer, J. M. Abzug, R. Cornwall, T. O. Wyrick, and D. S. Bae, "Pediatric scaphoid fractures," *Instructional Course Lectures*, vol. 66, pp. 429–436, 2017.

[2] I. Ahmed, F. Ashton, W. K. Tay, and D. Porter, "The pediatric fracture of the scaphoid in patients aged 13 years and under: an epidemiological study," *Journal of Pediatric Orthopaedics*, vol. 34, no. 2, pp. 150–154, 2014.

[3] J. C. Y. Liao and A. K. S. Chong, "Pediatric hand and wrist fractures," *Clinics in Plastic Surgery*, vol. 46, no. 3, pp. 425–436, 2019.

[4] O. Fabre, H. De Boeck, and P. Haentjens, "Fractures and nonunions of the carpal scaphoid in children," *Acta Orthopaedica Belgica*, vol. 67, no. 2, pp. 121–125, 2001.

[5] A. A. Williams and H. V. Lochner, "Pediatric hand and wrist injuries," *Current Reviews in Musculoskeletal Medicine*, vol. 6, no. 1, pp. 18–25, 2013.

[6] J. J. Gholson, D. S. Bae, D. Zurakowski, and P. M. Waters, "Scaphoid fractures in children and adolescents: contemporary injury patterns and factors influencing time to union," *The Journal of Bone and Joint Surgery-American*, vol. 93, no. 13, pp. 1210–1219, 2011.

[7] S. J. Rhemrev, D. Ootes, F. J. P. Beeres, S. A. G. Meylaerts, and I. B. Schipper, "Current methods of diagnosis and treatment of scaphoid fractures," *International Journal of Emergency Medicine*, vol. 4, no. 1, p. 4, 2011.

[8] H. Mussbichler, "Injuries of the carpal scaphoid in children," *Acta Radiologica*, vol. 56, no. 5, pp. 361–368, 1961.

[9] S. A. A. Nafie, "Fractures of the carpal bones in children," *Injury*, vol. 18, no. 2, pp. 117–119, 1987.

[10] E. B. Wilson, T. F. Beattie, and A. G. Wilkinson, "Epidemiological review and proposed management of 'scaphoid' injury in children," *European Journal of Emergency Medicine*, vol. 18, no. 1, pp. 57–61, 2011.

[11] A. W. Anz, B. D. Bushnell, D. K. Bynum, G. D. Chloros, and E. R. Wiesler, "Pediatric scaphoid fractures," *Journal of the American Academy of Orthopaedic Surgeons*, vol. 17, no. 2, pp. 77–87, 2009.

[12] Đ. Gajdobranski, D. Živanović, A. Mikov et al., "Scaphoid fractures in children," *Srpski Arhiv za Celokupno Lekarstvo*, vol. 142, no. 7-8, pp. 444–449, 2014.

[13] A. Christodoulou and C. Colton, "Scaphoid fractures in children," *Journal of Pediatric Orthopedics*, vol. 6, no. 1, pp. 37–39, 1986.

[14] S. Toh, H. Miura, K. Arai, M. Yasumura, M. Wada, and K. Tsubo, "Scaphoid fractures in children: problems and treatment," *Journal of Pediatric Orthopedics*, vol. 23, no. 2, pp. 216–221, 2003.

[15] B. Henderson and M. Letts, "Operative management of pediatric scaphoid fracture nonunion," *Journal of Pediatric Orthopedics*, vol. 23, no. 3, pp. 402–406, 2003.

[16] F. Duteille and G. Dautel, "Non-union fractures of the scaphoid and carpal bones in children: surgical treatment," *Journal of Pediatric Orthopaedics, Part B*, vol. 13, no. 1, pp. 34–38, 2004.

[17] C. Mintzer, P. Waters, and B. Simmons, "Nonunion of the scaphoid in children treated by Herbert screw fixation and bone grafting. A report of five cases," *The Journal of Bone and Joint Surgery British*, vol. 77, no. 1, pp. 98–100, 1995.

[18] J. J. Jauregui, E. W. Seger, K. Hesham, S. E. Walker, R. Abraham, and J. M. Abzug, "Operative management for pediatric and adolescent scaphoid nonunions: a meta-analysis," *Journal of Pediatric Orthopedics*, vol. 39, no. 2, pp. e130–e133, 2019.

[19] L. Böhler, E. Trojan, and H. Jahna, "The results of treatment of 734 fresh, simple fractures of the scaphoid," *The Journal of Hand Surgery*, vol. 28, no. 4, pp. 319–331, 2003.

[20] A. M. Herneth, A. Siegmeth, T. R. Bader et al., "Scaphoid fractures: evaluation with high-spatial-resolution US—initial results," *Radiology*, vol. 220, no. 1, pp. 231–235, 2013.

[21] J. C. Hunter, E. M. Escobedo, A. J. Wilson, D. P. Hanel, G. C. Zink-Brody, and F. A. Mann, "MR imaging of clinically suspected scaphoid fractures," *American Journal of Roentgenology*, vol. 168, no. 5, pp. 1287–1293, 1997.

[22] K. J. Johnson, S. F. Haigh, and K. E. Symonds, "MRI in the management of scaphoid fractures in skeletally immature patients," *Pediatric Radiology*, vol. 30, no. 10, pp. 685–688, 2000.

[23] A. J. Evenski, M. J. Adamczyk, R. P. Steiner, M. A. Morscher, and P. M. Riley, "Clinically suspected scaphoid fractures in children," *Journal of Pediatric Orthopaedics*, vol. 29, no. 4, pp. 352–355, 2009.

[24] M. S. Taljanovic, A. Karantanas, J. F. Griffith, G. L. Desilva, J. D. Rieke, and J. E. Sheppard, "Imaging and treatment of scaphoid fractures and their complications," *Seminars in Musculoskeletal Radiology*, vol. 16, no. 2, pp. 159–174, 2012.

[25] A. Fotiadou, A. Patel, T. Morgan, and A. H. Karantanas, "Wrist injuries in young adults: the diagnostic impact of CT and MRI," *European Journal of Radiology*, vol. 77, no. 2, pp. 235–239, 2011.

[26] M. D. Murphey, K. L. Foreman, M. K. Klassen-Fischer, M. G. Fox, E. M. Chung, and M. J. Kransdorf, "From the radiologic pathology archives imaging of osteonecrosis: radiologic-pathologic correlation," *Radiographics*, vol. 34, no. 4, pp. 1003–1028, 2014.

# 18

# Progressive Back Pain due to *Aspergillus nidulans* Vertebral Osteomyelitis in an Immunocompetent Patient: Surgical and Antifungal Management

**Mark K. Lyons, Matthew T. Neal, Naresh P. Patel, and Holenarasipur R. Vikram**

*Department of Neurological Surgery, Mayo Clinic Arizona, 5777 East Mayo Boulevard, Phoenix, AZ 85054, USA*

Correspondence should be addressed to Mark K. Lyons; lyons.mark2@mayo.edu

Academic Editor: Eyal Itshayek

*Case Report. Aspergillus* osteomyelitis is a destructive and progressive infection that has been described both in immunosuppressed and in immunocompetent hosts. We describe a case of lumbar vertebral osteomyelitis in a 61-year-old immunocompetent patient due to *Aspergillus nidulans* that was successfully treated with a combination of extensive surgical debridement, spinal stabilization, and a prolonged course of antifungal therapy. Imaging demonstrated findings consistent with L3 discitis. The biopsy grew *Aspergillus* fungus and was treated with vorconizole. Imaging showed progressive destructive osteomyelitis at L3-L4. Patient underwent anterior L3 and L4 partial corpectomies, anterior interbody fusion L3-L5, and posterior T11-S2 pedicle screw and rod fixation. Antifungal treatment resulted in resolution of infection. *Aspergillus* markers remain negative. One year following definitive treatment, the patient's back pain remains resolved. *Conclusion.* Definitive surgical resection of the infection, spinal stabilization, and aggressive antifungal therapy were required to eradicate the infection.

## 1. Introduction

*Aspergillus* osteomyelitis is an uncommon extra pulmonary manifestation of invasive aspergillosis [1, 2]. Although *Aspergillus* osteomyelitis is rare, the vertebral bodies are the most commonly infected site followed by spondylodiscitis [1, 3, 4]. Immunocompromised hosts are more susceptible to invasive aspergillosis. They include solid organ recipients; severe and sustained neutropenia in patients with hematologic malignancies, following hematopoietic stem cell transplantation; and those receiving high-dose steroids. Other risk factors include poorly controlled diabetes mellitus, chronic obstructive pulmonary disease, and intravenous drug users [1, 3–7]. The presenting symptoms and imaging characteristics of fungal osteomyelitis are nonspecific with back pain being the predominant complaint. In immunocompetent hosts, either hematogenous infection or a prior spinal procedure has been implicated as the cause of aspergillosis osteomyelitis [4]. The excellent review by Gamaletsou et al. looking at the various reported cases of aspergillosis osteomyelitis, where the subtype of the fungus was identified, found only three cases of *Aspergillus nidulans* osteomyelitis in the literature search of aspergillosis spinal infections [1]. The most common subtype was *Aspergillus fumigatus* by far. The majority of patients with *Aspergillus* osteomyelitis require surgical debridement and antifungal treatment. The reported fatality rate in patients with *Aspergillus* osteomyelitis was 23% in 86 patients culled from the reported literature [1]. This case highlights the importance of adequate tissue sampling for culture, histopathology, and noninvasive fungal studies to establish a timely etiologic diagnosis that leads to correct diagnosis and aggressive surgical and prolonged antifungal therapy with resolution of infection.

## 2. Case Report

A 61-year-old male in good health with a history of mild low back pain over several years began developing subacute onset of worsening of back pain and lower extremity pain over six weeks. He had a lumbar steroid injection 18 months prior. He was initially evaluated at an outside institution where a magnetic resonance (MR) imaging study of the spine was obtained which was interpreted as normal. Due to unremitting back pain, he presented to our institution where a repeat MR imaging study was obtained demonstrating abnormal intradiscal signal between the L3 and L4 vertebral bodies consistent with disc space infection and adjacent vertebral osteomyelitis (Figure 1). In addition, a small amount of enhancing phlegmon was noted. The patient underwent a CT-guided biopsy of the disc space which was nondiagnostic with negative cultures. At the time of his initial presentation, his white count was 7.2 with C-reactive protein of 84 and a sedimentation rate of 84. Blood cultures were obtained and were negative. The patient was initially placed on broad-spectrum antibiotics. With ongoing symptoms and no identifiable pathogen, an open L3 disc space biopsy was performed three days later. Fungal culture revealed growth of *Aspergillus nidulans*. Susceptibility testing was performed. Serum *Aspergillus* antigen and Fungitell assays were significantly elevated. He was started on voriconazole 200 mg orally twice per day with excellent serum levels.

Initially, the patient's back pain began to improve. However, 4 weeks after the disc space biopsy and initiation of antifungal treatment, his symptoms rapidly progressed. The patient's laboratory studies revealed a sedimentation rate greater than 100 and his C-reactive protein was elevated at 25. His *Aspergillus* antigen was 3.75 which was a slight increase from his level of 3.37 about 4 weeks earlier. In addition, his voriconazole level was 0.9 which was down from 4.1 3 weeks prior. A follow-up MR demonstrated persistent T1 and STIR sequence signal abnormalities involving the L3 and L4 vertebral bodies. There was progressive bony destruction of the L3 and L4 vertebral bodies as well as focal progressive kyphosis. In addition, new wedge compression deformities of L1, L2, and L5 had developed in the interim. Presumably these were related to poor bone density. Although the patient had only undergone six weeks of antifungal therapy, the progression of symptoms, laboratory markers, and radiographic deterioration prompted recommendation for surgical intervention. The significant risk of mortality with *Aspergillus nidulans* spinal osteomyelitis treatment was the key factor in the recommendation for surgical debridement [1–8]. Treatment recommendations for spinal osteomyelitis and suspected treatment failure may be guided by unchanged or increasing inflammatory markers after four weeks of treatment [9, 10]. Infectious Disease Society of America recommendations in cases of suspected treatment failure include follow-up MR imaging and additional tissue samples [9]. In cases of radiographic evidence of treatment failure, surgical debridement should be considered [9]. Given that all of these findings were present in our patient, aggressive surgical debridement and spinal stabilization was advised. The patient underwent an anterior lumbar discectomy at L3-L4 with partial corpectomies of the adjacent L3 and L4 vertebral bodies. After complete debridement of the infected disk and adjacent bone, an expandable titanium corpectomy cage was used for reconstruction. It was noted that the L3 disc material was very fibrotic, and intraoperative microbiology testing confirmed fungal hyphae consistent with aspergillosis. Anterior lumbar fusion procedures were also performed at L4-5 and L5-S1 using lordotic polyether-

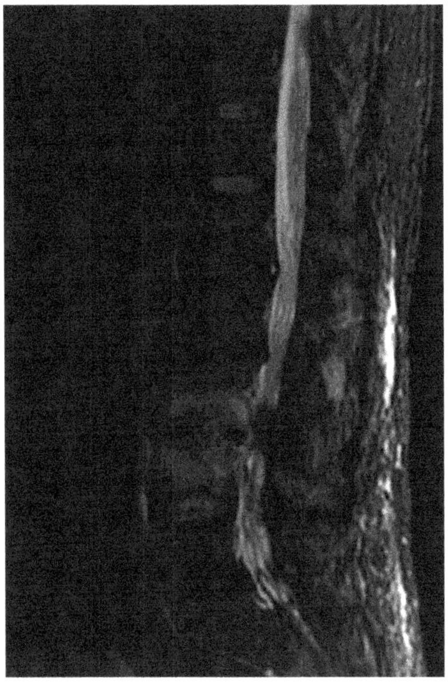

FIGURE 1: Sagittal STIR MR demonstrating signal abnormality in the L3 disc space with endplate irregularity.

etherketone cages containing integrated screws. The anterior fusion construct corrected lumbar lordosis-pelvic incidence mismatch, stabilized the anterior and middle spinal columns, and provided a favorable arthrodesis environment. Circumferential spinal fixation was also desired due to the patient's poor bone quality and placement of the expandable cage (Figures 2(a) and 2(b)). The patient was repositioned and then underwent a posterior bilateral pedicle screw and rod fixation from T11 S2 with iliac screws. We recommended a multilevel anterior and posterior fusion in order to maximize the chance of successful arthrodesis and reduce the chance of the need for further stabilization in the setting of this potentially fatal disease. The patient tolerated the surgical procedure well and reported immediate improvement in his back and leg pain. After surgery, he was initiated on voriconazole 300 mg twice daily along with caspofungin 50 mg daily for 6 weeks.

After 6 weeks, caspofungin was stopped and he received oral voriconazole at 300 mg twice daily for 7 months with adequate serum levels. Voriconazole was subsequently discontinued after the patient developed severe photosensitivity, and posaconazole 300 mg per day was initiated. Follow-up MR studies demonstrated resolution of the signal abnormality at the L3-L4 level without evidence of residual or recurrent infection. There was no evidence of spinal canal compromise. Due to the severity of the patient's pain on presentation, the patient could not tolerate standing X-rays preoperatively. However, standing spine X-rays at one year confirms good sagittal balance. The study demonstrated T11-S1 posterior fusion with pedicle screws and posterior stabilization rods with bilateral iliac screws, anterior discectomy with interbody grafts at L4-5 and L5-S1, and partial L3 and L4 corpectomies with an expandable cage. Imaging at

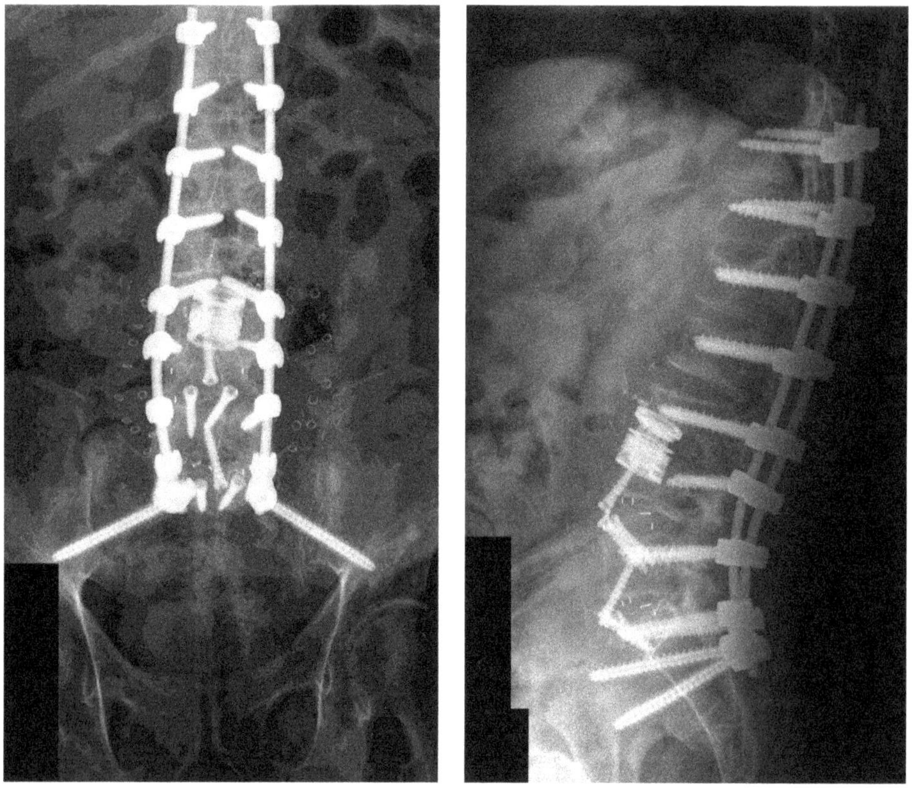

(a) (b)

Figure 2: (a, b) Standing anterior-posterior and lateral X-rays demonstrating T11-S2 bilateral pedicle screw and rod fixation with bilateral iliac screws. Anterior interbody L4 and L5 PEEK graft. Anterior L3 intradiscal expandable cage and bone graft.

two and three years is planned for deformity correction assessment. Serum *Aspergillus* antigen and Fungitell assay trended down and have normalized. His sedimentation rate and C-reactive protein levels are also normal. His back pain has significantly improved without any residual neurologic defects. Since he is now a year out from his extensive surgery without any evidence of persistent or recurrent infection, the plan is to discontinue posaconazole and monitor him closely.

## 3. Discussion

*Aspergillosis* osteomyelitis is an uncommon condition, and *Aspergillus nidulans* is a rare species of the fungus reported in the literature. In the limited number of vertebral aspergillosis cases reported in the literature, the complete response rate to treatment is approximately 50% of patients [1]. Chronic granulomatous disease is the most common immunodeficiency-related condition associated with *Aspergillus* osteomyelitis, especially in the pediatric population [11]. It is generally believed that the mechanism of infection is hematologic spread or direct inoculation, particularly in the immunocompromised population. However, as in our patient, nonimmunocompromised patients are also a population at risk for *Aspergillus* osteomyelitis [4, 12]. Studemeister and Stevens reported on a literature review of *Aspergillus* vertebral osteomyelitis in immunocompetent hosts [4]. The most common presenting symptom was back pain with *Aspergillus fumigatus* being the most common subtype identified. They identified 21 cases with the majority acquired by hematogenous spread; however, only 25% of those cases occurred after a spinal operation [4]. The mortality rate was 20% in those combined cases. The vertebral bodies are the most common infected site in *Aspergillus* osteomyelitis. The route of infection can occur by transpleural extension into adjacent vertebral bodies, by direct inoculation, and by hematogenous spread. And in our patient, given that the infection was at the L3 interspace, it is more likely that this was a hematogenous spread of the organism.

Inflammatory markers are often elevated in patients with *Aspergillus* osteomyelitis. However, these are nonspecific markers and underscored the importance of serum *Aspergillus* antigen testing in patients considered at risk for this disease. The management of *Aspergillus* osteomyelitis includes surgical debridement and antifungal therapies. The report by Gamaletsou et al. on the epidemiology and management of *Aspergillus* osteomyelitis supports this conclusion [1]. There is a significant reduction in the reported frequency of relapse in patients undergoing surgical debridement [1, 3, 12, 13]. The relatively low number of patients prevents categorizing risk by fungal subtype. It appears that the overall response rates to the various antifungal agents are similar. As in our case, the patient required aggressive surgical debridement, spinal stabilization, and a course of prolonged antifungal therapy in order to successfully treat his infection. The optimal duration of antifungal therapy is not known in *Aspergillus* osteomyelitis. The duration of treatment needs to be based on the potential cumulative nephrotoxicity as well as the morbidity of prolonged therapy in aspergillosis osteomyelitis [14]. However, our patient required discontinuation of the voriconazole secondary to severe photosensitivity side effect. He was able to start on posaconazole and has tolerated that medication well. Although the number of cases of *Aspergillus* osteomyelitis treated with posaconazole is limited, the available information suggests similar clinical response [15].

*Aspergillus* osteomyelitis is a severe infection that if not aggressively treated can potentially be fatal [1, 3, 4]. The relapse rate does appear to be higher without aggressive surgical intervention despite adequate and appropriate antifungal therapies. When clinical and anatomical considerations allowed for safe surgical intervention, it appears that aggressive surgical debridement and appropriate spinal stabilization followed by antifungal therapy may offer the best chance for the patient to have a good clinical outcome.

## References


[1] M. N. Gamaletsou, B. Rammaert, M. A. Bueno et al., "*Aspergillus* osteomyelitis: epidemiology, clinical manifestations, management, and outcome," *Journal of Infection*, vol. 68, no. 5, pp. 478–493, 2014.

[2] F. C. Vinas, P. K. King, and F. G. Diaz, "Spinal Aspergillus osteomyelitis," *Clinical Infectious Disease*, vol. 28, no. 6, pp. 1223–1229, 1999.

[3] E. Gabrielli, A. W. Fothergill, L. Brescini et al., "Osteomyelitis caused by *Aspergillus* species: a review of 310 reported cases," *Clinical Microbiology and Infection*, vol. 20, no. 6, pp. 559–565, 2014.

[4] A. Studemeister and D. A. Stevens, "*Aspergillus* vertebral osteomyelitis in immunocompetent hosts: role of triazole antifungal therapy," *Clinical Infectious Disease*, vol. 52, no. 1, pp. e1–e6, 2011.

[5] P. A. Barnwell, L. F. Jelsma, and M. J. Raff, "Aspergillus osteomyelitis Report of a case and review of the literature," *Diagnostic Microbiology and Infectious Disease*, vol. 3, no. 6, pp. 515–519, 1985.

[6] C. J. Corrall, W. G. Merz, K. Rekedal, and W. T. Hughes, "*Aspergillus* osteomyelitis in an immunocompetent adolescent: a case report and review of the literature," *Pediatrics*, vol. 70, pp. 455–461, 1982.

[7] C. Castelli, F. Benazzo, F. Mimoli, P. Marone, R. Seghazzi, and C. N. Carlizzi, "Aspergillus infection of the L3-L4 disc space in an immunosuppressed heart transplant patient," *Spine*, vol. 15, no. 12, pp. 1369–1373, 1990.

[8] S. Sethi, F. Siraj, K. L. Kaira, and P. Chopra, "Aspergillus vertebral osteomyelitis in immunocompetent patients," *Indian Journal of Orthopaedics*, vol. 46, no. 2, pp. 246–250, 2012.

[9] E. F. Berbari, S. S. Kanj, T. J. Kowalski et al., "2015 Infectious Diseases Society of America (IDSA) clinical practice guidelines for the diagnosis and treatment of native vertebral osteomyelitis in adults," *Clinical Infectious Diseases*, vol. 61, no. 6, pp. e26–e46, 2015.

[10] L. Gentile, F. Benazzo, F. De Rosa et al., "A systematic review: characteristics, complications and treatment of spondylodiscitis," *European Review for Medical and Pharmacological Sciences*, vol. 23, Supplement 2, pp. 117–128, 2019.

[11] S. D. Heinrich, T. Finney, R. Craver, L. Yin, and M. M. Zembo, "*Aspergillus* osteomyelitis in patients who have chronic granulomatous disease. Case report," *Journal of Bone and Joint Surgery*, vol. 73, no. 3, pp. 456–460, 1991.

[12] K. A. Asare, M. Jahng, J. L. Pincus, L. Massie, and S. A. Lee, "Sternal osteomyelitis caused by *Aspergillus fumigatus* following cardiac surgery: case and review," *Medical Mycology Case Reports*, vol. 2, pp. 4–6, 2013.

[13] S. Govender and K. P. Kumar, "Aspergillus spondylitis in immunocompetent patients," *International Orthopaedics*, vol. 25, no. 2, pp. 74–76, 2001.

[14] C. J. Hodiamont, K. M. Dolman, I. J. Ten Berge, W. J. Melchers, P. E. Verweij, and D. Pajkrt, "Multiple-azole-resistant *Aspergillus fumigatus* osteomyelitis in a patient with chronic granulomatous disease successfully treated with long-term oral posaconazole and surgery," *Medical Mycology*, vol. 47, no. 2, pp. 217–220, 2009.

[15] B. A. Lodge, E. D. Ashley, M. P. Steele, and J. R. Perfect, "Aspergillus fumigatus empyema, arthritis, and calcaneal osteomyelitis in a lung transplant patient successfully treated with posaconazole," *Journal of Clinical Microbiology*, vol. 42, no. 3, pp. 1376–1378, 2004.

19

# Bilateral Destructive Hip Disease from Untreated Juvenile Idiopathic Arthritis

**Arash Calafi,[1] Alton W. Skaggs,[2] Trevor J. Shelton,[3] and Brian M. Haus[3,4]**

[1]University of Washington Department of Orthopaedics and Sports Medicine, 1959 N.E. Pacific St., Box 356500 Seattle, WA 98195, USA
[2]School of Medicine at University of California at Davis, Sacramento, CA 95817, USA
[3]Department of Orthopaedic Surgery, University of California at Davis, 4860 Y Street, Suite 3800, Sacramento, CA 95829, USA
[4]Shriners Hospital for Children, Northern California, 2425 Stockton Blvd., Sacramento, CA 95817, USA

Correspondence should be addressed to Trevor J. Shelton; trevorjshelton@gmail.com

Academic Editor: Elke R. Ahlmann

We report a novel case of a pediatric patient with bilateral hip destruction from untreated Juvenile idiopathic arthritis (JIA). She was presented at the age of 9 with hip pain associated with bilateral acetabular dysplasia and a dislocated left femoral head. Only 1.5 years later, the patient developed complete destruction of the left femoral head and dislocated right femoral head. The authors have not identified literature describing a similar case report of bilateral femoral head destruction resulting from Persistent Oligoarticular JIA. Pediatric patients presenting with rapidly evolving destructive process should be evaluated for rheumatologic, infectious, and spinal etiologies.

## 1. Introduction

Juvenile idiopathic arthritis (JIA) is an umbrella term used to describe arthritis of unknown origin in greater than one joint, lasting greater than 6 months in patients with disease onset prior to age of 16 [1]. JIA is a diagnosis of exclusion, considered only after more common etiologies including septic joint, trauma, malignancy, or other immunologic disorders are ruled out. Presently, JIA consists of six categories with distinct clinical and laboratory features (Table 1) [2].

While specific pathophysiologic processes of JIA categories may differ, T-cell-mediated destruction of joint spaces leading to a significant loss of function, pain, stiffness, fatigue, joint effusion, reduced range of motion, erythema, and growth alterations is the prevailing cause of morbidity in these patients [3, 4]. Impacted joints of serious consequence are the knee, hip, and temporomandibular joint and may require surgical intervention [5, 6]. Hip involvement in those with JIA is reported between 20%-40%, and early identification of hip involvement in these patients may lead to more aggressive early treatment before hip joint destruction occurs [7]. However, when it does occur at a young age, it becomes challenging to treat and manage. Here, we present a case of a 10-year-old Mexican female who developed destructive bilateral hip disease in the setting of untreated Persistent Oligoarticular JIA.

*1.1. Case Presentation.* The patient was initially presented to our clinic at the age of 9 with a chief complaint of limping. Her developmental history was notable for developmental delay without underlying genetic or autoimmune conditions and low infantile weight for which she had a gastric tube. Family history was negative for any neuromuscular disease, hip dysplasia, or autoimmune disease. She had recently moved from Mexico with her family to the United States.

Her initial exam revealed a Trendelenburg gait and sign, left hip pain-free range-of-motion with 100° internal rotation, 50° external rotation, 135° flexion, 20 extension, and 70° abduction. Her right hip revealed pain-free range-of-motion with 90° internal rotation, 50° external rotation, 135° flexion, and 60° abduction. The comparison of both hips revealed a positive Galeazzi sign with a leg-length difference of 2 cm

TABLE 1: Six categories and definitions of juvenile idiopathic arthritis [2].

| Categories of juvenile idiopathic arthritis | Definitions |
|---|---|
| Systemic arthritis | Arthritis in one or more joints with or preceded by fever ≥ 2 weeks' duration and accompanied by one or more of the following:<br>(1) Evansecent (nonfixed) erythematous rash<br>(2) Generalized lymph node enlargement<br>(3) Hepatomegaly and/or splenomegaly<br>(4) Serositis |
| Psoriatic arthritis | Arthritis and psoriasis or arthritis and ≥2 of the following:<br>(1) Dactylitis<br>(2) Nail and pitting or onycholysis<br>(3) Psoriasis in a first-degree relative |
| Enthesitis-related arthritis | Arthritis and enthesitis or arthritis or enthesitis with ≥2 of the following:<br>(1) Presence of or a history of sacroiliac joint tenderness and/or inflammatory lumbosacral pain<br>(2) Presence of HLA-B27 antigen<br>(3) Onset of arthritis in a male >6 years of age<br>(4) Acute (symptomatic) anterior uveitis<br>(5) History of ankylosing spondylitis, enthesitis-related arthritis, sacroiliitis with inflammatory bowel disease, Reiter's syndrome, or acute anterior uveitis in a first-degree relative |
| Oligoarticular | Arthritis affecting 1-4 joints during the first 6 months of disease. Two subcategories:<br>Persistent oligoarthritis: affecting ≤4 joints throughout the disease course<br>Extended oligoarthritis: affecting >4 joints after the first 6 months of disease |
| Polyarthritis | Rheumatoid factor negative: arthritis affecting ≥5 joints during the first 6 months of disease; RF test is negative<br>Rheumatoid factor positive: arthritis affecting ≥5 joints during the first 6 months of disease; 2 or more tests for RF at least 3 months apart during the first 6 months of disease are positive |
| Undifferentiated arthritis | Arthritis that fulfills criteria in no category or in 2 or more of the above categories |

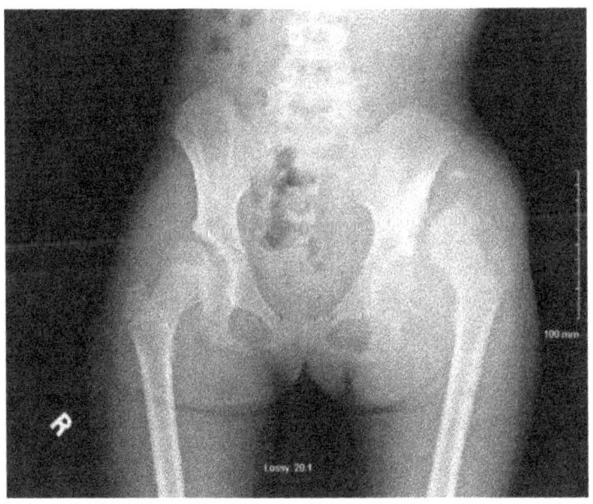

FIGURE 1: Plain AP radiograph performed in April 2014 shows dislocation of the left hip and pseudoacetabulum.

and normal bilateral reflexes. Imaging demonstrated bilateral hip dysplasia with left hip dislocation with pseudoacetabuli (Figures 1 and 2). At this time, the working diagnosis was untreated bilateral hip dysplasia, and we discussed surgical options including fusion, pelvic and femoral osteotomies, and total hip arthroplasty (THA). Given the chronicity of her dislocation and severity of her dysplasia, it was determined that any surgical treatment on the unilateral left hip dislocation was unlikely to provide a significant benefit and may make her worse. We recommended proceeding with a possible THA versus fusion in her teenage years when pain warranted treatment. For the right hip, we recommended a future periacetabular osteotomy (PAO) once her triradiate cartilage closed and her hip became symptomatic, possibly in a few years.

She was unfortunately lost to follow-up and did not receive additional treatment during this time but represented to our clinic 1.5 years later with progressive decrease in ambulation requiring a wheelchair and walker and bilateral left greater than right hip pain. On exam, both hips had painful range-of-motion with the development of a 5° hip flexion contracture on the left and increased flexion, abduction, and internal rotation on the right. Her limp was significantly worse, but her leg-length discrepancy decreased to 0.5 cm. Imaging demonstrated erosive changes of the bilateral femoral heads with infiltrative destructive patterns to the bilateral acetabula, hip effusions, and synovial thickening (Figures 3 and 4). In addition, she developed a new dislocation of the right hip. She was directly admitted from clinic for further work-up. On the day of admission, she had bilateral hip aspirations which showed unremarkable inflammatory fluid changes (left hip: 20 mL of cloudy, turbid, straw-colored fluid, cell count 908, polymorphonuclear cells 2%; right hip: 80 mL of bloody, cloudy fluid, cell count 359, polymorphonuclear cells 49%). Crystal exam, gram stain, and cultures were negative. Synovial fluid cytology demonstrated numerous benign reactive synovial cells without identification of malignant cells.

Given the severity of the destruction, a possible spinal etiology including tumor syrinx resulting in Charcot joint was suspected. Magnetic resonance imaging of the brain and

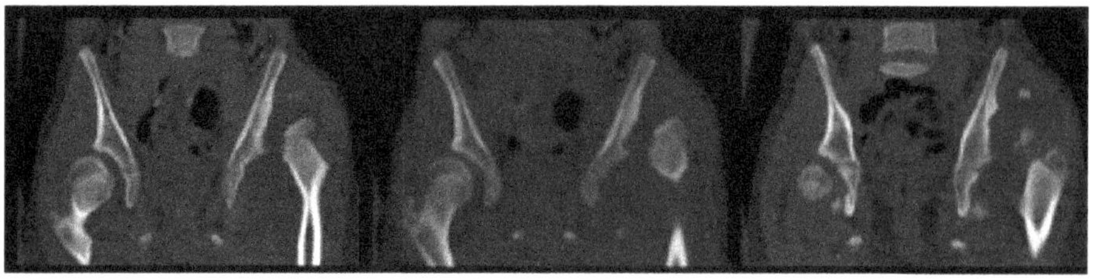

FIGURE 2: Coronal cuts of CT scan shows bilateral acetabular dysplasia with dislocated left femoral head localized in the anterosuperior aspect of the acetabulum with development of pseudoacetabulum.

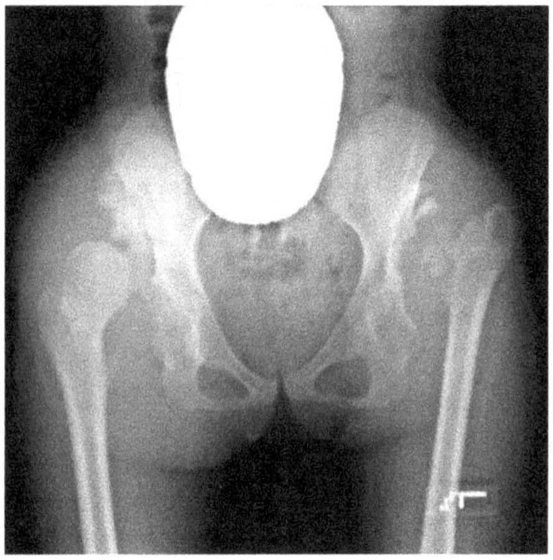

FIGURE 3: Plain AP radiograph performed on admission shows bony destruction of the bilateral acetabula and rapid progression of the left proximal femur with early cortical erosion of the right femoral head.

cervical/thoracic/lumbar spine was within normal limits. Other etiologies including bacterial, fungal, and viral infection were considered. Coccidioidomycosis and histoplasmosis titers and Lyme disease antibodies were negative. To evaluate for tuberculosis, a chest X-ray was obtained within normal limit while CT demonstrated a 4 mm nodule in the right middle lobe that was noncalcifying and believed to be postinfectious. AqQuantiFERON-TB gold test was negative. A complete blood count, basic metabolic panel, CRP (0.3 mg/dL), and ESR (7 mm/hr) were within normal limits with the exception of elevated platelets (550). Compliment fixation serum and immunodiffusion serum tests were negative. Autoimmune etiologies were also considered. Extensive serologic testing was performed including dilute Russel's viper venom time, lupus anticoagulant, anti-CCP, anticentromere, antimitochondrial, anti-double-stranded DNA, antinuclear antibody, anti-SSA, SSB antibody panel, rheumatoid factor (RF), and HLA-B27 which were all negative.

Because of the unusual and severe presentation of the disease and the lack of a diagnosis, on hospital day 10, she was taken to the operating room for bilateral hip arthrocentesis and bilateral hip arthroscopy for biopsy of the bone and synovium. A synovial biopsy was obtained to examine the tissue visually and histologically to confirm the diagnosis of an inflammatory arthritis. Intraoperative findings demonstrated right capsular destruction with unusual appearing and inflamed and reddened synovium with erosive destruction of the articular surface of the femoral head and acetabulum. On the left, there was a free-floating femoral head with multiple moderate-sized osteochondral loose bodies grossly inflamed synovium, intact labrum, no clearly discernable joint capsule, and near-complete absence of cartilage within the acetabulum and overlying the femoral head (Figure 5). Following the diagnostic component of the arthroscopy, she underwent a left femoral head arthroscopic resection, bilateral synovial and bone biopsies, and bilateral Kenalog intra-articular injections for pain relief. Biopsy results demonstrated synovial hyperplasia with chronic inflammatory changes. Postoperative X-rays showed left femoral head resection (Figure 6).

Given the results of the arthroscopic findings and synovial biopsy, we subsequently referred the patient to a board-certified pediatric rheumatologist for further evaluation. Additionally, she was found to have moderate arthropathy of her right calcaneocuboid and bilateral 1$^{st}$ metatarsophalangeal joints. Given these clinical findings, she was given the diagnosis of Persistent Oligoarticular JIA characterized by negative RF, CCP, and HLA-B27 and was subsequently started on methotrexate and folic acid.

At 3-year postoperatively, she has continued erosion of the right femoral head (Figure 7). A genetics consult was obtained, and comprehensive screening was negative. She remains nonweight bearing with the plan for bilateral THAs once she becomes a teenager. However, this could result in multiple challenges if the patient becomes nonambulatory, has limited acetabular bone stock, if the hip dysplasia requires femoral shortening, or if custom implants are needed due to the small size and deformity.

## 2. Discussion

Oligoarticular JIA (≤4 joints involved) is the most common subgroup of JIA and constitutes approximately 50% of JIA cases. It is subdivided into persistent oligoarthritis (no additional joint involvement after the first six months) and extended oligoarthritis (involvement of additional joints after the first six months) [2]. Typically, oligoarticular JIA affects females more than males, rarely presents after 10 years of age and generally affects large joints (most commonly knees and ankles) [8]. Initial symptoms in the hip are very rare in oligoarticular JIA and should raise concern for other etiology including Legg-Calve-Perthes, infection, spondyloarthropathy, neoplasm, or slipped capital femoral epiphysis. Although the hips are rarely involved, when they are, it is associated

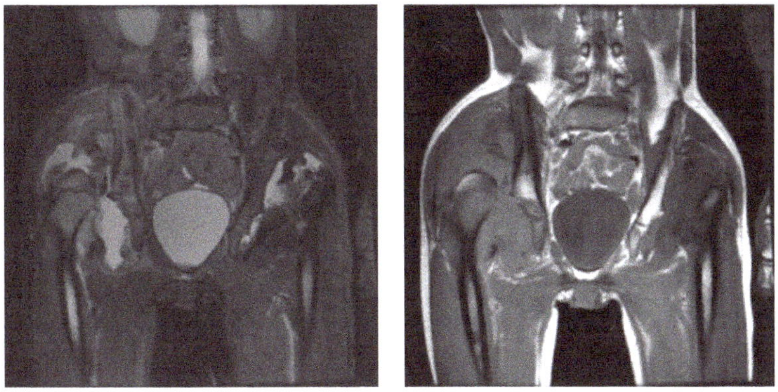

(a) (b)

Figure 4: MRI pelvis with coronal T1 (a) and coronal STIR (b) of pelvis performed on admission shows bilateral dislocated hips with right greater than left joint effusions, synovial thickening, and rice body formation.

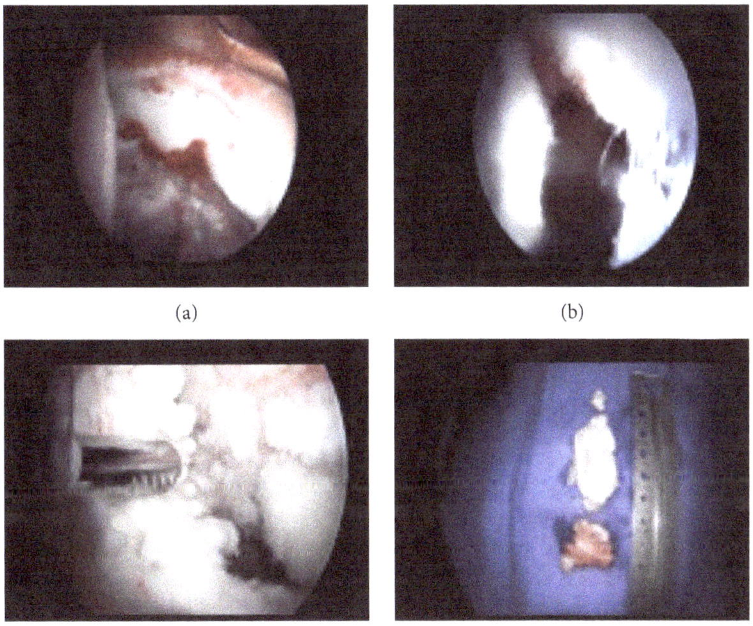

(a) (b) (c) (d)

Figure 5: Left hip arthroscopic imaging shows (a) intact labrum with destruction of the acetabulum, (b) destroyed joint capsule, (c) cartilaginous destruction of the femoral head and acetabulum, and (d) loose bodies removed from the left hip.

with a poor prognosis prior to starting treatment [9]. The diagnosis of oligoarticular JIA is made based on the presence of arthritis in ≤4 joints during the first six months of the disease after other causes have been excluded [2].

Treatment of oligoarticular JIA requires a multidisciplinary approach involving rheumatologist, physiotherapy, psychosocial support, pharmacologic therapy, and if warranted, surgical intervention. However, nearly 50% of the patient's symptoms will persist into adulthood [10]. Therefore, pharmacologic treatment prioritizes early and aggressive preservation of joint tissue. As such, disease-modifying antirheumatic drugs are the mainstay of JIA treatment. In addition, agents to control inflammation such as nonsteroidal anti-inflammatory drugs and corticosteroids are commonly prescribed. Biologics, including anti-TNF agents, may also be useful in patients with refractory JIA [1, 11]. Close follow-up is therefore essential, as combined immunosuppressive agents increase the risk of serious opportunistic infections.

Approximately 22% of patients with JIA will require major surgical intervention during their lifetime [12]. From 1991 to 2005, the average age of joint replacement performed in patients with JIA increased from 30.9 to 36.7 while the overall rate of arthroscopies dropped nearly 50% [13]. This trend is likely from more aggressive and early use of immunomodulating agents, helping to slow the disease course. While the knee, elbow, and ankle are more commonly affected in patients with JIA, hip destruction is associated

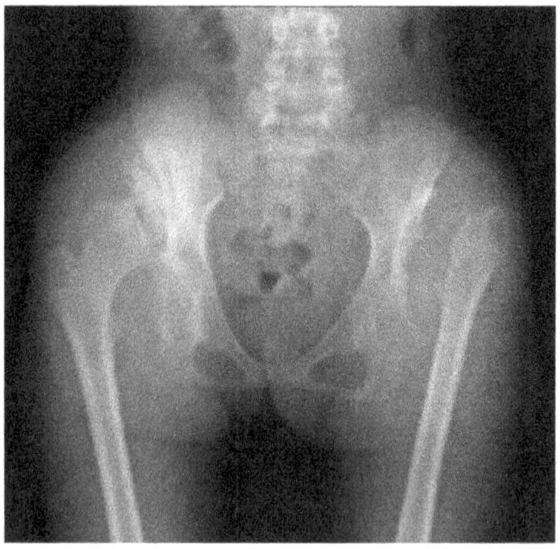

Figure 6: Plain AP radiograph performed 6 weeks after surgery shows interval resection of the femoral head that was fragmented. There is also resection of bony fragmentation adjacent to the acetabulum.

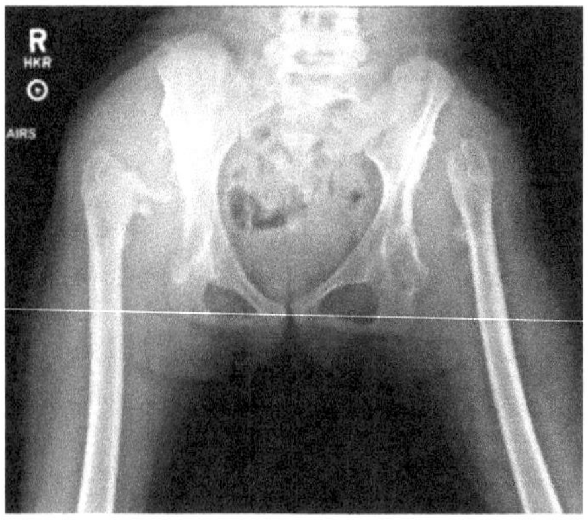

Figure 7: Plain AP radiograph performed one year after arthroscopic removal of femoral heads shows interval erosion of the right femoral head.

with greater functional deficits and morbidity [14]. Hip involvement in those with JIA is 20%-40%, but it is rarely the initially affected joint. Rather, hip symptoms typically manifests within 7 years after the initial diagnosis [7]. Typically, with the aid of immunomodulating agents, patients do not develop hip destruction necessitating joint replacement until the third or fourth decade [15]. Known predictors of early hip destruction include increased joint involvement, systemic symptoms associated with JIA, elevated immunoglobulins, increased platelet count, and hip involvement early in the disease course [7].

Patients with hip destruction and severe impairment may require a THA if physiotherapy and pharmacologic treatments fail. However, optimal timing for THA is controversial. It has been shown that implant survival is significantly better in young patients over the age of 25 at the time of THA [16]. THA in younger patients is technically challenging and complicated due to several factors. The femoral medullary canal can be excessively narrow and fragile, increasing the risk for fracture and prosthetic failure. There may also be deformities such as femoral and acetabular anteversion as well as the presence of flexion contractures. Moreover, bone stock can be depleted due to immunologic destruction and prolonged use of corticosteroid [5, 6, 17]. The use of immunosuppressants also increases the risk of postoperative infection and poor wound closure [14]. Finally, when considering THA in younger patients, growth status must also be considered. Premature physeal closure and growth retardation are common in JIA due to pain-related disuse of the affected limb, cachexia secondary to chronic inflammation (increased TNF-a and IL-1), osteopenia from chronic corticosteroid use, and malnutrition secondary to increased metabolic demand and pharmacologic side effects [4, 18]. Despite these risks, THA is considered a reasonable treatment modality in patients with refractory JIA and is associated with significant improvement in joint pain and mobility with a 10-year implant survival rate of 80-85% and 20-year implant survival of approximately 35% [16].

## Consent

The patient/family was informed that data concerning the case would be submitted for publication, and they provided consent.

## References

[1] P. J. Kahn, "Juvenile idiopathic arthritis: what the clinician needs to know," *Bulletin of the Hospital for Joint Diseases*, vol. 71, no. 3, pp. 194–199, 2013.

[2] R. E. Petty, T. R. Southwood, P. Manners et al., "International League of Associations for Rheumatology classification of juvenile idiopathic arthritis: second revision, Edmonton, 2001," *The Journal of Rheumatology*, vol. 31, no. 2, pp. 390–392, 2004.

[3] D. A. Chistiakov, K. V. Savost'anov, and A. A. Baranov, "Genetic background of juvenile idiopathic arthritis," *Autoimmunity*, vol. 47, no. 6, pp. 351–360, 2014.

[4] J. E. Weiss and N. T. Ilowite, "Juvenile idiopathic arthritis," *Pediatric Clinics of North America*, vol. 52, no. 2, pp. 413–442, 2005.

[5] P. J. Gowdie and S. M. Tse, "Juvenile idiopathic arthritis," *Pediatric Clinics of North America*, vol. 59, no. 2, pp. 301–327, 2012.

[6] P. B. Kitsoulis, K. S. Stafilas, A. Siamopoulou, P. N. Soucacos, and T. A. Xenakis, "Total hip arthroplasty in children with juvenile chronic arthritis: long-term results," *Journal of Pediatric Orthopaedics*, vol. 26, no. 1, pp. 8–12, 2006.

[7] M. Batthish, B. M. Feldman, P. S. Babyn, P. N. Tyrrell, and R. Schneider, "Predictors of hip disease in the systemic arthritis subtype of juvenile idiopathic arthritis," *The Journal of Rheumatology*, vol. 38, no. 5, pp. 954–958, 2011.

[8] C. Macaubas, K. Nguyen, D. Milojevic, J. L. Park, and E. D. Mellins, "Oligoarticular and polyarticular JIA: epidemiology

and pathogenesis," *Nature Reviews Rheumatology*, vol. 5, no. 11, pp. 616–626, 2009.

[9] T. Beukelman, N. M. Patkar, K. G. Saag et al., "2011 American College of Rheumatology recommendations for the treatment of juvenile idiopathic arthritis: initiation and safety monitoring of therapeutic agents for the treatment of arthritis and systemic features," *Arthritis Care & Research*, vol. 63, no. 4, pp. 465–482, 2011.

[10] M. Espinosa and B. S. Gottlieb, "Juvenile idiopathic arthritis," *Pediatrics in Review*, vol. 33, no. 7, pp. 303–313, 2012.

[11] H. Jennings, K. Hennessy, and G. J. Hendry, "The clinical effectiveness of intra-articular corticosteroids for arthritis of the lower limb in juvenile idiopathic arthritis: a systematic review," *Pediatric Rheumatology*, vol. 12, no. 1, p. 23, 2014.

[12] M. Zak and F. K. Pedersen, "Juvenile chronic arthritis into adulthood: a long-term follow-up study," *Rheumatology*, vol. 39, no. 2, pp. 198–204, 2000.

[13] C. Mertelsmann-Voss, S. Lyman, T. J. Pan, S. M. Goodman, M. P. Figgie, and L. A. Mandl, "US trends in rates of arthroplasty for inflammatory arthritis including rheumatoid arthritis, juvenile idiopathic arthritis, and spondyloarthritis," *Arthritis & Rheumatology*, vol. 66, no. 6, pp. 1432–1439, 2014.

[14] M. P. Abdel and M. P. Figgie, "Surgical management of the juvenile idiopathic arthritis patient with multiple joint involvement," *Orthopedic Clinics of North America*, vol. 45, no. 4, pp. 435–442, 2014.

[15] X. A. Li, S. Iyer, M. B. Cross, and M. P. Figgie, "Total joint replacement in adolescents: literature review and case examples," *Current Opinion in Pediatrics*, vol. 24, no. 1, pp. 57–63, 2012.

[16] I. Swarup, A. C. Marshall, Y. Y. Lee, and M. P. Figgie, "Implant survival and patient-reported outcomes after total hip arthroplasty in young patients with developmental dysplasia of the hip," *Hip International*, vol. 26, no. 4, pp. 367–373, 2016.

[17] S. B. Goodman, K. Hwang, and S. Imrie, "High complication rate in revision total hip arthroplasty in juvenile idiopathic arthritis," *Clinical Orthopaedics and Related Research*, vol. 472, no. 2, pp. 637–644, 2014.

[18] J. S. Daurka, A. K. Malik, D. A. Robin, and J. D. Witt, "The results of uncemented total hip replacement in children with juvenile idiopathic arthritis at ten years," *The Journal of Bone and Joint Surgery British volume*, vol. 94-B, no. 12, pp. 1618–1624, 2012.

# 20

# Thoracic Radicular Pain Caused by Extravertebral Gas and Fluid Collections Associated with Osteoporotic Vertebral Fracture Containing a Vacuum Cleft

**Kazunobu Kida,[1] Toshikazu Tani,[1] Tateo Kawazoe,[1] and Michio Toda[2]**

[1]*Department of Orthopaedic Surgery, Kubokawa Hospital, 902-1 Mitsuke, Shimanto-cho, Takaoka-gun, Kochi 786-0002, Japan*
[2]*Department of Orthopaedic Surgery, Kurashiki Medical Center, 250 Bakuro-cho, Kurashiki City, Okayama 710-8522, Japan*

Correspondence should be addressed to Kazunobu Kida; kazugonkochi@gmail.com

Academic Editor: Taketoshi Yasuda

The present study documents a phenomenon, which has received little attention despite its potential clinical importance. An 87-year-old woman presented with barely reported extravertebral gas and fluid collections probably originating from the contents of the adjacent cleft within the T10 collapsed osteoporotic vertebra. Her chief complaint was intractable pain radiating over the left thorax suggestive of intercostal neuralgia. The pain intensified when sitting up from a lateral decubitus position, correlating with a posture-related radiologic change of the intravertebral cleft, which appeared with a decubitus position and disappeared with a sitting position. Because these extravertebral collections were located where the 10th thoracic nerve root just exits the intervertebral foramina, her chest pain of a posture-dependent nature most likely resulted from nerve root compression by extravertebral gas and fluid forced out of the vertebral cleft. Posterior spinal fusion with pedicle screw instrumentation resulted in a complete resolution of the chest pain with disappearance of the extravertebral gas and fluid accumulations. An awareness of the possibility that the intravertebral cleft could communicate with the extravertebral space close to the nerve root will help avoid neurologic complications caused by bone cement leakage during vertebroplasty.

## 1. Introduction

A radiolucent area within the collapsed vertebra seen after osteoporotic vertebral fracture (OVF) usually contains gas and/or fluid, not necessarily representing a true vacuum, despite the common designation, intravertebral "vacuum" phenomenon [1] or the intravertebral "vacuum" cleft (IVC) [2].

As previously demonstrated, in some cases, in which the intravertebral and intradiscal clefts coexisted, the gas and/or fluid could migrate between the two adjacent clefts through the fractured endplate [1, 3]. Some reports also showed that symptomatic gaseous cysts could arise in the epidural or intradural space, presumably originating from the adjacent degenerated intervertebral disc [4, 5]. However, to the best of our knowledge, only a single study in the past reported on the radiologic appearance of extravertebral gas bubbles and edematous effusions secondary to the OVF containing IVC [6]. Unlike a simple radiologic observation in the previous report, the current study documents a patient who developed an intractable chest pain, not responding to conservative therapy, as a sign of the T10 nerve root compression by the localized extravertebral gas and fluid collections associated with the IVC inside the T10 collapsed vertebral body. The patient and her family provided written informed consent for publication of this case report and accompanying images.

## 2. Case Report

An 87-year-old woman with an intractable pain radiating over the left chest, suggestive of intercostal neuralgia, was referred to our spine center for further evaluation and management. Five weeks earlier, she experienced a ground-level

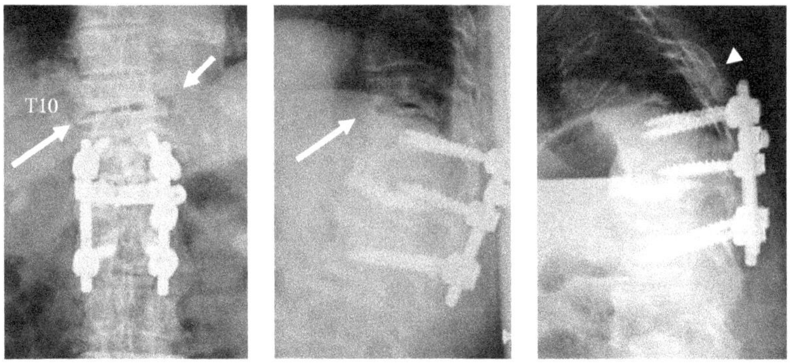


(a) (b) (c)

FIGURE 1: Preoperative thoracolumbar spine radiographs in the supine (a, b) and sitting (c) positions, showing intravertebral vacuum cleft (long arrows), extravertebral gas (short arrow), and the fracture line of T10 extending to posterior fusion mass bone (arrow head) grafted 8 years ago.

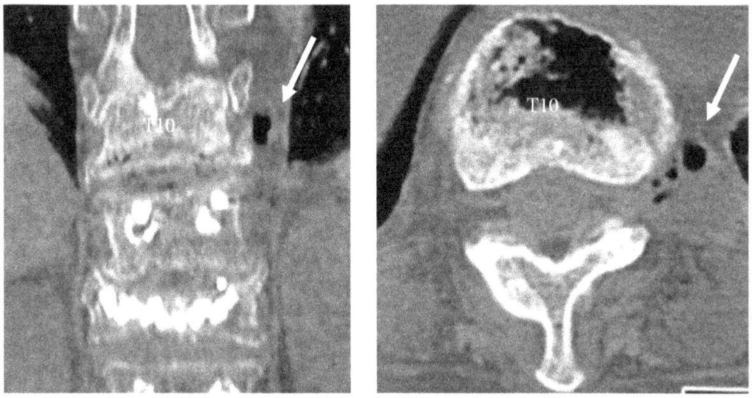


(a) (b)

FIGURE 2: Preoperative coronal (a) and axial (b) computed tomographies of the thoracic spine obtained in the supine position, more clearly showing the gas and fluid collections (arrows) just below the left 10th rib head in (a) and the T10-T11 extraforaminal zone in (b).

fall, causing severe back pain. According to the initial evaluation conducted elsewhere, she was diagnosed as having OVF of the T10 vertebral body and managed conservatively with a brace and pain medication for one month. Her chief complaint gradually changed from bilateral back pain to an aching pain extending to the left thorax before her first visit to our hospital. What is noteworthy about the history of this case is that 8 years previously, she had had a painful OVF of the T12 vertebral body at the age of 79 years, which was treated with vertebroplasty using hydroxyapatite (HA) blocks and posterior pedicle screw instrumentation followed by iliac bone graft fusion from T11 to L1 at another hospital [7].

On clinical examination at our hospital, the patient had no neurologic deficits, complaining of nothing but reporting a position-dependent severe chest pain on the left side, which intensified when sitting up from a supine position. Imaging studies revealed neither rib fractures nor abnormal findings of the chest cavity as a possible cause of the chest pain.

On the plain radiographs of the thoracic spine (Figure 1), the anteroposterior (AP) views and the lateral views taken in the supine position showed the IVC within the T10 collapsed vertebral body as a gas-like radiolucent area, which disappeared on the lateral view obtained in the sitting position (i.e., the opening-closing phenomenon) most likely indicating an OVF of nonneoplastic and noninfectious origin [8, 9]. The lateral radiograph in the sitting position also demonstrated that the fracture line extended through the posterior fusion mass bone, grafted 8 years ago, indicating a potentially unstable flexion-distraction injury. Close observation of the AP radiograph obtained in the supine position revealed a gas-like radiolucency at the extravertebral space just lateral to the T10 collapsed vertebral wall ipsilateral to the side of her chest pain. The computed tomography (CT) scans, which have a higher sensitivity in detecting gas than radiography and magnetic resonance imaging (MRI) scans, more clearly showed an accumulation of gas located just below the head of the left 10th rib, the place radiologically termed the T10-T11 extraforaminal zone (Figure 2).

In terms of the IVC contents of radiolucency on the plain radiographs, sagittal MRI revealed a gas-like signal void within the T10 collapsed vertebral body. Corresponding to the extravertebral area of radiolucency shown by the AP radiograph and the CT, both T1- and T2-weighted axial MRI showed combined gas-like and fluid-like signal

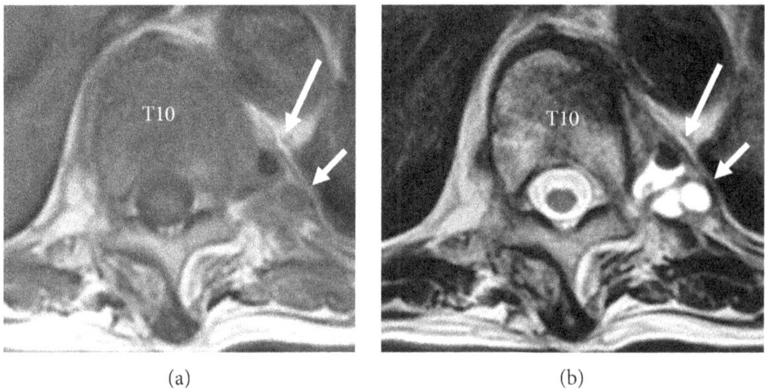


FIGURE 3: Preoperative axial T1-weighted (a) and T2-weighted (b) magnetic resonance imaging, showing the gas (long arrows pointing T1-low and T2-low signal intensity areas) and fluid (short arrows pointing T1-iso and T2-high signal intensity areas) collections just below the left 10th rib head.

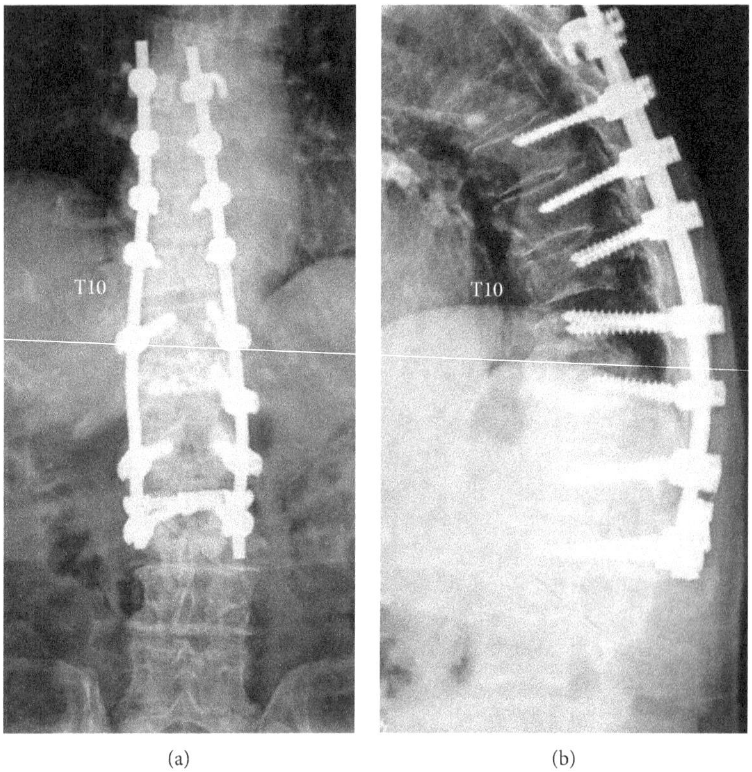


FIGURE 4: Anteroposterior (a) and lateral (b) radiographs of the thoracolumbar spine at the 2-year follow-up after surgery, showing posterior spinal fusion from T7 to L2 with pedicle screw instrumentation performed for the T10 osteoporotic vertebral fracture involving three columns.

intensities; i.e., a gas-like low signal intensity area with a fluid-like iso-signal intensity area on the T1-weighted image and a gas-like low signal intensity area with a fluid-like high signal intensity area on the T2-weighted image (Figure 3).

All these findings from the imaging studies suggested that the patient's chest pain probably resulted from T10 nerve root compression at the T10-T11 extraforaminal zone by a mixed accumulation of gas and fluid, which most likely originated from the adjacent IVC within the collapsed T10 vertebral body as a result of the "force pumping mechanism," as previously postulated [6].

Because of the unstable nature of the fracture involving all structural components from anterior through posterior spinal columns, in addition to her persistent disabling pain not responding to conservative therapy, we carried out posterior spinal fusion from T7 to L2 with pedicle screw instrumentation followed by iliac bone graft (Figure 4). Immediately after the surgical stabilization, the patient reported a complete resolution of the pain. This patient had no history of antiosteoporosis medications before the referral to our spine center. We administered pharmacological treatments postoperatively, consisting of teriparatide injections initially, followed by oral bisphosphonates. At a 2-year follow-up, she remained asymptomatic, and CT scans showed neither a gas accumulation nor a fluid collection both inside and outside of the T10 vertebral body.

## 3. Discussion

The IVC, initially shown by plain radiographs as a radiolucent space within the affected vertebral bodies after OVF, has been much more commonly identified by CT and MRI than previously thought. In clinical practice, the IVC, if demonstrated radiologically, serves as a fairly reliable sign that the vertebral collapse is not due to spinal neoplasm or infection [8, 9]. The presence of IVC usually indicates fracture nonunion; many studies showed a painful posture-related change of IVC, tending to widen with extension or supine position and narrow with flexion or an upright position. More recently, the advent of a new surgical technique for OVF, percutaneous vertebroplasty, has drawn increasing attention from spine surgeons to the IVC, which they need to fill with polymethylmethacrylate (PMMA) by injection with special care to avoid heat injury of the nerve by its leakage outside the vertebral body during vertebroplasty [10–12].

The current report described a patient who developed an intractable chest pain unilaterally associated with the T10 OVF containing the IVC. The pain intensified at the moment of sitting up from a decubitus position. This posture-dependent change of the pain intensity correlated with the radiographic changes of the IVC within the T10 collapsed vertebral body, appearing in a decubitus position and disappearing in a sitting position.

Importantly, we found the extravertebral small areas of gas-like radiolucency near the head of the 10th rib, ipsilateral to the side of the patient's chest pain, shown by the plain AP radiograph and more clearly by the CT. This location corresponded to the extraforaminal zone, where the 10th thoracic nerve root just exits the T10-T11 intervertebral foramina. On MRI, the signal intensities of the contents of these extravertebral radiolucent areas indicated a mixture of gases and fluids, which supports the MRI evidence commonly shown for the contents within the IVC.

To our knowledge, only one other study by Coulier [6] reported on the radiologic observation of extravertebral gas bubbles and edematous effusions associated with the OVF without any mention of the clinical symptoms. Our findings from the imaging studies coupled with the position-dependent change of the patient's pain intensity suggested that the chest pain most likely resulted from T10 nerve root compression by the extravertebral gases and fluids, which, as postulated by Coulier, could be forced out of the IVC as a consequence of increased pressure inside the IVC from the negative pressure values in the supine position to the positive values in the sitting position, the phenomenon called "force pumping mechanism." The T10 radicular lesion may have resulted from instability of the T10 fractured vertebral body itself, but in our case, there was a lack of radiological evidence of compressive bony fragments to suggest this possibility.

To treat this elderly patient through surgery, we opted to employ a long posterior spinal fusion from T7 to L2 with pedicle screw instrumentation, not only because the patient had had a posterior spinal fusion at T11-L1 in the past but also because she had an unstable OVF involving three columns. Had it not been for the possible communication between the IVC within the T10 collapsed vertebral body and the extravertebral space close to the T10 nerve root, we could have added the T10 vertebroplasty using bone cement without concern for iatrogenic damage to the nerve root.

The fact that the extravertebral extrusion of gas and/or fluid from the IVC has rarely been reported is somewhat counterintuitive. This is because vertebral fractures, if simply accompanied by the surrounding soft tissue disruptions, as is commonly the case, involving the periosteum and the ligamentous structures attached to the fractured vertebral body surface, could communicate with the extravertebral spaces. This dissociation may suggest that the communication between inside and outside of the IVC either requires some additional key factors for its generation or escapes radiological detection by casual imaging studies without dynamic observations or both. Regardless of the underlying mechanisms of this phenomenon, its incidence rate requires further confirmation.

## 4. Conclusion

This case report indicates that the cleft within the collapsed osteoporotic vertebra could communicate with the extravertebral space close to the nerve root. An awareness of this possibility underscores the need for adequate imaging studies before vertebroplasty and kyphoplasty, which, although considered minimally invasive and low-risk procedures, may place the nerve roots at risk with bone cement leakage not only into the epidural space but also at the extraforaminal zone.

## References

[1] P. Lafforgue, C. Chagnaud, V. Daumen-Legré, L. Daver, M. Kasbarian, and P. C. Acquaviva, "The intravertebral vacuum phenomenon ("vertebral osteonecrosis"). Migration of intradiscal gas in a fractured vertebral body?," *Spine*, vol. 22, no. 16, pp. 1885–1891, 1997.

[2] A. M. Wu, Y. L. Chi, and W. F. Ni, "Vertebral compression fracture with intravertebral vacuum cleft sign: pathogenesis, image, and surgical intervention," *Asian Spine Journal*, vol. 7, no. 2, pp. 148–155, 2013.

[3] T. Armingeat, T. Pham, V. Legre, and P. Lafforgue, "Coexistence of intravertebral vacuum and intradiscal vacuum," *Joint Bone Spine*, vol. 73, no. 4, pp. 428–432, 2006.

[4] Y. Kakitsubata, S. J. Theodorou, D. J. Theodorou et al., "Symptomatic epidural gas cyst associated with discal vacuum phenomenon," *Spine*, vol. 34, no. 21, pp. E784–E789, 2009.

[5] A. Sei, M. Mizutamari, T. Fujimoto, T. Taniwaki, and H. Mizuta, "Gas-filled intradural cysts of the lumbar spine and the possible pathogenesis," *The Spine Journal*, vol. 9, no. 7, pp. E6–E8, 2009.

[6] B. Coulier, "Extravertebral gas and fluid effusions associated with vertebral collapse containing a vacuum cleft possibly result from a pumping phenomenon: a new evidence of the dynamic hydro-pneumatical nature of the so-called vacuum phenomenon," *Journal of the Belgian Society of Radiology*, vol. 96, no. 1, pp. 10–16, 2013.

[7] K. Nishioka, S. Imae, M. Kitayama, J. I. Miki, T. Okawa, and T. Itakura, "Percutaneous vertebroplasty using hydroxyapatite blocks for the treatment of vertebral body fracture," *Neurologia Medico-Chirurgica*, vol. 49, no. 11, pp. 501–506, 2009.

[8] S. W. Feng, M. C. Chang, H. T. Wu, J. K. Yu, S. T. Wang, and C. L. Liu, "Are intravertebral vacuum phenomena benign lesions?," *European Spine Journal*, vol. 20, no. 8, pp. 1341–1348, 2011.

[9] J. Malghem, B. Maldague, M. A. Labaisse et al., "Intravertebral vacuum cleft: changes in content after supine positioning," *Radiology*, vol. 187, no. 2, pp. 483–487, 1993.

[10] M. J. Nieuwenhuijse, A. R. van Erkel, and P. D. S. Dijkstra, "Cement leakage in percutaneous vertebroplasty for osteoporotic vertebral compression fractures: identification of risk factors," *The Spine Journal*, vol. 11, no. 9, pp. 839–848, 2011.

[11] J. Ding, Q. Zhang, J. Zhu et al., "Risk factors for predicting cement leakage following percutaneous vertebroplasty for osteoporotic vertebral compression fractures," *European Spine Journal*, vol. 25, no. 11, pp. 3411–3417, 2016.

[12] M. J. Nieuwenhuijse, C. S. P. van Rijswijk, A. R. van Erkel, and S. P. D. Dijkstra, "The intravertebral cleft in painful long-standing osteoporotic vertebral compression fractures treated with percutaneous vertebroplasty: diagnostic assessment and clinical significance," *Spine*, vol. 37, no. 11, pp. 974–981, 2012.

# 21

# Atraumatic Left Distal Radial Artery Aneurysm

**Joseph Maalouly,[1] Dany Aouad,[1] Elias Saidy,[1] Antonios Tawk,[2] Georges Baaklini,[3] and Chawki Cortbawi[1]**

[1]*Department of Orthopedic Surgery and Traumatology, Saint Georges University Medical Center, Balamand University, P.O.Box 166378, Achrafieh, Beirut 1100 2807, Lebanon*
[2]*Saint Georges University Medical Center, Balamand University, P.O.Box 166378, Achrafieh, Beirut 1100 2807, Lebanon*
[3]*Department of Vascular Surgery, Saint Georges University Medical Center, Balamand University, P.O.Box 166378, Achrafieh, Beirut 1100 2807, Lebanon*

Correspondence should be addressed to Dany Aouad; dany.kh.aouad@gmail.com

Academic Editor: Eyal Itshayek

Distal radial artery aneurysms are an uncommon pathological entity in the field of surgery. Moreover, distal radial artery aneurysms of idiopathic etiology are even rarer. Herein, we present a rare case of idiopathic/atraumatic left radial artery aneurysm. A 73-year-old female patient presented with a chief complaint of a pulsatile mass located on her left wrist. Radiological imaging showed the presence of a distal radial artery aneurysm which was successfully surgically excised with subsequent ligation of the radial artery. Some of the etiologies and operative management of distal radial artery aneurysm in the anatomical snuffbox to what is in accordance with the literature are discussed. Distal radial artery aneurysms are rare. Hence, their misdiagnosis may lead to wrongful management and increase in morbidity. The appropriate management of distal radial aneurysm is almost always surgical.

## 1. Introduction

Arterial aneurysms of the upper extremity form an extremely rare pathological entity encountered in the surgical field. The rarest form of upper extremity arterial aneurysm is the distal radial artery aneurysm, while the most common form is the distal ulnar artery aneurysm. The majority of radial artery aneurysm cases reported in the literature are secondary to a traumatic event, with the anatomical snuffbox being the most common anatomical location [1, 2]. Other upper extremity arterial aneurysm etiologies reported in the literature include mycotic [3], arteriosclerotic [4, 5], idiopathic [6], and underlying vasculopathy [7]. The rarest etiology of radial artery aneurysm is the idiopathic etiology accounting for only nine cases in the literature [8]. A true aneurysm is when there is dilatation of the artery, usually occurring secondary to weakening of the arterial wall. Thus, the dilatation contains all the components of the arterial wall. A false aneurysm or a pseudoaneurysm is when there is a protrusion of a sac-like structure from an otherwise normal artery. Pseudoaneurysms are usually secondary to a disruption of the arterial wall [9]. Herein, we report a case of idiopathic distal radial artery aneurysm.

## 2. Case Presentation

A 73-year-old female patient with a past medical and surgical history positive for hypertension, dyslipidemia, and thrombocytopenia status postsplenectomy presented with a chief complaint of a pulsatile mass located on her left wrist. The patient denied any family history of aneurysms, any traumatic event to the hand, any recurrent punctures or arterial cannulation, and any surgeries. The patient reported that she is a nonsmoker. The patient started noticing the mass

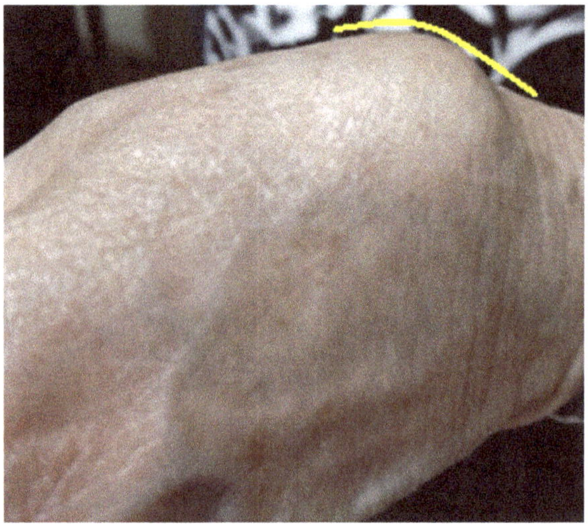

FIGURE 1: A mass located at the snuffbox area of the left hand.

one year prior to her presentation. She describes her mass as small at the beginning and gradually increasing in size. Upon physical examination, we noticed an irregular dark grey focally congested membranous fragment associated with a separate rubbery to firm beige tissue fragment (Figure 1). The mass was pulsatile, but no bruit was heard upon auscultation. The finding on Allen's test was positive. Upon further full body inspection and auscultation, no evidence of other aneurysms in other parts of the body was found. A laboratory workup was preformed, and results were negative for any evidence of systemic inflammation or disease of autoimmune etiology.

Computed Tomography Angiography (CTA) with IV contrast showed a $15 \times 9 \times 11$ mm aneurysm of the distal radial artery as it forms the dorsal arch (Figure 2). The radial and ulnar arteries were normally opacified and patent. There was no evidence of blood supply compromise at the level of the hand with intact superficial and deep palmar arches. The CT scan showed mild degenerative changes of the radioulnar joint, radiocarpal joint, and first carpometacarpal joint.

However, there were no evidence of trauma, previous fractures, or bone lesions.

Taking into consideration of various complications of an aneurysm from a thromboembolic event to rupture, surgical intervention was decided. The surgery was a joint surgery between the vascular surgery department and the orthopedic surgery department.

Under local anesthesia, the surgeons made an incision at the aneurysm site and established a primary control of the proximal and distal artery to the aneurysm using vessel loops. The aneurysm was dissected from the surrounding neurologic structures, and the artery was clamped (Figure 3). The aneurysm was then excised, and primary repair with end-to-end anastomosis was done.

The patient was followed postoperatively for two days before her discharge with an uneventful hospital stay.

The histopathology report of the excised mass described features compatible with an aneurysm filled with nonorganized fibrin thrombus. The report also described the aneurysm macroscopically as an irregular, dark-grey, focally congested membranous tissue fragments measuring $3 \times 1 \times 0.7$ cm associated with a separate rubbery to firm beige tissue fragment measuring $1.3 \times 1 \times 0.2$ cm.

## 3. Discussion

Upper extremity aneurysms are extremely rare encounters in the surgical field with radial aneurysms being the rarest with a prevalence of 2.9% among all aneurysms affecting the upper extremities [2]. This rarity is attributed to the fact that the radial artery has a small lumen. Thus, there is a low probability for an aneurysm to form based on Laplace's law since vessels with small lumen require higher pressures for the aneurysm to enlarge [9, 10]. The most common location for a distal radial artery aneurysm is at the level of the anatomical snuffbox.

In this presented case, our patient presented with a chief complaint of a pulsatile mass located on her left forearm with no associated pain or paresthesia. The diagnosis of the distal radial artery aneurysm was made clinically with physical exam findings of a pulsatile mass along with radiologic modalities used for the visualization of the mass. The diagnosis was later confirmed with postoperative pathological studies. Due to the potential complications of an aneurysm, surgical intervention was advised as the appropriate management of the distal radial artery aneurysm. Rupture of the aneurysm is a rare complication. Other complications include thromboembolism formation with subsequent distal ischemia due to vessel occlusion or nerve compression due to expanding mass [6, 11]. Based on physical exam and imaging finding, a reconstructive approach was taken. The aneurysm was surgically excised with subsequent radial artery ligation via a primary end-to-end anastomosis. The postoperative course of the patient was uneventful, and the patient was discharged two days postoperation.

## 4. Conclusion

Atraumatic or idiopathic distal radial artery aneurysms are extremely rare encountered medical conditions. The misdiagnosis of an upper extremity aneurysm for a ganglion, a neuroma, a lipoma, or a synovial cyst leads to wrongful management, and it is associated with increased morbidity. The appropriate diagnosis of a distal radial artery aneurysm in the above patient was the combination of the clinical picture painted with the patient's history and physical examination and the radiologic modalities used for better visualization. Due to the various complications of an upper extremity aneurysm that can range from a thromboembolic event to rupture, surgery is usually indicated as it is the case with our patient. The operative management of our patient included the surgical excision of the distal radial artery aneurysm on the left upper extremity with subsequent ligation of the radial artery via end-to-end anastomosis.

However, which surgical approach to use remains controversial as the literature does not contain clear guidelines

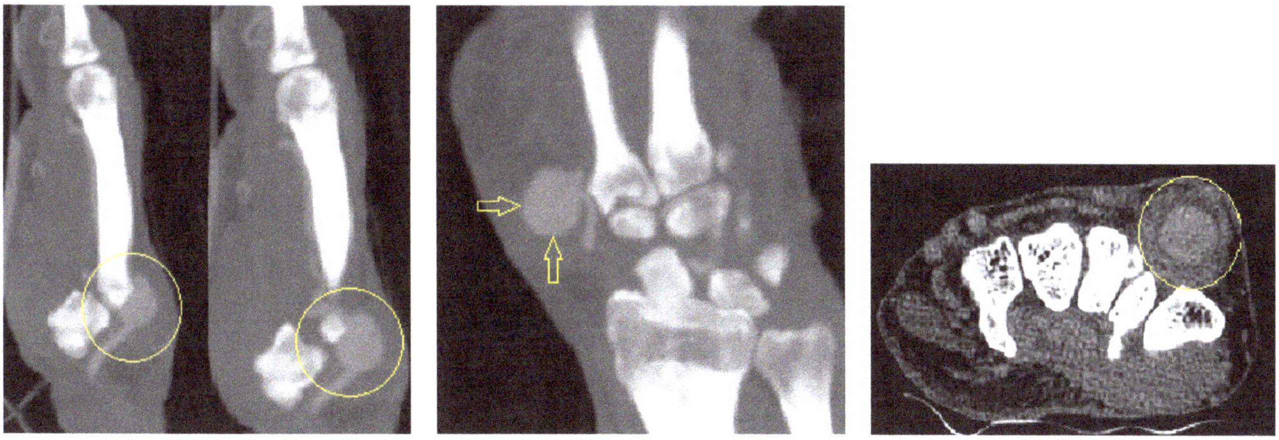

(a) (b) (c)

FIGURE 2: Computed Tomography Angiography shows the 15 × 9 × 11 mm distal radial artery aneurysm (yellow circles and arrows) in sagittal (a), coronal (b), and transverse (c) sections.

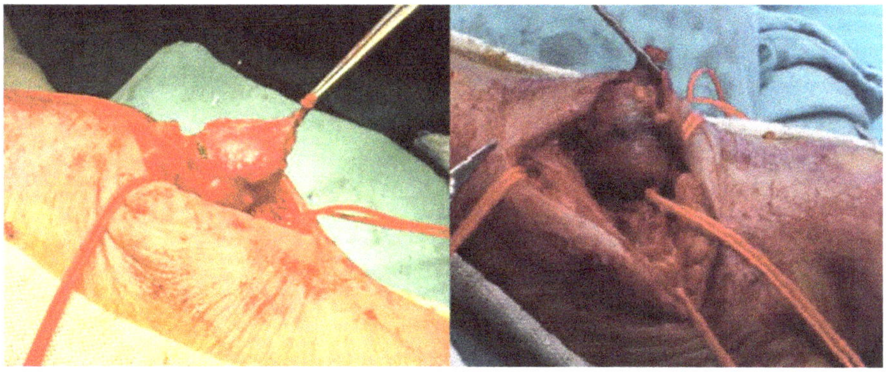

FIGURE 3: Exploration of the aneurysm with the radial artery controlled with vessel loops proximally and distally.

for the operative management of such pathology since distal radial artery aneurysm at the anatomical snuffbox are uncommon entities reported as case reports in the literature [8, 12, 13].

## Consent

Full consent from the patient was obtained for publishing this article and images.

## References


[1] P. K. Ho, A. J. Weiland, M. A. McClinton, and E. F. S. Wilgis, "Aneurysms of the upper extremity," *The Journal of Hand Surgery*, vol. 12, no. 1, pp. 39–46, 1987.

[2] J. A. Ogeng'o and B. Otieno, "Aneurysms in the arteries of the upper extremity in a Kenyan population," *Cardiovascular Pathology*, vol. 20, no. 1, pp. e53–e56, 2011.

[3] R. A. Poirier and H. C. Stansel Jr., "Arterial aneurysms of the hand," *The American Journal of Surgery*, vol. 124, no. 1, pp. 72–74, 1972.

[4] S. Thorrens, O. H. Trippel, and J. J. Bergan, "Arteriosclerotic aneurysms of the hand: excision and restoration of continuity," *Archives of Surgery*, vol. 92, no. 6, pp. 937–939, 1966.

[5] S. Malt, "An arteriosclerotic aneurysm of the hand," *Archives of Surgery*, vol. 113, no. 6, pp. 762-763, 1978.

[6] Y. Yamamoto, T. Kudo, K. Igari, T. Toyofuku, and Y. Inoue, "Radial artery aneurysm in the anatomical snuff box: a case report and literature review," *International Journal of Surgery Case Reports*, vol. 27, pp. 44–47, 2016.

[7] Y. Umeda, Y. Matsuno, M. Imaizumi, Y. Mori, H. Iwata, and H. Takiya, "Bilateral radial artery aneurysms in the anatomical snuff box seen in Marfan syndrome patient: case report and literature review," *Annals of Vascular Diseases*, vol. 2, no. 3, pp. 185–189, 2009.

[8] N. Al-Zoubi, "Idiopathic true aneurysm of distal radial artery: case report," *Vascular Health and Risk Management*, vol. 14, pp. 279–281, 2018.

[9] S. Turner, C. B. Howard, and N. S. Dallimore, "A case report of a true aneurysm of a digital artery," *Journal of Hand Surgery*, vol. 9, no. 2, pp. 205-206, 1984.

[10] S. B. Erdogan, S. Akansel, N. T. Selcuk, and S. A. Aka, "Reconstructive surgery of true aneurysm of the radial artery: a case report," *Northern Clinics of Istanbul*, vol. 5, no. 1, pp. 72–74, 2018.

[11] J. Dawson and R. Fitridge, "Update on aneurysm disease: current insights and controversies: peripheral aneurysms: when to intervene–is rupture really a danger?," *Progress in Cardiovascular Diseases*, vol. 56, no. 1, pp. 26–35, 2013.

[12] L. E. Meira Jr., T. M. Gouvêa, and T. J. D. Macedo, "Idiopathic radial artery aneurysm: case report," *Jornal Vascular Brasileiro*, vol. 10, no. 4, pp. 315–318, 2011.

[13] N. P. Walton and F. Choudhary, "Idiopathic radial artery aneurysm in the anatomical snuff box," *Acta Orthopaedica Belgica*, vol. 68, no. 3, pp. 292–294, 2002.

22

# Mask-Related Glasses Fogging: A Predisposing Mechanism of Falls during the COVID-19 Pandemic

**John F. Dankert and Mandeep S. Virk**

*Department of Orthopedic Surgery, NYU Langone Health, New York, New York, USA*

Correspondence should be addressed to Mandeep S. Virk; mandeep.virk@nyulangone.org

Academic Editor: Werner Kolb

Fogging is a relatively infrequent, yet annoying, issue encountered by individuals who wear glasses. With the arrival of COVID-19, glasses fogging is more common due to the ubiquitous use of face masks. Individuals are stuck wrestling between leaving their mask off or trying to navigate their day-to-day lives with fogged glasses and risk falling. We report a case of an olecranon fracture sustained due to reduced visibility secondary to mask-related fogging during the COVID-19 pandemic. The recommendations included here will provide health care providers with the necessary information to educate patients regarding prevention of mask-related glass fogging.

## 1. Introduction

Orthopedic surgeons have encountered unique challenges in providing patient care during the COVID-19 pandemic. One of the immediate threats from the virus was its impact on patients undergoing both emergent and elective orthopedic surgery. Previous work demonstrated that an active symptomatic COVID-19 infection predicted poor outcomes for patients with a traumatic musculoskeletal injury [1]. Indeed, infection with the virus was found to increase mortality and complication rates for patients admitted with a hip fracture [2]. Communities have focused on implementing societal changes to limit the impact of COVID-19.

Hand hygiene, social distancing, and masks have all become a recommended part of daily routines to reduce the spread of COVID-19. However, the near ubiquitous use of masks has left many elderly and visually impaired patients who use prescription glasses struggling with glasses fogging. Mask-related fogging can result in a fall via mechanisms including tripping, slipping, and misjudging step depth. Over 3 million geriatric patients are brought to an emergency department in the United States every year for a fall-related injury [3]. One out of every 5 falls has been reported to lead to a musculoskeletal injury in this population. During the COVID-19 pandemic, we have cared for multiple patients who have attributed their fall to impaired sight after their glasses became fogged. Off the shelf masks, commonly used in the community setting, are notorious for glasses fogging. This issue, combined with gait instability and poor bone quality, as often observed in a geriatric population, can contribute to serious fall-type musculoskeletal injuries requiring surgical treatment.

We present this case report to draw attention to mask-related glasses fogging as a mechanism for falling during the COVID-19 pandemic. This report provides information for health care professionals to apply in everyday practice with the goal of educating patients regarding the risk and prevention of falls with mask-related glasses fogging.

## 2. Case Presentation

Our patient was a 70-year-old female who presented with left elbow pain after falling while walking outside. She reported that her glasses were fogged due to an ill-fitting mask causing her to misjudge her step on a raised section of the sidewalk. She landed on the point of her left elbow and complained of pain and swelling over the impact site. On physical examination, she was tender to palpation over her left olecranon with limited elbow range of motion secondary to pain. Orthogonal imaging of the left elbow demonstrated a

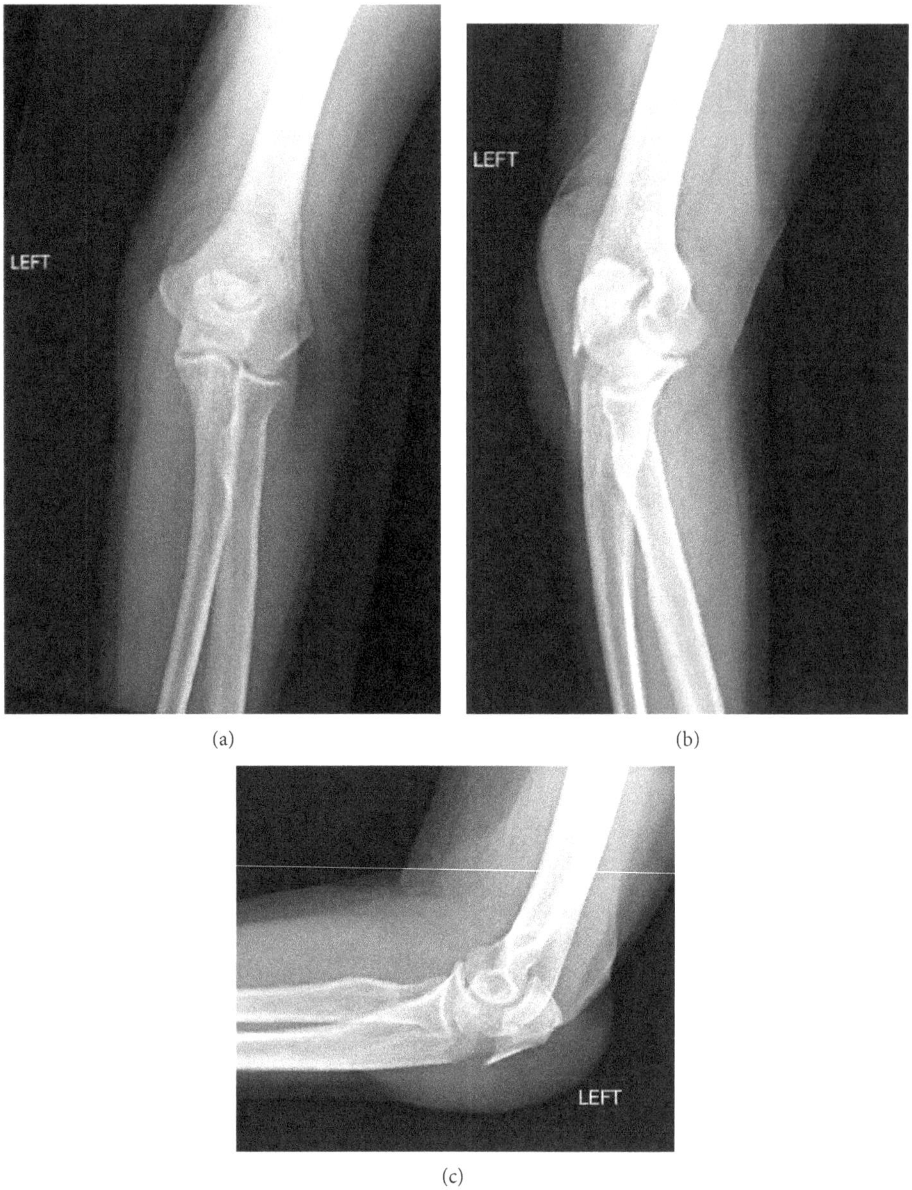


FIGURE 1: Preoperative AP (a), oblique (b), and lateral (c) radiographs demonstrating a displaced and comminuted left olecranon fracture.

displaced comminuted olecranon fracture (Figure 1). She was indicated for and subsequently underwent surgical repair of the olecranon fracture without any complications. At the 5-month follow-up visit, she reported only minimal pain with mild stiffness (Figure 2). She could actively flex-extend through a 10°-140° arc of motion with 80° of maximum pronation and 80° of maximum supination. Due to COVID-19 restrictions limiting her access to supervised physical therapy programs, a home exercise therapy program was prescribed to continue assisting her with reobtaining her preinjury level of function.

## 3. Discussion

Glasses fogging has been previously recognized as a problem for glasses wearers. It is considered an occupational hazard for people who wear safety glasses at work and a risk factor for eye injuries [4]. Fogging can occur from either moisture in the environment or from an individual's breath. This effect is especially apparent in cold weather because the moisture evaporates slowly from cold surfaces. When the warmer water vapor encounters a colder glass lens, it converts into a layer of droplets and results in fogging. Glasses fogging may be accentuated when wearing a mask as moisture-laden breath is directed towards the glass lenses.

We performed an extensive literature search on available solutions for preventing or minimizing glasses fogging related to mask wear. A poorly fitting mask was the primary reason for mask-related fogging in any environment [5]. Several techniques have been described to assist glasses wearers with fogging issues. These interventions are primarily based on improving the mask fit on the face or reducing the fogging phenomenon on the lenses via the application of chemical agents.

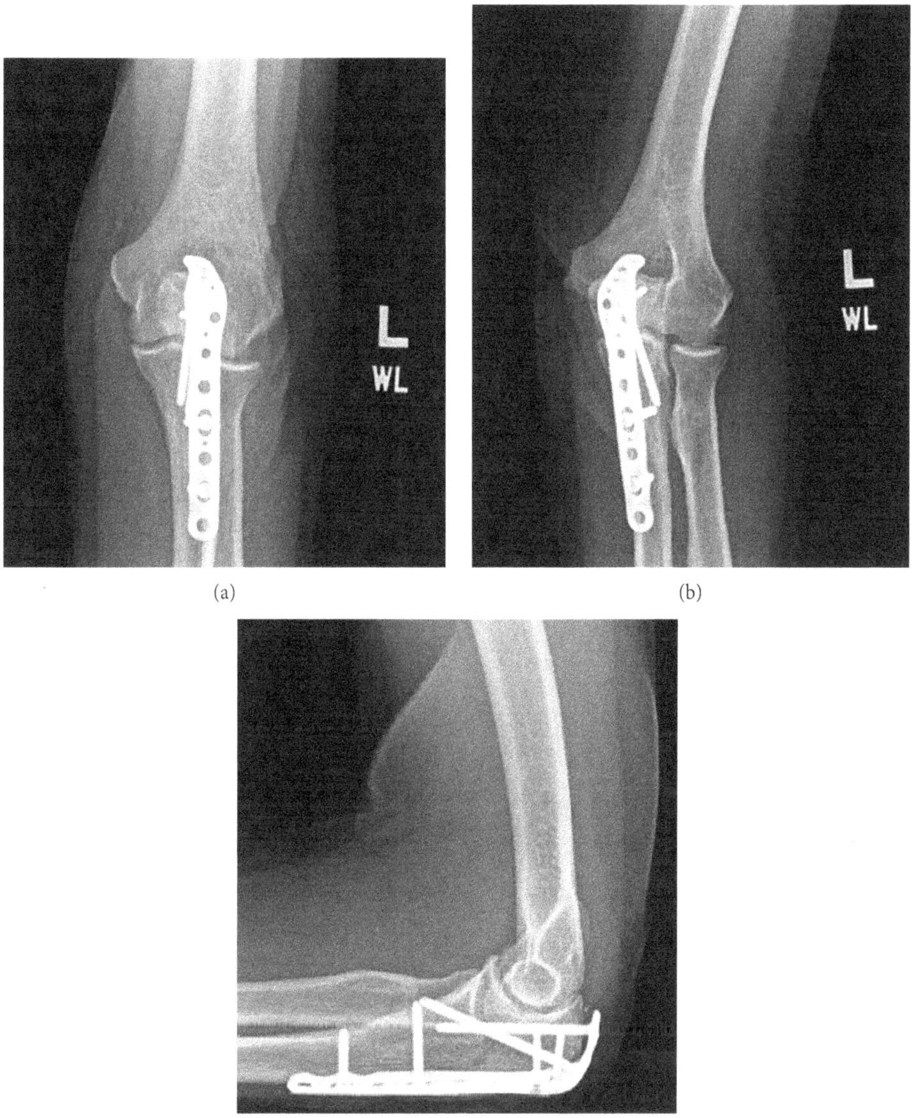


(a) (b) (c)

FIGURE 2: AP (a), oblique (b), and lateral (c) radiographs of the patient's left olecranon at the 3-month follow-up visit after operative fixation.

Size, shape, and accessory modifications contribute to a mask's overall fit. N95, loose-fitting surgical, and cloth masks are produced in multiple sizes to better match anatomic variations [6]. Surgical-type and cloth masks have been more popular during the COVID-19 pandemic, in part, due to the general public's lack of access to the in-demand N95 masks and the associated fit testing training required to correctly use N95 masks [7, 8]. All of these mask types often include a metal clip that may be molded over the nasal bridge. This metal clip improves the mask seal and prevents warm breath from leaking towards the glass lenses. However, the pressure from the clip can cause skin reactions after long wear times [9]. Alternatively, self-adhesive silicone pads may be placed inside a surgical-type or cloth mask to increase the seal against the patient's nose and upper maxilla. Applying an adhesive tape along the top border of the mask and adjacent skin is another trick that has been used by surgeons for years to prevent glasses fogging during procedures [5, 10]. Importantly, the repeated use of adhesive tape can cause a rash on sensitive skin and leave an area of hyperpigmentation with chronic application [11]. Alternatively, commercial masks with a built-in one-way valve to allow for the egress of breath can be helpful, but this feature increases the price of the mask [12]. Regarding the mask material, selecting a more absorbent fabric (e.g., cotton) will trap breath moisture and reduce fogging [13]. Finally, the American Academy of Ophthalmology has recommended sliding glasses down over the mask to pinch the upper part of the mask with the glasses nose pads [14]. The best method will likely depend on trial-and-error and patient preference.

Both professional and "at-home" chemical coatings are available to minimize glasses fogging. Dish soap or soap solutions, if not thoroughly washed from the lenses, can form a thin layer of antifogging coating [5]. However, too much soap residue can itself impede vision, and its antifog effect is not long-lasting. Antifog solutions are also commercially available, but these sprays and gels again require repeat application and may be expensive [15]. Finally, permanent antifog coatings are an option for select types of lenses [5]. Consultation with an optometrist or ophthalmologist will help patients in identifying an appropriate solution for their needs.

Multiple studies have investigated participants' heart rates, oxygen saturation, carbon dioxide levels, and symptoms while wearing masks. FFP2 masks covered with a surgical mask were found to be associated with increases in heart rate and nonclinically relevant drops in arterial oxygen saturation when evaluated over different wear time periods [16]. When compared to not wearing a mask, FFP2 masks were similarly found to result in significant, but not clinically relevant, increases in carbon dioxide partial pressure and decreases in oxygen saturation at different work levels [17]. When N95 and surgical masks were compared, N95 masks led to a larger increase in perioral surface temperature and higher reported sensations of humidity, heat, breathing difficulty, discomfort, and mask touching after one hour of wear [18]. Other reported symptoms included dizziness and headaches [16–18]. Assisting patients with mitigating the negative effects of mask wearing is necessary to ensure adequate protection from the COVID-19 virus.

## 4. Conclusion

Mask-related fogging has become a commonly reported menace for glasses wearers during the COVID-19 pandemic. Reduced visibility due to glasses fogging is an additional risk factor for falls especially in the elderly population where other fall predisposing risk factors like balance issues, gait disturbances, and walking aids are commonly present. The information provided in this report will allow orthopedic surgeons and other health care professionals, who may not wear glasses and not be aware of this potential issue, better assist their glasses-wearing patients with identifying solutions to reduce glasses fogging.

## Consent

No written consent has been obtained from the patient as there is no patient identifiable data included in the case report.

## References

[1] S. R. Konda, R. A. Ranson, S. J. Solasz et al., "Modification of a validated risk stratification tool to characterize geriatric hip fracture outcomes and optimize care in a post-COVID-19 world," *Journal of Orthopaedic Trauma*, vol. 34, no. 9, pp. e317–e324, 2020.

[2] K. A. Egol, S. R. Konda, M. L. Bird et al., "Increased mortality and major complications in hip fracture care during the COVID-19 pandemic: a New York City perspective," *Journal of Orthopaedic Trauma*, vol. 34, no. 8, pp. 395–402, 2020.

[3] 2020, 2021, http://cdc.gov/, https://www.cdc.gov/injury/features/older-adult-falls/index.html/.

[4] 2013, 2021, http://cdc.gov/, https://www.cdc.gov/niosh/topics/eye/toolbox-eye.html/.

[5] P. Agarwal and D. Sharma, "How to prevent fogging of spectacle glasses when wearing a face mask," *The Indian Journal of Surgery*, pp. 1-2, 2021.

[6] E. O'Kelly, A. Arora, S. Pirog, J. Ward, and P. J. Clarkson, "Comparing the fit of N95, KN95, surgical, and cloth face masks and assessing the accuracy of fit checking," *PLoS One*, vol. 16, no. 1, article e0245688, 2021.

[7] J. J. Bartoszko, M. A. M. Farooqi, W. Alhazzani, and M. Loeb, "Medical masks vs N95 respirators for preventing COVID-19 in healthcare workers: a systematic review and meta-analysis of randomized trials," *Influenza and Other Respiratory Viruses*, vol. 14, no. 4, pp. 365–373, 2020.

[8] E. McMahon, K. Wada, and A. Dufresne, "Implementing fit testing for N95 filtering facepiece respirators: practical information from a large cohort of hospital workers," *American Journal of Infection Control*, vol. 36, no. 4, pp. 298–300, 2008.

[9] S. R. Desai, C. Kovarik, B. Brod et al., "COVID-19 and personal protective equipment: treatment and prevention of skin conditions related to the occupational use of personal protective equipment," *Journal of the American Academy of Dermatology*, vol. 83, no. 2, pp. 675–677, 2020.

[10] K. G. Ramamoorthy, "Anti-fogging techniques as part of personal protective equipment (PPE)," *Indian Journal of Anaesthesia*, vol. 64, no. 12, pp. 1085-1086, 2020.

[11] D. Bonamonte, C. Foti, G. Gullo, and G. Angelini, "Hyperpigmentation, Hypopigmentation and Discolorations Due to Contactants," in *Clinical Contact Dermatitis*, G. Angelini, D. Bonamonte, and C. Foti, Eds., Springer, Cham, 2021.

[12] R. J. Roberge, "Are exhalation valves on N95 filtering facepiece respirators beneficial at low-moderate work rates: an overview," *Journal of Occupational and Environmental Hygiene*, vol. 9, no. 11, pp. 617–623, 2012.

[13] S. Beesoon, N. Behary, and A. Perwuelz, "Universal masking during COVID-19 pandemic: Can textile engineering help public health? Narrative review of the evidence," *Preventive Medicine*, vol. 139, article 106236, 2020.

[14] V. Hazanchuk, *How to wear a face mask without fogging your glasses*, American Academy of Ophthalmology, 2021, 2021, https://www.aao.org/eye-health/tips-prevention/face-mask-foggy-glasses-coronavirus-covid.

[15] M. Madan, N. Malhotra, N. Gupta, S. Ish, and P. Ish, "Fogging of goggles in PPE during COVID-19 pandemic. A practical problem with multiple possible solutions," *Advances in Respiratory Medicine*, vol. 88, no. 6, pp. 636-637, 2020.

[16] A. Scarano, F. Inchingolo, B. Rapone, F. Festa, S. Rexhep Tari, and F. Lorusso, "Protective face masks: effect on the oxygenation and heart rate status of oral surgeons during surgery," *International Journal of Environmental Research and Public Health*, vol. 18, no. 5, p. 2363, 2021.

[17] C. Georgi, A. Haase-Fielitz, D. Meretz, L. Gäsert, and C. Butter, "The impact of commonly-worn face masks on physiological parameters and on discomfort during standard work-related physical effort," *Deutsches Ärzteblatt International*, vol. 117, no. 40, pp. 674-675, 2020.

[18] A. Scarano, F. Inchingolo, and F. Lorusso, "Facial skin temperature and discomfort when wearing protective face masks: thermal infrared imaging evaluation and hands moving the mask," *International Journal of Environmental Research and Public Health*, vol. 17, no. 13, p. 4624, 2020.

# 23

# Pediatric Infectious Prepatellar Bursitis with *Kingella kingae*

**Charles C. Pitts, Walter R. Smith, and Michael J. Conklin**

*Department of Orthopaedic Surgery, University of Alabama at Birmingham, USA*

Correspondence should be addressed to Walter R. Smith; smithwalt1@gmail.com

Academic Editor: Bayram Unver

We present the first reported case of septic prepatellar bursitis with *Kingella kingae* in a 2-year-old female. Although it is a well-established cause of osteoarticular infections in the pediatric population, *K. kingae* has never been reported as the etiology for septic bursitis. A high index of suspicion is required for the diagnosis given that this organism is difficult to culture and isolate using standard laboratory methods. Our diagnosis was established through bursal fluid analysis, though oropharyngeal polymerase chain reaction (PCR) may be also be considered. Our case also builds upon prior literature suggesting that the pathophysiology of septic bursitis in children differs from that of the adult and may be more comparable to that of pediatric osteomyelitis. As an organism of increasing prevalence, *K. kingae* should remain high on the differential for osteoarticular or periarticular infections when cultures fail to isolate a distinct pathogen. Early diagnosis and a formal irrigation and debridement, if warranted, are crucial in preventing devastating complications of untreated septic bursitis.

## 1. Introduction

*Kingella kingae* is a Gram-negative bacterium originally described in the 1960s. While clinical interest was minimal for the first thirty years following its discovery, *K. kingae* is now recognized as an important pathogen in the pediatric population. It is the leading cause of osteoarticular infections in children aged six to thirty-six months, including septic arthritis and osteomyelitis, with the first series of cases being described by Ceroni et al. and Kiang et al [1, 2].

Oropharyngeal carriage of *K. kingae* has previously been shown to have a strong association with osteoarticular infections in children [3]. The cytotoxin RTX (repeat-in-toxin) facilitates spread of the pathogen to the bloodstream and other surrounding tissues [1]. *K. kingae* osteoarticular infections usually have a mild presentation. Diagnosis is often challenging, as fever, leukocytosis, positive Gram stain, and elevations in erythrocyte sedimentation rate (ESR) and C-reactive protein (CRP) can be absent. Due to aforementioned reasons, oropharyngeal polymerase chain reaction (PCR) has gained popularity as a useful diagnostic modality when *Kingella* infection is suspected [4, 5]. Although *K. kingae* is susceptible to a variety of antibiotics including beta lactams, a high clinical suspicion and early diagnosis are keys in management of the disease [1, 2, 6].

Prepatellar bursitis, or infectious bursitis of any kind, is a relatively rare condition in the pediatric population. One series by Paisley showed that the infection was usually preceded by an injury, traumatic event, or local infection, with *S. aureus* and *S. pyogenes* being the most common causative organisms [7]. All patients recovered uneventfully when treated with aspiration, incision and drainage, antibiotics, or a combination of these modalities.

We present a case of a *K. kingae* infection resulting in prepatellar septic bursitis in a 2-year-old female. Although *K. kingae* is a well-established cause of osteoarticular infections in this age group, it has not been reported in the literature as the etiology for a case of septic bursitis.

## 2. Case Report

A 2-year, 5-month-old girl presented to the pediatric orthopaedic clinic for evaluation of left knee pain of about 3 weeks duration. The patient had no medical problems except for an upper respiratory infection approximately 1 month prior to the onset of her symptoms. Reportedly, the patient struck her knee against a bed frame, and this event developed into anterior knee swelling and difficulty bearing weight over the next four days. When her parents noted difficulty with ambulation, she was brought to the emergency department (ED) for evaluation.

While in the ED, the patient had an erythematous and swollen anterior knee that was warm to the touch. She had pain-free range of motion but walked with a slight limp. She was afebrile with stable vital signs, and parents denied any fever or constitutional symptoms since her injury. Plain radiographs of the left knee were normal with the exception of prepatellar soft tissue edema (Figure 1). Laboratory studies revealed CRP of 0.2 mg/dL (0.0-0.5 mg/dL), ESR 29 mm/hr (0-20 mm/hr), and white blood cell (WBC) count of 6.46 cells $\times 10^3/\mu$L ($4.8 - 13.2 \times 10^3/\mu$L). Her symptoms at that time were considered by the ED physician to be posttraumatic with low concern for infectious etiology, and she was discharged without medication.

Her symptoms failed to resolve, and she was evaluated in the orthopaedic clinic two weeks after her ED presentation. She had no constitutional symptoms. She had full passive range of motion of the knee with little pain, but she walked with her left knee held in slight flexion, resulting in a limp. She continued to show swelling and erythema with fluctuance of the prepatellar area that was painful to touch. Her temperature was 98.3 degrees Fahrenheit. Laboratory studies revealed a CRP level of 0.2 mg/dL, ESR 39 mm/hr, and WBC 8.5 cells $\times 10^3/\mu$L. An ultrasound of the knee revealed a collection of fluid within the prepatellar bursa (Figure 2). Due to the elevated ESR and prolonged course of symptoms, there was concern for an infectious prepatellar bursitis. Aspiration with possible irrigation and debridement of the prepatellar bursa was recommended.

The patient was brought to the operating room and general anesthesia was induced. Aspiration of the prepatellar bursa yielded thick, blood-tinged, purulent fluid. A small, transverse incision over a Langer's line was made over the prepatellar bursa, and irrigation and debridement were carried out. Bursal fluid was inoculated into a blood culture bottle. Intravenous clindamycin was given, and a stat cell count on the bursal fluid disclosed 74,740 WBC/$\mu$L with 83% polymorphonuclear cells (PMNs). Gram stain was negative. The patient was discharged on oral clindamycin.

On postoperative day 3, *Kingella kingae* was isolated from the culture and the patient was called in for follow-up. She was no longer walking with a limp, had full range of motion of the left knee, and had no drainage from her incision. Infectious Disease was consulted and they recommended a 21-day course of oral cephalexin. She was seen again on postoperative day 19 and continued to be asymptomatic and compliant with antibiotic treatment. Her gait was normal, and there was no erythema or fluctuance in the prepatellar area. Repeat ESR, CRP, and WBC count had decreased to within the normal ranges. Radiographs showed no periosteal reaction to suggest osteomyelitis. The patient did not appear for her 6 week follow-up appointment, as her parents had called to inform us that she was having no further symptoms.

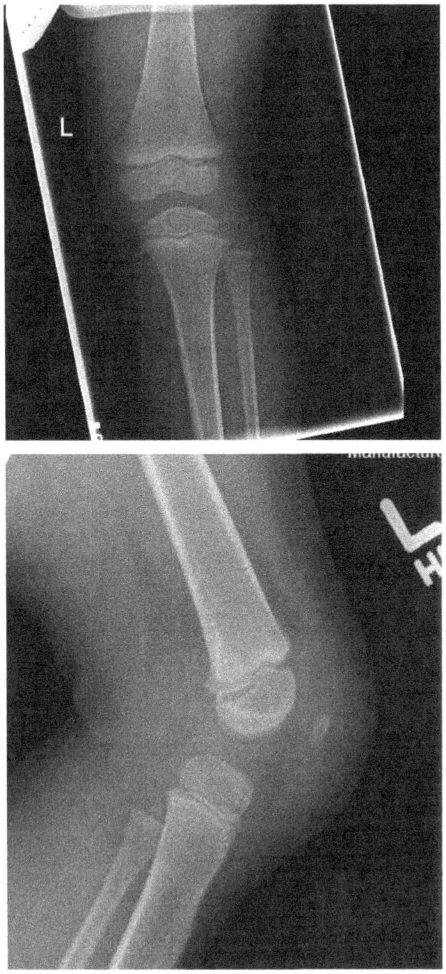


Figure 1: AP and lateral radiograph of the affected knee shows no obvious bony injury or effusion but notable prepatellar soft tissue swelling.

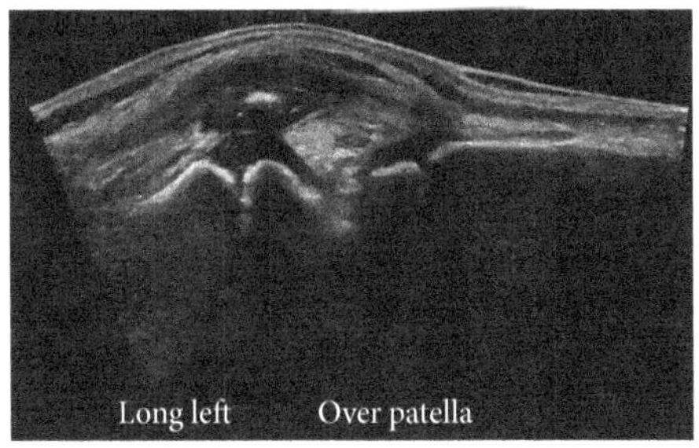


Figure 2: Ultrasound of the affected knee confirms a collection of fluid within the prepatellar bursa.

## 3. Discussion

While not uncommon in the adult population, septic bursitis is rarely reported in children [7]. There have been few reported cases in the literature, none of which have isolated *K. kingae* as the causative organism. Harwell and Fisher reported on ten cases of septic bursitis in children less than sixteen years old, all of which had predisposing trauma similar to our case [8]. However, *Staphylococcus aureus* and

*Streptococcus pyogenes* were the only two organisms isolated from the infected bursae [8]. Another series of ten patients over a twenty-five-year span showed similar results with all cultures yielding *S. aureus* or *S. pyogenes*. The prepatellar bursa was identified as the most common site of occurrence in both series [7, 8].

*Kingella kingae* is particularly evasive of laboratory culture and difficult to isolate using standard methods. An early series described by Yagupsky and Dagan showed growth of *Kingella kingae* on a standard culture medium in only 2 of 25 cases [9]. For this reason, *Kingella* should remain on the differential diagnosis for osteoarticular or periarticular infections even when cultures fail to isolate a distinct pathogen. Therefore, we feel that the current case report is important for delineating *Kingella* as a possible pathogen in pediatric septic bursitis.

The generally accepted pathophysiologic sequence for the development of septic bursitis in adults is repetitive trauma to the area which allows bacterial inoculation through the skin. However, in our case and in previously published series, infection in children is preceded by an acute traumatic event. As previously suggested, this bears resemblance to the pathophysiology of osteomyelitis in the pediatric population. Bacteria leading to osteomyelitis typically spread hematogenously after a minor trauma, suggesting that septic bursitis may develop in a similar fashion. This is also consistent with the fact that *K. kingae* is known to disseminate via the bloodstream as opposed to direct invasion through a compromise in the epidermal barrier [10].

The differential diagnosis for a swollen knee in a child is quite broad. Possible etiologies include trauma, intra- or extra-articular infection, and inflammatory arthropathies. A notable physical exam finding that may help distinguish septic arthritis from septic bursitis is severe pain with range of motion, which is generally minimal or absent in septic bursitis. With infection of the prepatellar bursa, there may be pain at extremes of flexion, but generally there is a reasonable arc of motion without pain. Ultrasonography is useful to assess for a fluid collection involving either the joint or the bursa. Routine radiographs should be performed initially and at follow-up to ensure infection of the bone was not missed. Complete blood count with differential and inflammatory markers should be obtained if an infectious etiology is suspected. However, these markers are often insensitive for septic bursitis as demonstrated in our case. Bursal fluid analysis should be sent for laboratory testing. It is important to note that oropharyngeal PCR should be considered if cultures fail to yield an organism, as this has been shown in multiple studies to be predictive of *Kingella kingae* infection [4, 5]. Additionally, it may significantly shorten the time-to-detection. We chose to forego PCR in this scenario due to the fact that bursal fluid yielded an organism within 72 hours.

In summary, we present the first reported case of septic bursitis with *K. kingae*. Understanding that *K. kingae* may be a cause of septic bursitis is important because it is often difficult to culture. Our case builds upon prior literature suggesting that the pathophysiology of septic bursitis in children differs from that of the adult and may be similar to that of pediatric osteomyelitis. If left untreated, septic prepatellar bursitis may progress to patellar osteomyelitis or septic arthritis of the knee [7]. Early diagnosis and a high index of suspicion is crucial in preventing these complications which may lead to significant bony and cartilaginous destruction.

## References

[1] D. Ceroni, A. Cherkaoui, S. Ferey, A. Kaelin, and J. Schrenzel, "Kingella kingae osteoarticular infections in young children: clinical features and contribution of a new specific real-time PCR assay to the diagnosis," *Journal of Pediatric Orthopaedics*, vol. 30, no. 3, pp. 301–304, 2010.

[2] K. M. Kiang, F. Ogunmodede, B. A. Juni et al., "Outbreak of osteomyelitis/septic arthritis caused by Kingella kingae among child care center attendees," *Pediatrics*, vol. 116, no. 2, pp. e206–e213, 2005.

[3] J. Gravel, D. Ceroni, L. Lacroix et al., "Association between oropharyngeal carriage ofKingella kingaeand osteoarticular infection in young children: a case–control study," *CMAJ*, vol. 189, no. 35, pp. E1107–E1111, 2017.

[4] P. Yagupsky, "Diagnosing Kingella kingae infections in infants and young children," *Expert Review of Anti-Infective Therapy*, vol. 15, no. 10, pp. 925–934, 2017.

[5] D. Ceroni, V. Dubois-Ferriere, A. Cherkaoui et al., "Detection of Kingella kingae osteoarticular infections in children by oropharyngeal swab PCR," *Pediatrics*, vol. 131, no. 1, pp. e230–e235, 2013.

[6] G. Dubnov-Raz, M. Ephros, B. Z. Garty et al., "Invasive pediatric Kingella kingae Infections," *The Pediatric Infectious Disease Journal*, vol. 29, no. 7, pp. 639–643, 2010.

[7] J. W. Paisley, "Septic bursitis in childhood," *Journal of Pediatric Orthopedics*, vol. 2, no. 1, pp. 57–61, 1982.

[8] J. Harwell and D. Fisher, "Pediatric septic bursitis: case report of retrocalcaneal infection and review of the literature," *Clinical Infectious Diseases*, vol. 32, no. 6, pp. e102–e104, 2001.

[9] P. Yagupsky and R. Dagan, "Kingella kingae: an emerging cause of invasive infections in young children," *Clinical Infectious Diseases*, vol. 24, no. 5, pp. 860–866, 1997.

[10] P. Yagupsky, "Kingella kingae: carriage, transmission, and disease," *Clinical Microbiology Reviews*, vol. 28, no. 1, pp. 54–79, 2015.

# 24

# A Technical Nuance to Avoid Lumbar Five Radiculopathy with Anterior Lumbar Fusion and Posterior Instrumentation

**Matthew T. Neal, Maziyar A. Kalani, and Mark K. Lyons**

*Department of Neurologic Surgery, Mayo Clinic College of Medicine and Science, 5777 East Mayo Boulevard, Phoenix, AZ 85054, USA*

Correspondence should be addressed to Mark K. Lyons; lyons.mark2@mayo.edu

Academic Editor: Taketoshi Yasuda

The anterior lumbar interbody fusion (ALIF) is a well-established procedure used to treat a multitude of spinal pathologies. When performed at the L5-S1 level, the ALIF is often supplemented with posterior pedicle screw and rod fixation. Because the interbody device can restore disk and foraminal height, one benefit of the ALIF procedure is indirect neural decompression in the spinal canal and neural foramina. If the contour of the posterior rod is not matched to the exact position of the tulip heads on the pedicle screws, spondylolisthesis can be introduced, leading to foraminal stenosis and nerve compression. This concern is particularly germane when the posterior instrumentation is placed percutaneously without any direct foraminal decompression. In this report, we describe a patient who had an L4-S1 ALIF, resulting in new L5-S1 retrolisthesis and worsening L5 radiculopathy. Technical nuances and avoidance strategies are discussed.

## 1. Introduction

The anterior lumbar interbody fusion (ALIF) is a popular procedure and is being performed by spinal surgeons at an increasing rate [1]. The procedure can be used to treat diverse pathologies and has many benefits. Demonstrated radiographic advantages include effective restoration of disk height, reduction of spondylolisthesis, and improved spinopelvic parameters [2, 3]. The approach allows for a complete discectomy and placement of a large interbody cage, resulting in solid anterior column support and fusion rates in excess of 90% [4]. The ALIF has also been associated with improved patient-reported outcome measures [2, 5].

Posterior instrumentation is commonly added to augment the ALIF. Posterior instrumentation is particularly helpful in cases with high sacral slope or isthmic spondylolisthesis to avoid instrumentation failure or pseudoarthrosis [6]. To minimize devascularization of paraspinal musculature, delayed muscle atrophy, disruption of muscular insertion to the spinous processes, and other approach-related injury, ALIF is often combined with percutaneous rod and screw fixation inserted through paramedian incisions [7, 8].

The ALIF procedure has been associated with diverse complications such as vascular injuries, injuries to other structures in the peritoneal compartment, fractures, pseudoarthrosis, and neural injury [9–13]. At the L5-S1 level, the ALIF has been associated with L5 radiculopathies [14, 15]. Most commonly, L5 radiculopathy has been contributed to a stretch neuropraxia.

In this report, we discuss another source of postoperative L5 radiculopathy following L5-S1 ALIF with posterior instrumentation. We describe a scenario where preexisting L5-S1 foraminal stenosis was exacerbated when the rods were inserted and retrolisthesis was introduced. Strategies to avoid this complication are discussed.

## 2. Case Presentation

The 61-year-old male patient presented with chronic low back pain and progressive bilateral thigh pain following both lumbar 4 and 5 dermatomal distributions. He also described subjective bilateral lower extremity weakness and numbness in the left foot. He experienced a progressive functional decline, despite extensive conservative treatment modalities.

X-ray and magnetic resonance imaging (MRI) demonstrated grade 1 spondylolisthesis at L4-5 and bilateral foraminal stenosis at both L4-5 and L5-S1 (Figures 1 and 2). The patient elected to pursue anterior lumbar fusions at L4-5 and L5-S1, followed by posterior percutaneous L4-S1 pedicle screw and rod fixation.

After a standard retroperitoneal exposure of the L4-5 and L5-S1 disk spaces, we performed meticuluous discectomies. We used disk space trials to determine the optimal size for the interbody cages. The interbody cages (Sovereign™ Spinal System, Medtronic Sofamor Danek USA, Inc., Memphis, TN) containing demineralized bone matrix were inserted at both levels and secured with integrated screws. X-rays (Figure 3) demonstrated good restoration of disk height at both levels. Anterolisthesis was reduced at the L4-5 level, and neutral sagittal alignment was maintained at L5-S1.

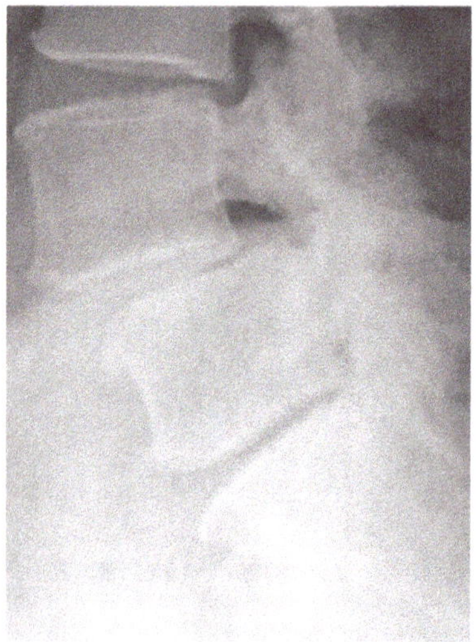

Figure 1: Preoperative lateral lumbar X-ray.

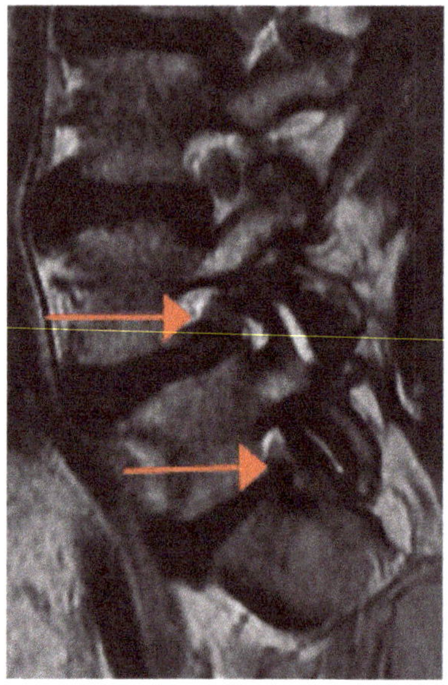

Figure 2: Preoperative T2 sagittal MRI demonstrating spondylolisthesis at L4-5 and foraminal stenosis at both L4-5 and L5-S1.

The patient was positioned prone for placement of posterior instrumentation. Using the StealthStation® S8® Navigation System, pedicle screws (CD Horizon™ Solera™ Voyager™ Awl-Tap Screws, Medtronic Sofamor Danek USA, Inc., Memphis, TN) were inserted bilaterally through paramedian incisions. Screw insertion was uncomplicated and supplemented by free-run electromyography (EMG) monitoring. Satisfactory positioning of the pedicle screws was confirmed intraoperatively using the O-arm™ imaging system (Medtronic, Minneapolis, MN).

Rods spanning from L4-S1 and set screws were then inserted utilizing the threaded, extended tabs attached to the tulip heads of the pedicle screws. The set screws were tightened with the appropriate torque, and the extended tabs were removed. Postoperative X-rays (Figure 4) were obtained.

Immediately following surgery, the patient experienced increased right-sided gluteal pain which was treated with a short course of oral steroids and gabinoids. However, at his second postoperative visit, 4 weeks after surgery, he had developed 4/5 weakness with right ankle dorsiflexion. A postoperative CT confirmed satisfactory positioning of the instrumentation. The postoperative MRI (Figure 5) and CT scan (Figure 6) demonstrated severe compression of the exiting L5 nerve root, which was wedged between the disk space anteriorly and the S1 superior articulating process posteriorly.

The patient was returned to the operating room for L5 laminectomy and complete right L5-S1 facetectomy. Six months following surgery, the patient was noted to have trace weakness with his right ankle dorsiflexion. Otherwise, he was neurologically intact. He denied significant back or leg symptoms. He was not requiring any pain medication, and he had resumed all normal activities.

## 3. Discussion

Complications can be associated with either the ALIF or the posterior instrumentation portions of the procedure. Reported complications are diverse and range from vascular injuries, bowel and ureter injuries, postoperative bleeding requiring reoperation, postoperative paralytic ileus, sacral insufficiency fracture, pseudoarthrosis, and neurological injury [9–13]. A review article on iatrogenic neurologic deficits after lumbar spine surgery reported a 4.1% rate of new-onset neurologic injury after anterior or lateral lumbar fusion surgery [10]. Postoperative L5 radiculopathies after L5-S1 ALIF procedures have been described [14, 15]. The postoperative deficit has most commonly been attributed to a stretch neuropraxia from over distraction of the disk L5-S1 space.

One potential complication of the L5-S1 ALIF with posterior instrumentation is exacerbation of foraminal stenosis when the tulip heads of pedicle screws are reduced to the rod. To the authors' knowledge, this complication has not been reported and discussed. Numerous studies have described the powerful phenomenon of indirect decompression of the neural elements using lateral or anterior interbody cages [16–18]. The reports describe

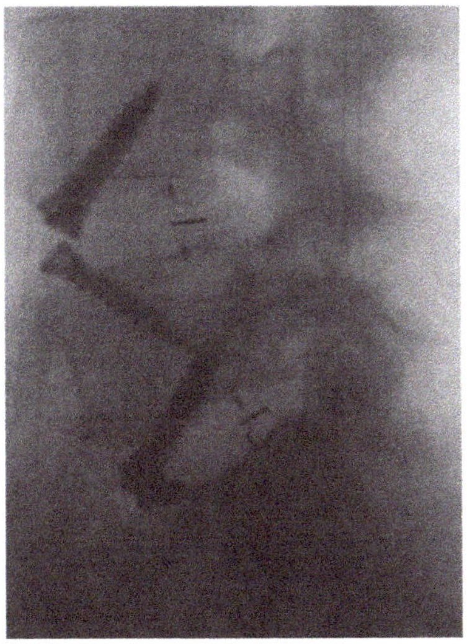

Figure 3: Intraoperative sagittal X-ray demonstrating anterior interbody grafts.

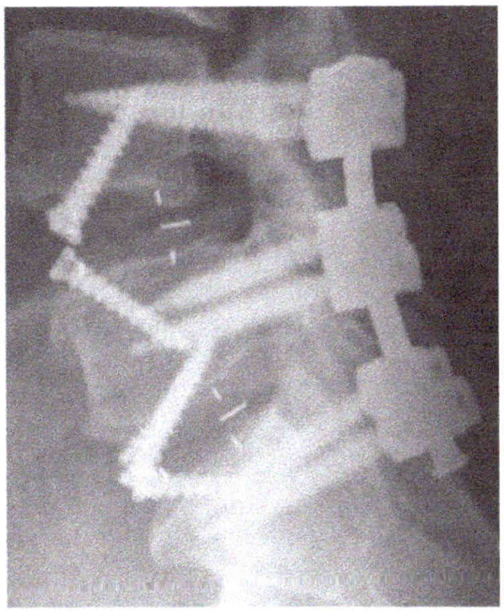

Figure 4: Postoperative lateral X-ray.

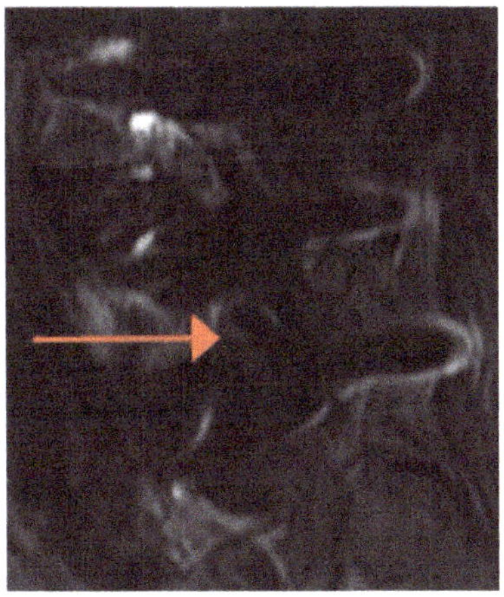

Figure 5: Postoperative sagittal T2 MRI demonstrating persistent L5 nerve compression in the L5-S1 foramen (arrow).

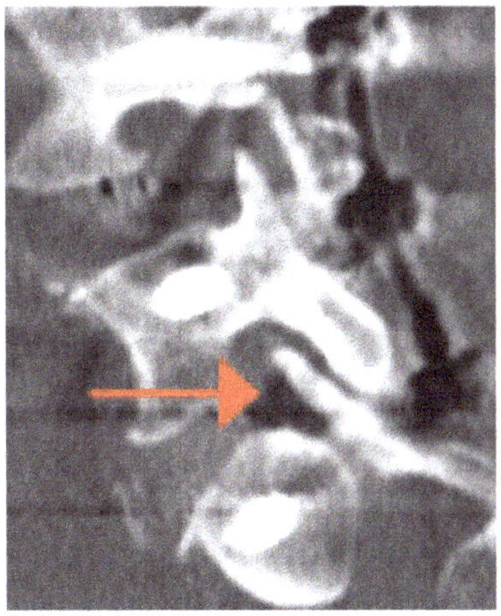

Figure 6: Postoperative sagittal CT scan demonstrating persistent L5 nerve root compression in the L5-S1 foramen (arrow).

how interbody cages can increase disk height, foraminal height, and cross-sectional area of the spinal canal and foramina. However, it is important to recognize that placement of spinal hardware, in particular rod and screw constructs, can introduce antero- or retrolisthesis, resulting in neural compression. In this case, the L5 pedicle screw vertebral body was inadvertently reduced to the rod, producing retrolisthesis of L5 on S1. The L5 root was compressed between the L5-S1 annulus and the superior articulating facet of S1, most significantly in the medial aspect of the lumbosacral tunnel.

Avoidance of this complication starts with careful analysis of the preoperative CT and MRI studies. In this case, the preoperative MRI (Figure 2) demonstrated high-grade foraminal stenosis in the anterior-posterior plane. Therefore, avoidance of any new retrolisthesis at this level would be critical to avoid worsening nerve compression. Direct nerve decompression should also have been considered.

As with any ALIF case, cautious technique is required during the cage trialing and cage insertion processes. Oversizing the graft and aggressive malleting with the cage trial should be avoided. These maneuvers have been associated with L5 radiculopathy after L5-S1 ALIF [14, 15]. The surgeon should also account for the geometric shape of the interbody cage. A hyperlordotic graft may actually reduce the anterior-posterior diameter and cross-sectional area of the foramen. In these cases, a posterior decompression may be needed.

When the posterior screws are placed, the position of the tulip heads on the pedicle screws should be noted. We now pay close attention to the relative positions of the tulip heads when we obtain our X-rays or O-arm™ (Medtronic, Minneapolis, MN) imaging studies. The contour of the rod and the position of the tulip heads should be matched such that the tulip heads are not reduced to the rod, unless this is the desired effect. Reduction of anterolisthesis or introduction of retrolisthesis may result L5 nerve compression in the lumbosacral tunnel. Another strategy to avoid undesired reduction of screws is to use a commercially available product such as Bendini® (Nuvasive, San Diego, CA). This product uses computer-assisted technology to bend rods precisely to match the tulip head locations.

Finally, intraoperative imaging studies obtained after rod placement should be studied carefully for new spinal malalignment which could result in neural compression.

## 4. Conclusion

During lumbar fusion surgery, securing rods to pedicle screws can introduce spondylolisthesis. When no direct nerve decompression is performed, surgeons must carefully match the rod contour to the screw positions to avoid exacerbation of foraminal stenosis and neural compromise.

## References

[1] K. Varshneya, Z. A. Medress, M. Jensen et al., "Trends in anterior lumbar interbody fusion in the United States," *Clinical Spine Surgery*, vol. 33, pp. 1–E30, 2020.

[2] K. Farah, T. Graillon, P. Rakotozanany, S. Pesenti, B. Blondel, and S. Fuentes, "Circumferential minimally invasive approach for low-grade isthmic spondylolisthesis: a clinical and radiological study of 43 patients," *Orthopaedics & Traumatology, Surgery & Research*, vol. 104, no. 5, pp. 575–579, 2018.

[3] M. Formica, E. Quarto, A. Zanirato et al., "ALIF in the correction of spinal sagittal misalignment. A systematic review of literature," *European Spine Journal*, vol. 30, no. 1, pp. 50–62, 2021.

[4] G. D. Schroeder, C. K. Kepler, P. W. Millhouse et al., "L5/S1 fusion rates in degenerative spine surgery: a systematic review comparing ALIF, TLIF, and axial interbody arthrodesis," *Clinical Spine Surgery: A Spine Publication*, vol. 29, no. 4, pp. 150–155, 2016.

[5] A. Y. Chan, B. V. Lien, E. H. Choi et al., "Back pain outcomes after minimally invasive anterior lumbar interbody fusion: a systematic review," *Neurosurgical Focus*, vol. 49, no. 3, article E3, 2020.

[6] L. L. Viglione, U. Chamoli, and A. D. Diwan, "Is stand-alone anterior lumbar interbody fusion a safe and efficacious treatment for isthmic spondylolisthesis of L5-S1?," *Global Spine Journal*, vol. 7, no. 6, pp. 587–595, 2017.

[7] J. A. Thomas, C. I. M. Thomason, B. A. Braly, and C. M. Menezes, "Rate of failure of indirect decompression in lateral single-position surgery: clinical results," *Neurosurgical Focus*, vol. 49, no. 3, article E5, 2020.

[8] J. Park, D. W. Ham, B. T. Kwon, S. M. Park, H. J. Kim, and J. S. Yeom, "Minimally invasive spine surgery: techniques, technologies, and indications," *Asian Spine Journal*, vol. 14, no. 5, pp. 694–701, 2020.

[9] J. Manunga, C. Alcala, J. Smith et al., "Technical approach, outcomes, and exposure-related complications in patients undergoing anterior lumbar interbody fusion," *Journal of Vascular Surgery*, vol. 73, no. 3, pp. 992–998, 2021.

[10] G. M. Ghobrial, K. A. Williams Jr., P. Arnold, M. Fehlings, and J. S. Harrop, "Iatrogenic neurologic deficit after lumbar spine surgery: a review," *Clinical Neurology and Neurosurgery*, vol. 139, pp. 76–80, 2015.

[11] A. Jaeger, D. Giber, C. Bastard et al., "Risk factors of instrumentation failure and pseudarthrosis after stand-alone L5-S1 anterior lumbar interbody fusion: a retrospective cohort study," *Journal of Neurosurgery Spine*, vol. 31, no. 3, pp. 338–346, 2019.

[12] J. M. Kolz, S. A. Mitchell, B. D. Elder, A. S. Sebastian, P. M. Huddleston, and B. A. Freedman, "Sacral insufficiency fracture following short-segment lumbosacral fusion: case series and review of the literature," *Global Spine Journal*, vol. 10, no. - article 219256822095033, 2020.

[13] J. F. Lastfogel, T. J. Altstadt, R. B. Rodgers, and E. M. Horn, "Sacral fractures following stand-alone L5-S1 anterior lumbar interbody fusion for isthmic spondylolisthesis," *Journal of Neurosurgery Spine*, vol. 13, no. 2, pp. 288–293, 2010.

[14] Q. Yue, T. Hale, A. Knecht, and J. Laidacker, "Intraoperative loss of tibialis anterior transcranial electrical motor evoked potentials predicted postoperative footdrop," *World Neurosurgery*, vol. 97, pp. 755.e1–755.e3, 2017.

[15] E. Dowlati, H. Alexander, and J. M. Voyadzis, "Vulnerability of the L5 nerve root during anterior lumbar interbody fusion at L5-S1: case series and review of the literature," *Neurosurgical Focus*, vol. 49, no. 3, article E7, 2020.

[16] G. X. Lin, G. Rui, S. Sharma, A. Mahatthanatrakul, and J. S. Kim, "The correlation of intraoperative distraction of intervertebral disc with the postoperative canal and foramen expansion following oblique lumbar interbody fusion," *European Spine Journal*, vol. 30, no. 1, pp. 151–163, 2021.

[17] H. Nakashima, T. Kanemura, K. Satake et al., "Patient-reported quality of life following posterior lumbar interbody fusion or indirect decompression using lateral lumbar interbody fusion," *Spine*, vol. 45, no. 18, pp. E1172–E1178, 2020.

[18] W. Limthongkul, T. Tanasansomboon, W. Yingsakmongkol, T. Tanaviriyachai, K. Radcliff, and W. Singhatanadgige, "Indirect decompression effect to central canal and ligamentum flavum after extreme lateral lumbar interbody fusion and oblique lumbar interbody fusion," *Spine*, vol. 45, no. 17, pp. E1077–E1084, 2020.

# 25

# Characteristic Poses in Ballet in the Case of a Retired Classical Ballerina after Bilateral THA: A Case Report and Review of Literature

**Futoshi Morio**[1] **Shigeo Fukunishi,**[2] **Tomokazu Fukui,**[1] **Makoto Kanto,**[1] **Kenta Amai,**[1] **Shinichi Yoshiya,**[2] **and Toshiya Tachibana**[1]

[1]*Department of Orthopaedic Surgery, Hyogo College of Medicine, Japan*
[2]*Nishinomiya Kaisei Hospital, Japan*

Correspondence should be addressed to Futoshi Morio; 2104morio.com@gmail.com

Academic Editor: Hiroshi Takahashi

*Background.* Ballet dance involves extreme range of motion (ROM) in the hip joint. This ROM can cause injuries including labral strain, tears, and subluxation episodes. *Case Presentation.* A 69-year-old female classical ballet dance instructor presented bilateral hip pain. The plain radiograph showed end-stage osteoarthritic change in the bilateral hip. She could neither dance nor perform daily activities. Bilateral hybrid total hip arthroplasty (THA) was performed. After surgery, she was able to demonstrate the split position on the floor as an active classical ballerina. The plain radiograph was taken in the split position, and the radiograph did not show any characteristics of impingement or subluxation of the femoral head. *Conclusion.* She was able to continue working as a classical ballet instructor after bilateral THA. Additionally, any characteristics of impingement or subluxation of the femoral head were not revealed in the postoperative radiograph in the split position.

## 1. Introduction

Ballerinas are often described as both artists and athletes. In recent years, the number of people who learn ballet has increased worldwide. Ballerinas' lower extremities leave them at risk of musculoskeletal injuries due to the unique demands in ballet. Previous studies have reported injury incidence rates of 67% to 95% among professional ballet dancers and 17% to 24% in modern dancers [1–6]. Ballet dance involves extreme hip abduction, flexion, and extension, as well as external rotation (i.e., turnout). This extreme range of motion can cause injuries, including labral strain, tears, and subluxation episodes [7, 8]. Hip injuries have been reported in multiple studies and comprises between 7% and 50% of injuries in dancers [9]. In a recent systematic review, hip/-groin injuries in professional dancers were recorded, at a rate of 27.7% [10]. There are few reports on performing total hip arthroplasty (THA) for ballerinas, as many orthopedic surgeons tend to choose arthroscopic or osteotomy surgery. Because of the risk of dislocation after THA, many orthopedic surgeons may hesitate to do THA. In this report, we present a rare case of a ballet dance instructor who sustained bilateral osteoarthritis of the hip and underwent bilateral THA. She was able to successfully go back to her previous dance activities after surgery. The purpose of this article is to describe the management of ballerina who sustained end-stage hip osteoarthritis. If surgeons understand the characteristic movement of a ballerina, we are considering that THA for ballerina is not a contraindication.

## 2. Case Presentation

This study was approved by the Institutional Review Board of Hyogo College of Medicine, and informed consent was obtained from the patient in the study.

A 69-year-old female ballet dance instructor presented discomfort and pain in her bilateral hip. She had danced ballet since childhood, had appeared on many stages, and played an active role as a professional ballerina. She noted the symptoms approximately 3 years before her initial visit to our institute without a history of hip trauma. Additionally, she had no other family history of acetabular dysplasia. Her initial physical examination revealed bilateral hip pain (L > R) with limitation in the range of motion (ROM). Hip pain was exacerbated by ballet movements, but it was possible to dance on the stage. The plain radiograph showed osteoarthritic change in both hips, and borderline acetabular dysplasia was suspected as a sharp angle (R°/L°) of 39°/41°, a center edge angle (R°/L°) of 25°/23°, and acetabular head index (R %/L %) of 82%/80% (Figure 1). Seven years after the initial visit, hip pain and limitation in ROM (R°/L°) progressed as follows: flection 100°/90°, external rotation 45°/30°, internal rotation 0°/0°, and abduction 20°/15°. The plain radiograph revealed end-stage osteoarthritis (OA) (Figure 2). At that time, she could neither dance nor perform daily activities. She had retired from being a ballerina and became an instructor. THA was performed on the left hip first, and subsequently, THA was performed on the right hip 9 months after the initial surgery. Both THA were performed with the modified Hardinge approach in the lateral position. A computed tomography- (CT-) based navigation system (CT-based hip navigation version 1.1, Stryker Navigation, Freiburg, Germany) was assisted for cup positioning. A cementless cup (Trident Acetabular Shell, Stryker Orthopedics, NJ, USA), a cemented stem (Exeter V40 Femoral Stem, Stryker Orthopedics, NJ, USA), a ceramic head (BIOLOX delta V40 Ceramic Head, Stryker Orthopedics, NJ, USA), and a nonelevated ultrahigh molecular weight polyethylene liner (Trident X3 insert, Stryker Orthopedics, NJ, USA) were implanted. For preoperative planning of cup placement in our surgical concept, radiographic cup inclination was fixed at 40 degrees while radiographic cup anteversion was aimed at approximately 20 degrees. However, sufficient cup coverage in the original acetabulum based on individual anatomy is given priority over the general target anteversion to ensure adequate cup coverage. Following the theory, preoperative target cup alignment is proceeded to prioritize avoiding anterior or posterior protrusion from acetabular edge over the target radiographic anteversion angle [11]. So, in the present case, preoperative planning was inclination 40° and anteversion (R°/L°) 22°/28°. During surgery, to avoid the implant-implant and implant-bone impingement and subsequent dislocation, we adjust stem anteversion using a cemented stem depending on the cases. Impingement was confirmed through the impingement test with flexion 120°, flexion 90° with internal rotation 60°, and extension 0° with maximum external rotation by the trial stem as our routine procedure. The implant-implant impingement and the bony impingement were not revealed. For the leg length adjustment, we gave priority to the joint stability in order to avoid impingement rather than leg lengthening. In the present case, we planned bilateral THA subsequently, and equalization of leg length could be achieved at the time of the second surgery (Figure 3). After implantation, the anterior capsule was repaired. The postoperative rehabilitation program was not special for the ballerina, and she underwent free mobilization and full-weight-bearing exercise one day after surgery. At the time of THA, we did not expect the patient to be able to give demonstrations of ballet dance during the coating period.

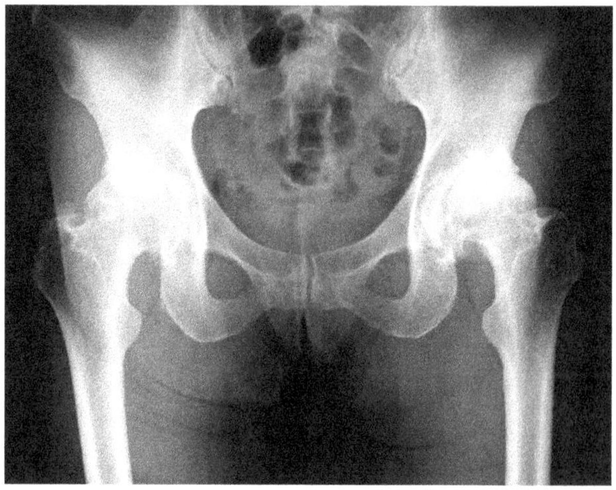

Figure 1: The plain radiograph of initial visit to our hospital at 7 years before surgery. Osteoarthritic changes in both hips without acetabular dysplasia were identified.

However, three years after surgery, she was able to continue working as an instructor. The ROM had improved as follows: flection 110°/115°, external rotation 45°/45°, internal rotation 30°/30°, and abduction 45°/45°. Amazingly, the patient was able to demonstrate the split position on the floor as an active classical ballerina (video (available here)). The plain radiograph was taken in the split position (Figure 4(a)) and left split position (Figure 4(b)), and the radiograph did not show any characteristics of impingement or tendency of dislocation.

## 3. Discussion

Ballet is a healthy activity which helps people to improve their quality of life. On the other hand, ballet is a "high-risk" activity with high incidence of musculoskeletal impairments. Duthon et al. and Jacobs et al. described that extreme range of motion of the hip can cause injuries, including labral strain, tears, and cartilage damage in the superior and posterosuperior areas of the acetabulum [7, 8]. The years of dancing can contribute to a ballerina developing pain secondary to OA in the hip due to repetitive extreme movements [12]. It has been reported that the practice of some dance movements could expose the dancer's hip to loss of joint congruence and recurrent impingements, which could lead to early OA. In the present case, it could be possible that borderline acetabular dysplasia participates in the progressed osteoarthritis; however, the repetitive extreme movements and the recurrent impingements in the characteristic motion of a ballerina could cause progressed osteoarthritis. Additionally, Buyls et al. [13] described that left hip pain was involved in all dancers with unilateral OA, which may reflect the tendency of ballerinas to use the left leg as the standing leg, and suggest that strenuous physical activity may lead to osteoarthritis. Just as in the present case, OA of the left hip was more progressed than that of the right hip. In surgical treatment of a hip disorder for the ballerina, when hip pain develops in a ballerina and conservative treatment fails, the

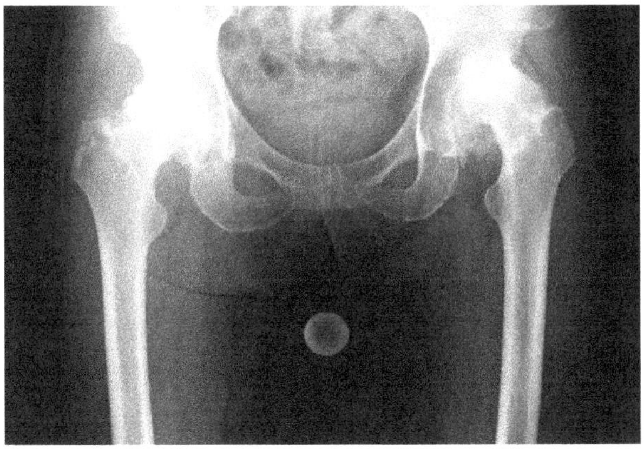

FIGURE 2: The plain radiograph before surgery. End-stage osteoarthritis was revealed in both hips.

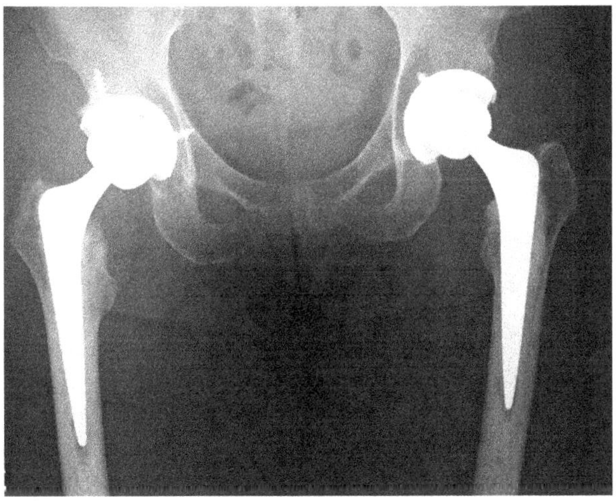

FIGURE 3: Postoperative plain radiograph. Hybrid THA was performed on both hips.

most common decision to be made by surgeons is whether the patient is a candidate for arthroscopic treatment of the hip or requires an open procedure, such as periacetabular osteotomy [14, 15]. Although there are many hip disorders in ballerinas epidemiologically, there are only two case reports on performing THA on ballerinas. This may be because many orthopedic surgeons are concerned about the risk of dislocation caused by implant-implant impingement and bony impingement due to the wide range of motion. Recently, Komiyama et al. [16] analyzed the dynamic hip kinematics of patients with recreational classical ballet who underwent THA and reported that no implant impingement was revealed during two typical postures. Regarding the characteristic poses and hyperflexibility of the hips in ballerinas, "turnout" is emphasized; this is the hip in external rotation with the knees in extension in ballet. The technique of classical ballet is based on "turnout" or outward rotation of the legs. Therefore, the movements of classical ballet must be executed in a "turnout" position. The ideal "turnout" demonstrates 180° of external rotation starting at the hips and results in the feet being easily placed in a 180° position on the floor. Therefore, ballerinas have increased range of motion of the hip in external rotation and decreased internal hip rotation compared to nondancers [17]. Normally, when measuring the abduction angle, the leg to be measured was maintained in a neutral rotation with the foot perpendicular to the floor. It was then abducted passively in the frontal plane to the extreme of range [18]. With this measurement method, the abduction angle showed to be lower than 45°. However, in ballerinas, hip abduction is combined with "turnout" and hip flexion is a movement used by ballet dancers during many movements at a standing position. Valenti et al. [19] stated that the more the dancer externally rotates the hip, the greater the hip abduction will be. In the present case, postoperative hip ROM was measured and showed flexion 110°/115°, external rotation 45°/45°, internal rotation 30°/30°, and abduction 45°/45° on the bed for medical examination. These values show a wider ROM as compared to normal patients, and we could not recognize the extreme wide range of motion of ballerinas; however, the patient was able to demonstrate her range of split position.-Surgeons and physical therapists should understand characteristic movements of ballerinas during surgery and physical therapy and keep in mind that ballerinas could achieve the nearly 90° abduction by combining maximum external rotation. As the matter of course, both soft tissue preservation and precise implant positioning are important to avoid impingement and dislocation for THA. On the other hand, we consider that a strict impingement test during surgery according to the characteristic posture of a ballerina which is hyperextension and hyperabduction with external rotation could be the important key management rather than combined anteversion as generally recommended. The postoperative radiograph with the patient in the split position showed the relationship of the acetabulum, femur, and implant. In this radiograph, the femur was externally rotated and the major trochanter takes the bottom direction. It could avoid the impingement between the greater trochanter and the posterior acetabular rim. Additionally, implant-implant impingement did not occur in this characteristic posture. Generally, orthopedic surgeons hesitate to do THA considering the risk of dislocation due to the wide range of motion in a ballerina. However, we could understand that characteristic movements of ballerinas with nearly 90° abduction by combining maximum external rotation is not a risk for impingement unexpectedly. On the other hand, Figure 4(b) shows the right hip in flexion with the knees in extension anteriorly and left hip hyperextended with the knee extended posteriorly. The radiograph did not show implant-implant impingement or subluxation of the femoral head. However, if the left hip will be hyperextended perfectly, it is possible that the liner-to-neck contact might develop. Following the results, implant-implant impingement and subluxation of the femoral head should be checked by conducting an impingement test with hyperextension of the hip, knee, and ankle in neutral positions during left hip THA for the ballerina.

There were some limitations in this study. First, the patient in the present study was a 69-year-old retired

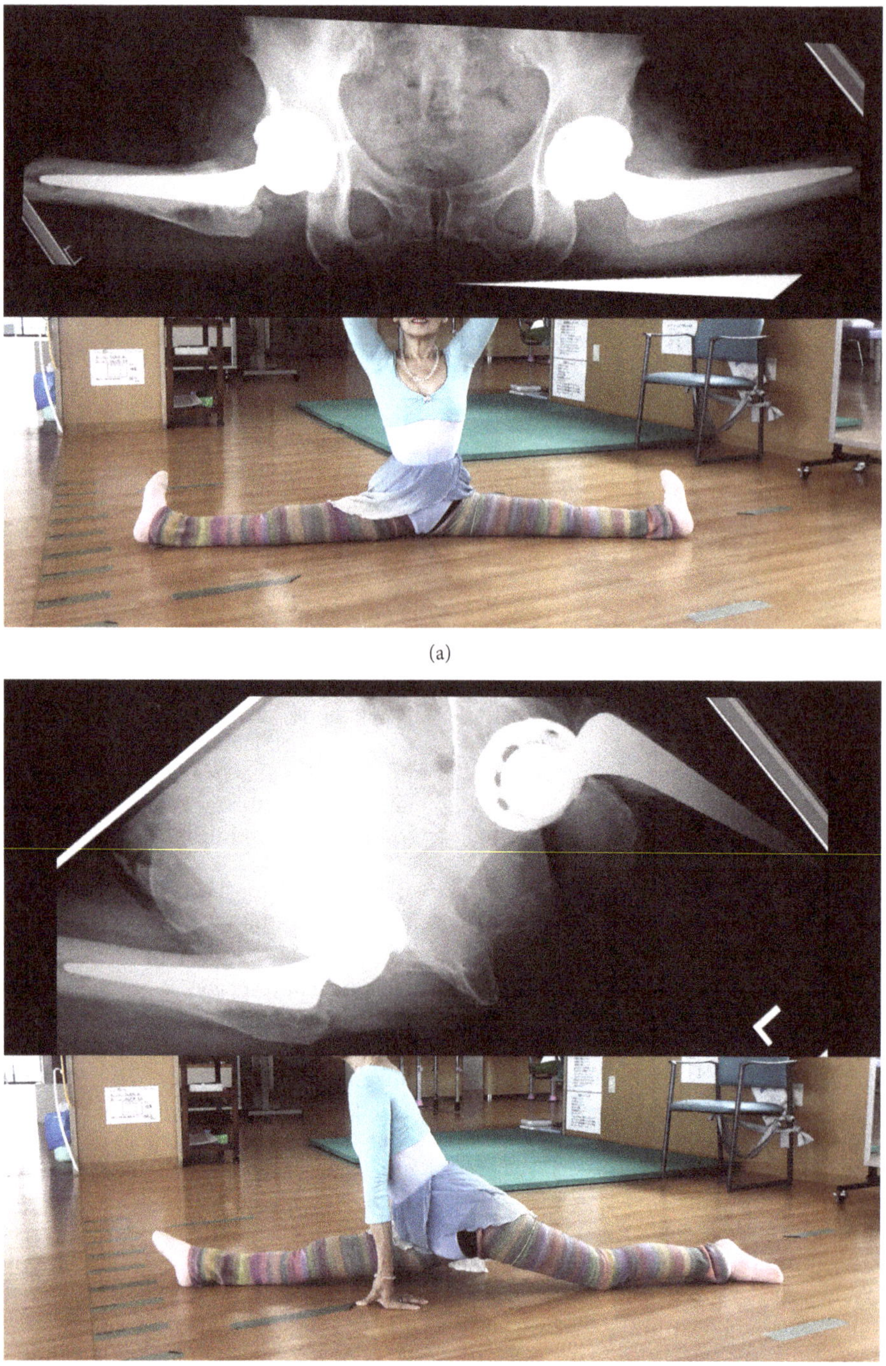

(a)

(b)

Figure 4: Postoperative radiograph with two types of characteristic postures in ballet. The patient was demonstrating the split position. These views were obtained with cassettes by getting as close as possible to the patient's back during the actual postures. The radiograph did not show any characteristics of bony impingement, implant-implant impingement, or subluxation of the femoral head: (a) split position; (b) left split position.

ballerina; therefore, the results may differ and the indication for THA may not be necessary for an active and younger ballerina. Age, sex, performance level, and pelvic alignment could be other factors for the indication of THA. Therefore, we could not recommend THA for all ballet dancers. Second, since only static analysis was performed in the present study, it is necessary to perform dynamic analysis in the future. Third, the postoperative follow-up period was quite short in this case report. The patient's wide range of motion and activity after THA might pose a risk of developing dislocation or polyethylene wear in the future. Therefore, future observation of progress is necessary.

## 4. Conclusion

The patient was able to continue working as a classical ballet instructor after bilateral THA. Additionally, any characteristics of impingement or subluxation of the femoral head were not revealed in the postoperative radiograph in the split position.

## Abbreviations

ROM: Range of motion
THA: Total hip arthroplasty
CT: Computed tomography.

## Consent

Written informed consent was obtained from the patient for the publication of this case report and any accompanying images. A copy of the written consent form is available for review by the editor-in-chief of the journal.

## Authors' Contributions

FM and SF contribute to the conception and design of the manuscript. All authors contribute to the data interpretation and preparation of the manuscript. All authors approved the final version of the manuscript.

## References

[1] S. Bronner, S. Ojofeitimi, and D. Rose, "Injuries in a modern dance company," *The American Journal of Sports Medicine*, vol. 31, no. 3, pp. 365–373, 2003.

[2] S. Byhring and K. Bø, "Musculoskeletal injuries in the Norwegian national ballet: a prospective cohort study," *Scandinavian Journal of Medicine & Science in Sports*, vol. 12, no. 6, pp. 365–370, 2002.

[3] J. G. Garrick and R. K. Requa, "Ballet injuries: an analysis of epidemiology and financial outcome," *The American Journal of Sports Medicine*, vol. 21, no. 4, pp. 586–590, 1993.

[4] J. G. Garrick, "Early identification of musculoskeletal complaints and injuries among female ballet students," *Journal of Dance Medicine & Science*, vol. 3, no. 2, pp. 80–83, 1999.

[5] C. Nilsson, J. Leanderson, and A. Wykman, "The injury panorama in a Swedish professional ballet company," *Knee Surgery, Sports Traumatology, Arthroscopy*, vol. 9, no. 4, pp. 242–246, 2001.

[6] E. R. Wiesler, D. M. Hunter, and D. F. Martin, "Ankle flexibility and injury patterns in dancers," *The American Journal of Sports Medicine*, vol. 24, no. 6, pp. 754–757, 1996.

[7] V. B. Duthon, C. Charbonnier, and F. C. Kolo, "Correlation of clinical and magnetic resonance imaging findings in hips of elite female ballet dancers," *Arthroscopy*, vol. 29, no. 3, pp. 411–419, 2013.

[8] C. L. Jacobs, C. A. Hincapie, and D. Cassidy, "Musculoskeletal injuries and pain in dancers, a systematic review update," *Journal of Dance Medicine & Science*, vol. 16, no. 2, pp. 74–84, 2012.

[9] B. R. Moser, "Hip pain in dancers," *Current Sports Medicine Reports*, vol. 13, no. 6, pp. 383–389, 2014.

[10] N. Trentacosta, D. Sugimoto, and L. J. Micheli, "Hip and groin injuries in dancers: a systematic review," *Sports Health*, vol. 9, no. 5, pp. 422–427, 2017.

[11] Y. Masumoto, S. Fukunishi, T. Fukui et al., "New combined anteversion technique in hybrid THA: cup-first procedure with CT-based navigation," *European Journal of Orthopaedic Surgery and Traumatology*, vol. 30, no. 3, pp. 465–472, 2020.

[12] M. Angioi, G. D. Maffulli, M. McCormack, D. Morrissey, O. Chan, and N. Maffulli, "Early signs of osteoarthritis in professional ballet dancers: a preliminary study," *Clinical Journal of Sport Medicine*, vol. 24, no. 5, pp. 435–437, 2014.

[13] I. R. Buyls, A. B. Rietveld, and T. Ourila, "Total hip replacement in dancers," *Clinical Rheumatology*, vol. 32, no. 4, pp. 511–514, 2013.

[14] E. N. Novais, S. Thanacharoenpanich, A. Seker et al., "Do young female dancers improve symptoms and return to dancing after periacetabular osteotomy for the treatment of symptomatic hip dysplasia?," *Journal of Hip Preservation Surgery*, vol. 5, no. 2, pp. 150–156, 2018.

[15] O. A. Sogbein, A. Shah, J. Kay et al., "Predictors of outcomes after hip arthroscopic surgery for femoroacetabular Impingement: A Systematic Review," *Orthopaedic Journal of Sports Medicine*, vol. 7, no. 6, article 232596711984898, 2019.

[16] K. Komiyama, S. Hamai, D. Hara et al., "Dynamic hip kinematics during recreational classical ballet and hula dance after total hip arthroplasty: two case reports," *Journal of Medical Case Reports*, vol. 13, no. 1, p. 11, 2019.

[17] A. Gupta, B. Fernihough, and G. Bailey, "An evaluation of differences in hip external rotation strength and range of motion between female dancers and non-dancers," *British Journal of Sports Medicine*, vol. 38, no. 6, pp. 778–783, 2004.

[18] N. Steinberg, I. Hershkovitz, and S. Peleg, "Range of joint movement in female dancers and nondancers aged 8 to 16 years," *The American Journal of Sports Medicine*, vol. 34, no. 5, pp. 814–823, 2006.

[19] E. E. Valenti, V. E. Valenti, C. Ferreira et al., "Evaluation of movements of lower limbs in non-professional ballet dancers: hip abduction and flexion," *Sports Medicine, Arthroscopy, Rehabilitation, Therapy & Technology: SMARTT*, vol. 3, no. 1, 2011.

# 26

# Pyogenic Lumbar Facet Joint Infection with Foot Drop

**Haruka Maehara[1,2] Toshihiro Sano,[1] Yuki Yanagawa,[1] Kyuichi Hashimoto,[1] and Nobuaki Tadokoro[1,3]**

[1]*Department of Orthopaedic Surgery, Kochi Prefectural Hata Kenmin Hospital, 3-1 Yoshina, Yamana-cho, Sukumo, Kochi 788-0785, Japan*
[2]*Department of Orthopaedic Surgery, Susaki Kuroshio Hospital, 4–30, Midorimachi, Susaki, Kochi 785-0036, Japan*
[3]*Department of Orthopaedic Surgery, Kochi Medical School, 185-1 Kohasu, Oko-cho, Nankoku, Kochi 783-8505, Japan*

Correspondence should be addressed to Haruka Maehara; xa-troy29@hotmail.co.jp

Academic Editor: Werner Kolb

Pyogenic facet joint infection (PFJI) is a relatively rare spinal infection. Clinical suspicion of this condition is a key for diagnosis. We report a case of PFJI which required decompression surgery for severe neurological dysfunction. The patient was a 44-year-old woman who had a previous history of orthotic therapy for idiopathic scoliosis. The patient was admitted to our hospital with a history of two days of high fever and severe low back pain. There was no neurologic deficit, and blood tests revealed high levels of inflammatory markers. There was a slight amount of fluid that had collected at L4/5 facet joint in lumbar MRI. She was admitted for examination and treatment of fever of unknown origin and low back pain. Antibiotic treatment started the day after hospitalization since the first report of the blood culture taken upon admission tested positive to gram-positive cocci. As low back pain and fever persisted, an MRI was taken again on the fifth day of hospitalization. Repeated MRI showed fluid extension from the left facet joint to paravertebral muscles and epidural space. She was diagnosed with PFJI, and facet joint puncture was performed. At this time, it became clear that she had foot drop on the right, the contralateral side of the PFJI. She underwent irrigation, debridement, and partial laminectomy. Methicillin-sensitive Staphylococcus aureus (MSSA) was detected in blood cultures at the time of hospitalization, in the puncture fluid and tissue collected during surgery. The patient recovered completely from foot drop after the operation and a three-month course of antibiotics. As the imaging findings may be inadequate in the early stages of onset and PFJI potentially causes neurologic deficit such as foot drop, neurological findings need to be carefully observed even after hospitalization and one should reexamine the MRI if symptoms or clinical findings did not improve or were aggravated.

## 1. Introduction

Pyogenic facet joint infection (PFJI) is a relatively rare spinal infection [1], which is reported to account for 4% of spinal infections overall. Compared with pyogenic spondylodiscitis, diagnostic information on PFJI is still insufficient due to its rarity. We report a case of PFJI which required decompression surgery for severe neurological dysfunction.

## 2. Case Presentation

A 44-year-old female presented at our emergency department with chief complaints of severe back pain and fever for the past two days. She had a previous history of orthotic therapy for idiopathic scoliosis and no immunosuppressive disease. Her body temperature was 41 degrees, and there was tenderness at the spinous processes of the lower level of the lumbar spine and no neurologic deficit. The white blood cell (WBC) count was 9,250 cells/$\mu$L, and C-reactive protein (CRP) was elevated to 13 mg/dL. Although scoliosis was observed on X-ray, no clear bone or joint destruction was confirmed. MRI showed a slight amount of fluid had collected at the left L4/5 facet joint; these findings are considered to be associated with degenerative changes (Figure 1). She was admitted for examination and treatment of fever of unknown origin and low back pain.

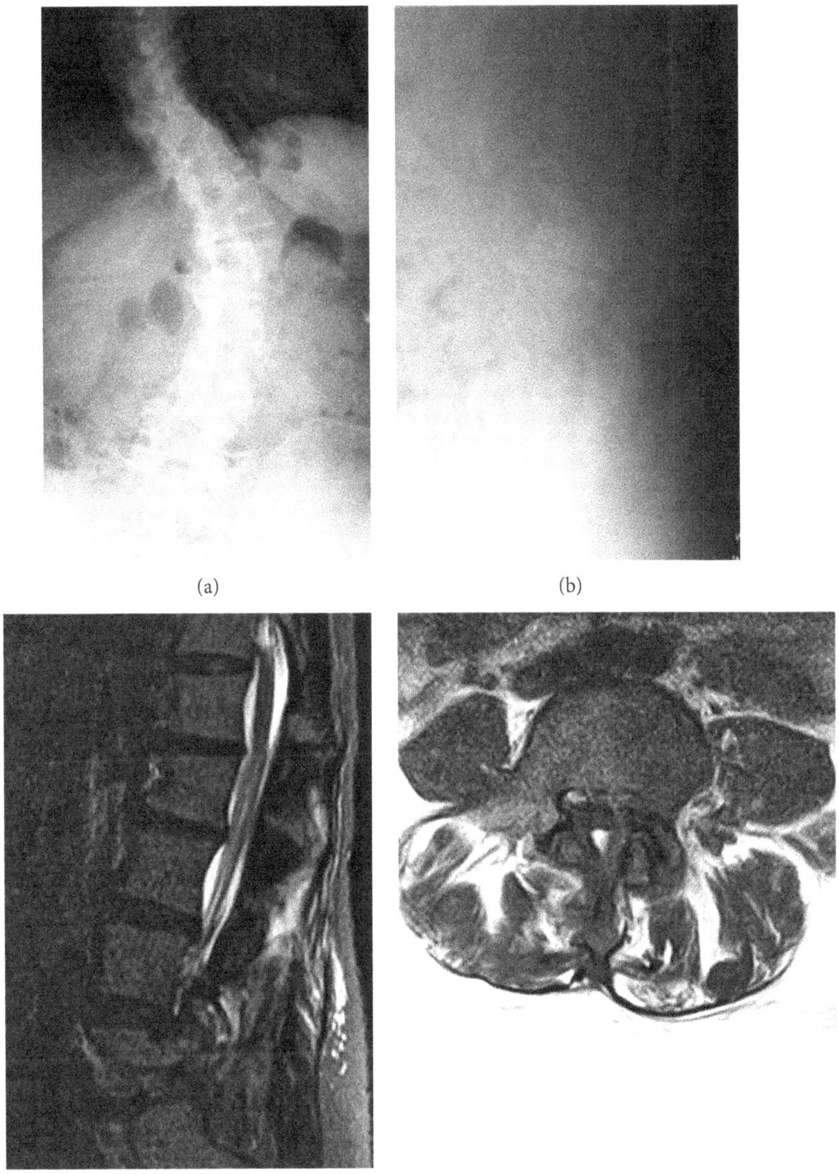

(a) (b) (c) (d)

FIGURE 1: Images of administration on the 5th day of hospitalization. X-ray (a, b) sagittal T2 short tau inversion recovery (T2-STIR) MRI (c), axial L4/5 T2-weighted MRI (d).

The first report of the blood culture taken upon admission tested positive to gram-positive cocci, and the patient was started on an intravenous course of sulbactam ampicillin (3 g every 6 hours) and vancomycin (1 g every 8 hours) as the empiric treatment of bacteremia on the second day of hospitalization. Methicillin-sensitive Staphylococcus aureus (MSSA) was isolated in the blood culture on the fourth day after admission, which was sensitive to cephazolin, levofloxacin, and many other antibiotic drugs. And the patient was put on an intravenous antibiotic course of cephazolin (2 g every 8 hours) and oral rifampicin (450 mg every day) for the MSSA bacteremia. On the fifth day after admission, the CRP level was 11 mg/dL, low back pain persisted, and fever was still approximately 38 degrees. Therefore, we took another MRI. The repeated MRI revealed continuous fluid from the facet joint to paravertebral muscles and epidural space (Figure 2). Other fever origins such as bacterial pneumonia and urinary tract infection were negative, and therefore, she was diagnosed with PFJI.

We performed a diagnostic facet joint puncture on the left L4/5 (Figure 3) on the 8th day; the culture tests detected MSSA and were negative for calcium pyrophosphate and uric acid crystals. Thus, we confirmed that it was indeed a pyogenic facet joint infection.

In response to the antibiotic treatment, the CRP level decreased and pain tended to improve, but we observed the right foot drop and MMT3 level muscle weakness in the iliopsoas and quadriceps the day after the puncture. As the atypical findings of lumbar radiculopathy coincided in this case; weakness in the contralateral side of the affected facet

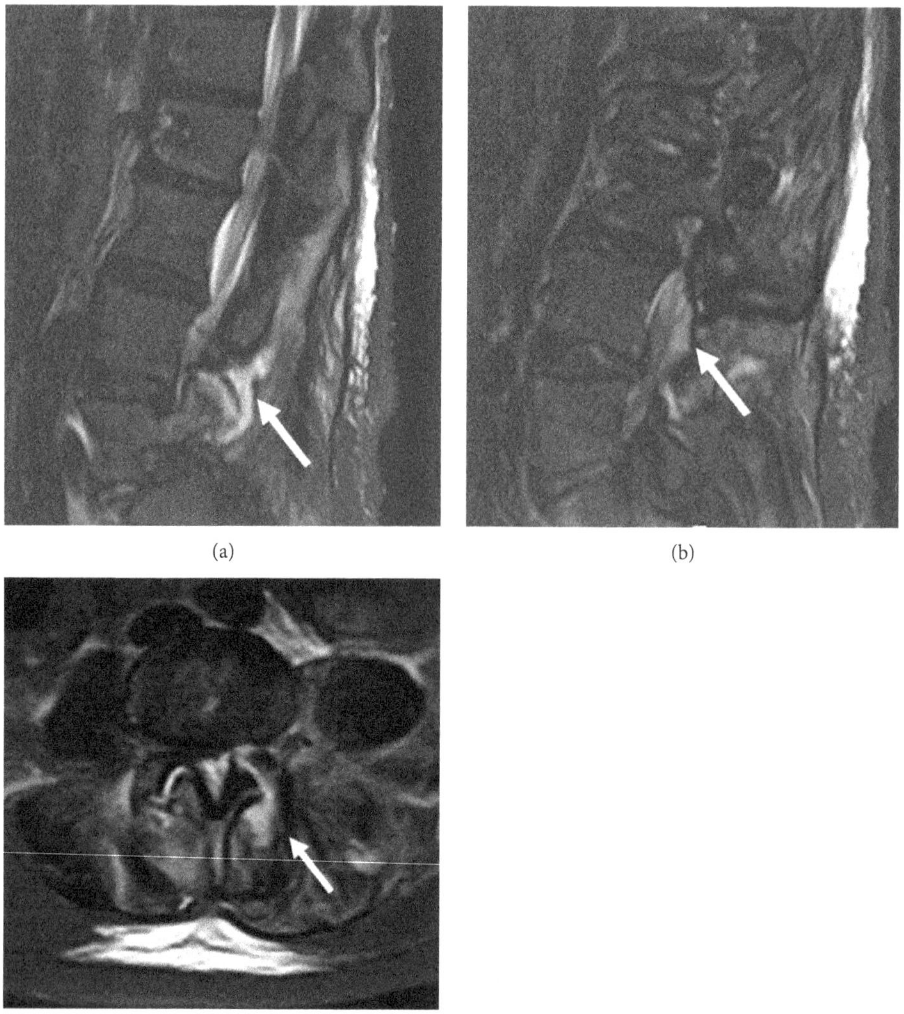

(a) (b) (c)

FIGURE 2: MRI images on the 5th day of hospitalization. Sagittal view (a and b) and axial view at L4/5 (c) of T2-STIR MRI showing an abscess from the facet joint to the paravertebral muscle (a, c) and epidural abscess (arrows).

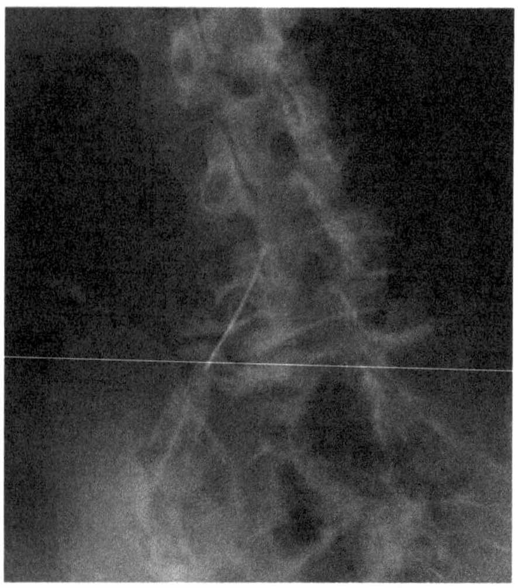

FIGURE 3: X-ray during left L4/5 facet puncture.

joint, and no leg sensory dysfunction including pain and numbness, we searched for other causes of paralysis such as cerebral infarction. However, none were clear, so we performed L4/5 and 5/S1 partial laminectomy and left L4/5 facet joint capsulotomy and irrigation debridement on the 11th day of admission. The epidural space and the left L4/5 facet joint were filled with inflammatory granulomatous tissue.

After the operation, the patient was continued on a course of antibiotics, CRP gradually decreased, and CRP became negative a month after hospitalization. Two weeks after surgery, we took a follow-up MRI, which showed signal changes at the left L5 pedicle and L4 and 5 vertebral bodies around the pedicle, which suggested osteomyelitis (Figure 4). Therefore, we changed the course of antibiotics to oral levofloxacin and rifampicin that has good penetration into the bone and joint [2], and the patient was discharged from our hospital. Muscle weakness in the right lower limbs, including the foot drop, also improved and reached MMT5 levels three months after the admission. Inflammatory changes in the paravertebral muscles and fluid retention in the facet joints had almost disappeared, and bone edema

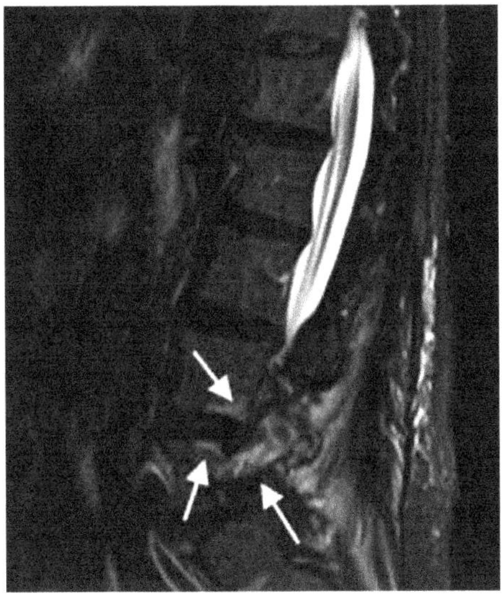

FIGURE 4: MRI image at two weeks after surgery. Sagittal view of T2-STIR MRI showing bone edema of the left L5 pedicle and L4 and 5 vertebral bodies around the pedicle (arrows).

had diminished. Therefore, we decided to discontinue the antibiotic treatment at this stage. The patient took antibiotics for a total of three months. At the one-year follow-up, there was no recurrence of either low back pain, lower limb muscle weakness, or elevated CRP, and no significant instability was observed on the lumbar dynamic X-ray.

## 3. Discussion

Pyogenic arthritis of the facet joint was first reported in 1987 by Halpin and Gibson [3]. It is considered to be a relatively rare disease [1]. However, PFJI was reported to account for 20% of pyogenic spinal infections in 2006 [3]. Compared with pyogenic spondylodiscitis involving disc and vertebral body complex, the facet joints damaged by PFJI are small. Thus, clinical suspicion of this condition is important in order to arrive at a diagnosis.

Symptoms are mainly severe low back pain not relieved by rest and fever. About 40% of patients have some kind of radiculopathy, but severe cases may involve paralysis or cauda equina syndrome, which account for approximately 10% of all cases [1, 4, 5]. The patient in our study also showed typical clinical symptoms of low back pain and fever. Although neurological deficit was not evident upon admission, a foot drop on the contralateral side developed after admission. The reported diverse neurological presentation including the peculiar neurological deficit of this patient might be explained by the varying degree of the abscess formation and the preexisting spinal stenosis. It has been reported that 32% of pyogenic vertebral osteomyelitis patients with severe neurological deficit experienced a deterioration of preexisting neurologic signs or the appearance of a new motor weakness after hospitalization, with a median time to exacerbation of 11 days [6]. As the present case also showed a new neurological deficit, it is necessary to carefully observe the neurological findings after hospitalization, as is the case with pyogenic spondylitis.

MRI is most effective in confirming the diagnosis of PFJI at an early stage [7], and a case has been reported in which effusion of a facet joint and edematous changes of the paravertebral muscle were observed two days after onset [8]. In this case, we can find MRI changes of the facet joint at two days after the onset of symptoms. However, it may be difficult to distinguish it from degenerative findings because there were fewer inflammatory findings in the tissue around the facet joints and the paravertebral muscle abscess and epidural abscess were unclear. Therefore, despite the typical clinical symptoms, the diagnosis was not made on the day of admission. Similarly, there was a case report in which a definitive diagnosis was not made at the first visit, and MRI was reexamined after one month when the symptoms persisted or relapsed [5]. Therefore, we recommend MRI reexamination if symptoms persist or relapse [9].

Paraspinal and/or epidural extension is seen in 81% of cases [4], and in this case as well, it was found to spread to the epidural and paravertebral muscles. Staphylococcus aureus was the most common etiologic organism, and it has been reported to account for approximately 80% of all cases [1, 4]. In our case, MSSA was also detected in blood cultures, facet joint fluid, and infectious tissues collected during surgery.

The focus of the treatment is antibiotic administration and drainage, and surgical treatment is mainly performed on severe neurologic dysfunction, like in this case [4]. The patient was treated with an intravenous course of cefazoline and oral rifampicin as a treatment for MSSA bacteremia and PFJI. The rationale behind this antibiotic treatment is a systematic review from 2014, in which the use of rifampicin as an adjunctive agent in treatment may improve outcomes of Staphylococcus aureus bacteremia [10]. However, in recent years, there have been some reports that the use of rifampicin as an adjunctive agent for Staphylococcus aureus bacteremia does not improve prognosis [11, 12], and therefore, it is necessary to carefully observe the side effects when it is used. No side effects were observed in this case. Although the optimal duration of antibiotic treatment for PFJI has not been defined, intravenous administration for two to four weeks or more followed by oral administration for a total of eight weeks or more is recommended [4, 5]. In this case, osteomyelitis became apparent during the course, and the antibiotic treatment lasted 3 months, because MRI showed a signal change resolution with the maintenance of negative CRP. The patient was treated with levofloxacin and rifampicin as the oral antibiotic drugs for PJFI and osteomyelitis. The combined use of oral levofloxacin and rifampicin is described in the IDSA guidelines for the treatment of vertebral osteomyelitis, and the drugs penetrated into the bone and joint effectively [2, 13].

## 4. Conclusion

We experienced a case of PFJI that required surgery due to foot drop. We need to take PFJI into account when we suspect spinal infection disease. Since the imaging findings may be inadequate in the early stages of onset and PFJI potentially causes neurologic deficit such as foot drop, it was considered necessary to follow-up carefully and reexamine the MRI if symptoms or clinical findings did not improve or became aggravated.

## References

[1] A. J. Muffoletto, L. M. Ketonen, J. T. Mader, W. N. Crow, and A. G. Hadjipavlou, "Hematogenous pyogenic facet joint infection," *Spine*, vol. 26, no. 14, pp. 1570–1576, 2001.

[2] A. K. Thabit, D. F. Fatani, M. S. Bamakhrama, O. A. Barnawi, L. O. Basudan, and S. F. Alhejaili, "Antibiotic penetration into bone and joints: an updated review," *International Journal of Infectious Diseases*, vol. 81, pp. 128–136, 2019.

[3] D. S. Halpin and R. D. Gibson, "Septic arthritis of a lumbar facet joint," *The Journal of Bone and Joint Surgery*, vol. 69-B, no. 3, pp. 457–459, 1987.

[4] J. Narváez, J. M. Nolla, J. A. Narváez et al., "Spontaneous pyogenic facet joint infection," *Seminars in Arthritis and Rheumatism*, vol. 35, no. 5, pp. 272–283, 2006.

[5] D. Klekot, A. Zimny, B. Czapiga, and M. Sąsiadek, "Izolowane zapalenie stawu międzykręgowego jako rzadka przyczyna ostrego i przewlekłego zespołu bólowego odcinka lędźwiowo-krzyżowego kręgosłupa - opis przypadku i przegląd literatury," *Polish Journal of Radiology*, vol. 77, no. 4, pp. 72–76, 2012.

[6] A. Lemaignen, I. Ghout, A. Dinh et al., "Characteristics of and risk factors for severe neurological deficit in patients with pyogenic vertebral osteomyelitis," *Medicine*, vol. 96, no. 21, article e6387, 2017.

[7] C. Michel-Batôt, H. Dintinger, A. Blum et al., "A particular form of septic arthritis: septic arthritis of facet joint," *Joint, Bone, Spine*, vol. 75, no. 1, pp. 78–83, 2008.

[8] A. Fujiwara, K. Tamai, M. Yamato, H. Yoshida, and K. Saotome, "Septic arthritis of a lumbar facet joint: report of a case with early MRI findings," *Journal of Spinal Disorders*, vol. 11, no. 5, pp. 452-453, 1998.

[9] K. W. Rhyu, S. E. Park, J. H. Ji, I. Park, and Y. Y. Kim, "Pyogenic arthritis of the facet joint with concurrent epidural and paraspinal abscess: a case report," *Asian Spine Journal*, vol. 5, no. 4, pp. 245–249, 2011.

[10] C. D. Russell, A. Lawson McLean, C. Saunders, and I. F. Laurenson, "Adjunctive rifampicin may improve outcomes in Staphylococcus aureus bacteraemia: a systematic review," *Journal of Medical Microbiology*, vol. 63, no. 6, pp. 841–848, 2014.

[11] G. E. Thwaites, M. Scarborough, A. Szubert et al., "Adjunctive rifampicin for _Staphylococcus aureus_ bacteraemia (ARREST): a multicentre, randomised, double-blind, placebo-controlled trial," *Lancet*, vol. 391, no. 10121, pp. 668–678, 2018.

[12] H. Ma, J. Cheng, L. Peng, Y. Gao, G. Zhang, and Z. Luo, "Adjunctive rifampin for the treatment of Staphylococcus aureus bacteremia with deep infections: a meta-analysis," *PLoS One*, vol. 15, no. 3, article e0230383, 2020.

[13] E. F. Berbari, S. S. Kanj, T. J. Kowalski et al., "2015 Infectious Diseases Society of America (IDSA) clinical practice guidelines for the diagnosis and treatment of native vertebral osteomyelitis in adults," *Clinical Infectious Diseases*, vol. 61, no. 6, pp. e26–e46, 2015.

27

# Metacarpal Stress Fracture is not an Uncommon Condition in Adolescent Racket Athletes

**Karen Nishikawa,[1] Yuka Kimura,[2] Daisuke Chiba,[2] Norihiro Sasaki,[2] Shizuka Sasaki,[2] Shinji Nishikawa,[3] and Yasuyuki Ishibashi[2]**

[1] *Hirosaki University School of Medicine, 5 Zaifu-cho, Hirosaki, Aomori, Japan 036-8562*
[2] *Department of Orthopaedic Surgery, Hirosaki University Graduate School of Medicine, 5 Zaifu-cho, Hirosaki, Aomori, Japan 036-8562*
[3] *Nishikawa Hand Surgery Orthopaedic Clinic, 2-2-12 Waseda, Hirosaki, Aomori, Japan*

Correspondence should be addressed to Yasuyuki Ishibashi; yasuyuki@hirosaki-u.ac.jp

Academic Editor: Koichi Sairyo

*Background.* Stress fractures of the metacarpal bones are considered uncommon. We report on 11 adolescent athletes with these stress fractures, successfully treated with cessation of sports activities. *Representative case presentation.* In case 1, a 15-year-old male tennis player presented with right hand pain of 4-week duration without an acute trauma history. Tenderness existed on palpation along the dorsal and proximal second metacarpal bone. Plain radiographs demonstrated a periosteal reaction on the proximal shaft of the second metacarpal. Racket swinging was suspended. He returned to competitive tennis 2 months after the initial visit and continues to participate without symptoms. In case 2, a 16-year-old male boxer presented with right hand pain of 2-week duration that arose while punching. Acute trauma history was absent. Tenderness existed on palpation over the third metacarpal of the right hand. Plain radiographs demonstrated no periosteal reaction or fracture line. MRI showed a high signal on the third metatarsal bone on fat suppression and a low signal on T2-weighted images. Nonoperative treatment was initiated without external fixation, and punching was suspended. He returned to boxing 1 month after the initial visit without symptoms. *Conclusions.* The current case series of metacarpal stress fractures demonstrate that this condition is not as rare as previously reported. Metacarpal stress fractures are generally ignored since the clinical and radiological findings are mostly unclear. If an athlete experiences hand pain without acute onset during sports activities, especially in racket sports, the presence of a metacarpal stress fracture should be assessed by MRI.

## 1. Background

Stress fractures are common overuse injuries in athletes and generally occur in the lumbar spine and lower extremities; those affecting the upper limbs are uncommon, accounting for 2.8-7.6% of all stress fractures [1, 2]. Because the number of sports-specific movements involving repetitive use of an upper limb has increased in sports such as racket sports, throwing sports, and boxing, the incidence of stress fractures in the upper limbs also may increase. Nevertheless, stress fractures of the metacarpal bones are considered relatively uncommon. We report on 11 adolescent athletes aged 13 to 24 years old with stress fractures of the metacarpal bones, successfully treated with cessation of sports activities.

## 2. Case Presentation

*2.1. Case Report 1.* A 15-year-old male tennis player presented to our institution with right hand pain of 4-week duration without an acute trauma history. His involved side was the racket-hand side. Physical examination revealed tenderness on palpation along the dorsal and proximal second metacarpal bone. No swelling, ecchymosis, mass, or deformity was seen in the hand. He had full range of motion of

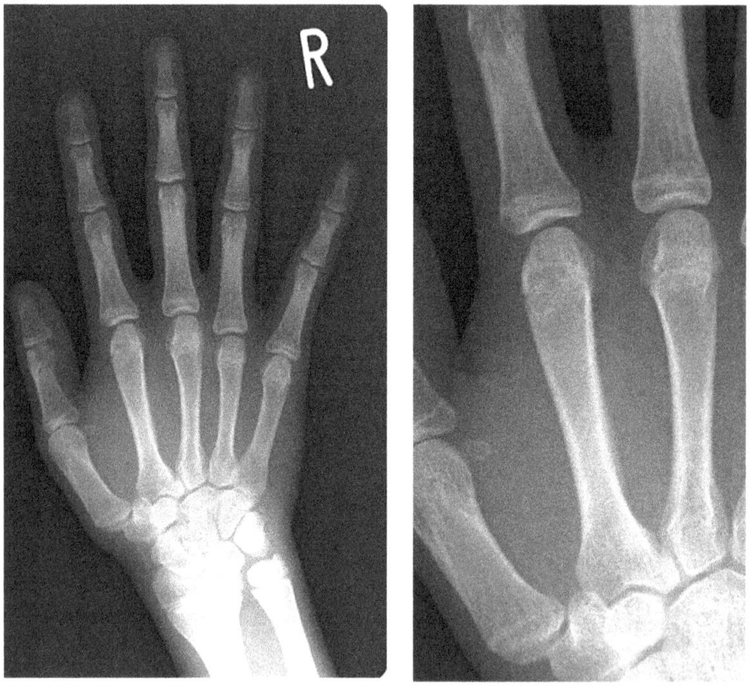


(a) (b)

Figure 1: Right hand radiograph showing a periosteal reaction at the ulnar side in the shaft of the second metacarpal.

the wrist and fingers in all planes without pain. Hand anteroposterior (A-P) radiographs demonstrated a periosteal reaction on the ulnar aspect of the proximal shaft of the second metacarpal (Figure 1). Second metacarpal stress fracture was diagnosed. Nonoperative treatment was initiated without external fixation. Racket swinging was suspended. He returned to competitive tennis 3 weeks after the initial visit and continues to participate without symptoms.

*2.2. Case Report 2.* A 16-year-old male boxer presented to our institution with right hand pain of 2-week duration that arose while punching. Acute trauma history was absent. Physical examination revealed tenderness on palpation over the third metacarpal of the right hand. Hand A-P radiographs demonstrated no periosteal reaction or fracture line (Figure 2(a)). Magnetic resonance imaging (MRI) showed a high signal on the third metatarsal bone on fat suppression and a low signal on T2-weighted images (Figure 2(b)). Third metacarpal stress fracture was diagnosed. Nonoperative treatment was initiated without external fixation, and punching was suspended. He returned to boxing 1 month after the initial visit and continues to participate without symptoms.

This case report included 11 athletes (six males and five females; mean age, 16.9 years; range, 13-24 years) diagnosed with the stress fractures of the metacarpal bones. The patient profiles and clinical results are shown in Table 1. Six patients played tennis, two played badminton, two boxed, and one bowled. Nine of the 11 patients injured the right hand and two injured the left hand. All those playing racket sports injured the dominant hand (racket-hand side). No patient had an acute trauma history. All patients except for one chronic patient had dorsal hand pain during sports activity for about 2 weeks from onset to initial visit. In ten patients, the second metacarpal bone was involved, and six patients had shaft and four had stress fractures at the base of the second metacarpal. Only one patient, who was a boxer, had a stress fracture at the shaft of the third metacarpal bone. Two of the 11 patients were diagnosed only using a plain radiograph of the hand, demonstrating periosteal or cortical stress reactions in the metacarpal bone, and nine patients underwent MRI in addition to plain radiography.

All patients were treated nonoperatively with rest and cessation of sports activity. After conservative therapy without external fixation such as a casting, the symptoms disappeared completely in all cases. Before returning to sports activity, the grip form of racket sports players was checked; if the players showed incorrect grip, their grip form was altered. In some cases, we advised to switch western grip over to eastern grip. Most patients returned to their sports activity within 6 months. All patients provided informed written consent for this study, and in particular, patients under 17 years old provided the consent with their guardian. The ethical committee of our institution approved this case report.

## 3. Discussion

Stress fractures in the metacarpal bones were previously considered to be rare; however, this report showed a relatively high number of cases. We found many metacarpal stress fractures because we could use MRI relatively easily.

The second metacarpal is the longest of all the metacarpals, with a broad base linked to the first and third metacarpals, trapezoid, trapezium, and capitate. The extensor carpi radialis longus inserts on the radial aspect of the base of the second metacarpal, and the flexor carpi radialis inserts on the anterior aspect of the base of the second metacarpal.

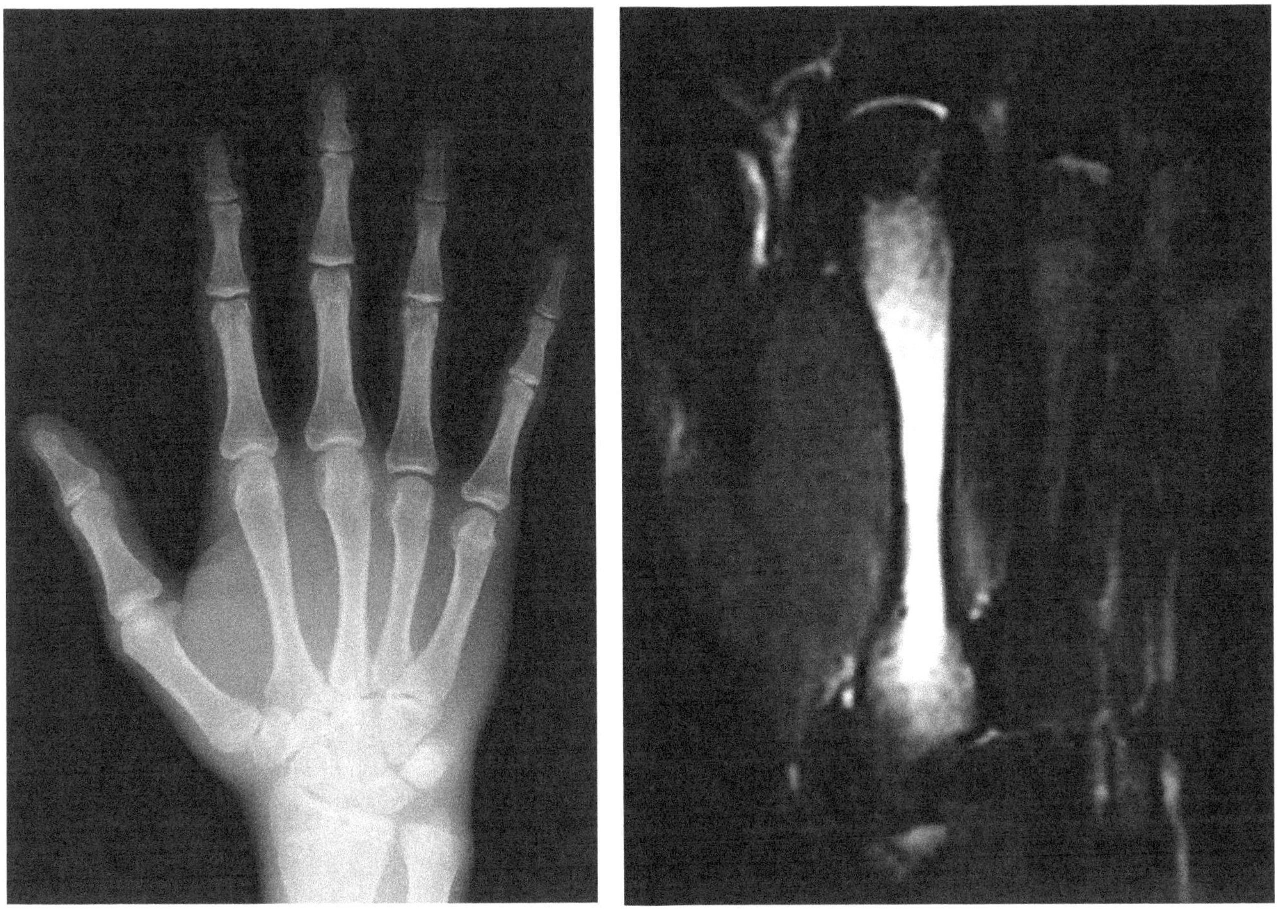

(a) (b)

FIGURE 2: (a) Left hand radiograph showing no periosteal reaction or fracture line in the metacarpal. (b) Fat-suppressed fast spin-echo T2-weighted magnetic resonance showing high signal intensity in the shaft of the left third metacarpal.

TABLE 1: Profile and clinical results in the eleven cases of metacarpal stress fracture.

| Case | Age (years) | Sex | Time from onset to initial visit (weeks) | Metacarpal | Location | Sports | Time from initial visit to return to sports (weeks) |
|---|---|---|---|---|---|---|---|
| 1 | 13 | F | 2 | Second | Shaft | Badminton | 4 |
| 2 | 14 | F | 1 | Second | Base | Soft tennis | 12 |
| 3 | 14 | M | 3 | Second | Base | Badminton | 4 |
| 4 | 15 | M | 4 | Second | Base | Tennis | 3 |
| 5 | 16 | M | 2 | Third | Shaft | Boxing | 4 |
| 6 | 16 | M | 2 | Second | Shaft | Tennis | 4 |
| 7 | 16 | F | 3 | Second | Base | Tennis | 10 |
| 8 | 18 | F | 1 | Second | Shaft | Tennis | 4 |
| 9 | 18 | M | 52 | Second | Shaft | Boxing | 5 |
| 10 | 22 | F | 1 | Second | Shaft | Tennis | 4 |
| 11 | 24 | M | 2 | Second | Shaft | Bowling | 4 |

Therefore, flexing and extending the wrist joint produce larger mechanical stress to the base of the second metacarpal and cause stress fractures distal to the insertion of these muscles.

The second metacarpal bone bears mechanical stress at the point where players hit the ball using a racket [3]. Knudson, using a 3D motion analysis system, demonstrated increased mechanical force on the base of the second

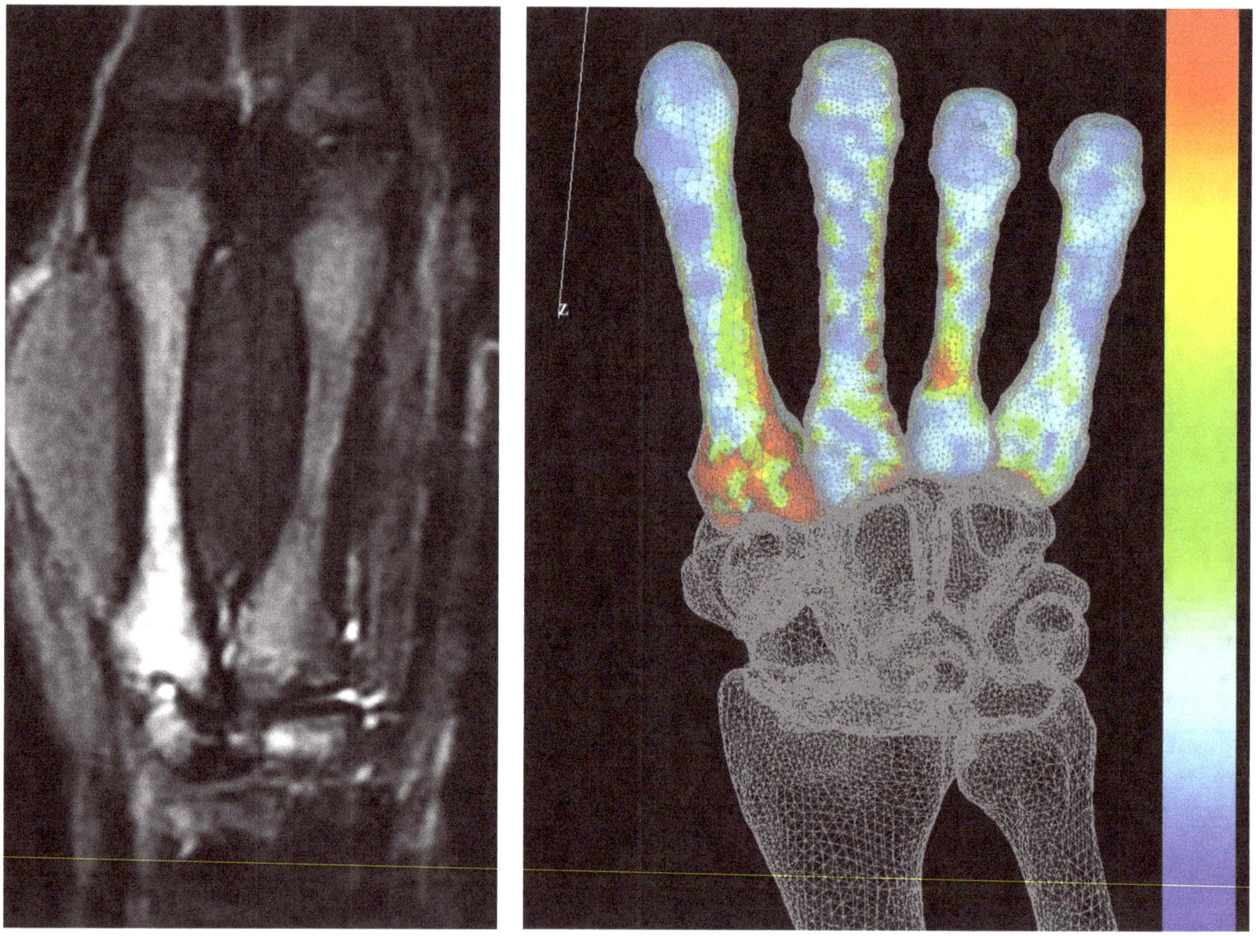


(a) (b)

Figure 3: (a) Fat-suppressed T2-weighted MRI showing high signal intensity in the base of the second metacarpal. (b) Finite element analysis showing the stress distribution of the second metacarpal. Maximum stress was present at the base of the second metacarpal bone.

metacarpal bone when tennis players hit the ball with the forehand stroke [4]. Stress fractures of metacarpal bones typically occur at the ulnar aspect [5–8] probably because both the ligaments and the joint congruence between the second and third metacarpals are greater than those between the first and second; biomechanically, the force produced by beating the racket is directed from radial to ulnar, with the greatest tension in the medial aspect of the metacarpal base [6, 9]. Our computed tomography- (CT-) based finite element analysis (FEA) software (Mechanical Finder, Research Center for Computational Mechanics, Tokyo, Japan) showed increased mechanical stress at the base and ulnar side of the second metacarpal (Figure 3), revealing one of the causes of stress fractures of the second metacarpal bone.

Eight of the 11 patients played racket sports. The grip style of the racket is related to the sports-specific mechanism of stress fracture. Balius et al. reported that six of seven tennis players with stress fractures of the second metacarpal were using the semiwestern or western grip [8]. In the western grip, the palm is parallel to the surface of the racket, and hence, the wrist joint requires pronation and supination motion during racket movement, delivering mechanical stress to the second metacarpal [7]. However, in the eastern grip, the palm is perpendicular to the surface the racket (Figure 4) [8]. Waninger and Lomnardo reported that changing the grip style from western to eastern would be effective to prevent stress fractures of the metacarpal bone [9]. In some cases, western style was actually switched over to eastern style. Moreover, if the racket sports players demonstrated incorrect grip form, we tried to alter their form. In particular, the incidence of stress fracture in metacarpal bone can be likely in teenagers based on the previous [8] and current data. Some teenagers seem to be inexperienced and demonstrate incorrect form despite practicing harder. For instance, we had them grab a racket along the line connecting the metaphalangeal joint of the index finger to the hypothenar eminence. Grip size was changed to make adequate space; one-finger breath is made between the index and the thumb finger while they grab a racket. Altering incorrect grip form to correct one and grip style have potential to reduce the stress of metacarpal bone.

Two patients in this series were boxers, and one had involvement of the third metacarpal bone. Because of the characteristics of the knuckle, where the third metacarpal head protrudes the most, repetitive punching might cause stress fractures of the third metacarpal. The mechanism of metacarpal stress fractures in boxing differs from that in racket sports. Metacarpal stress fractures in other

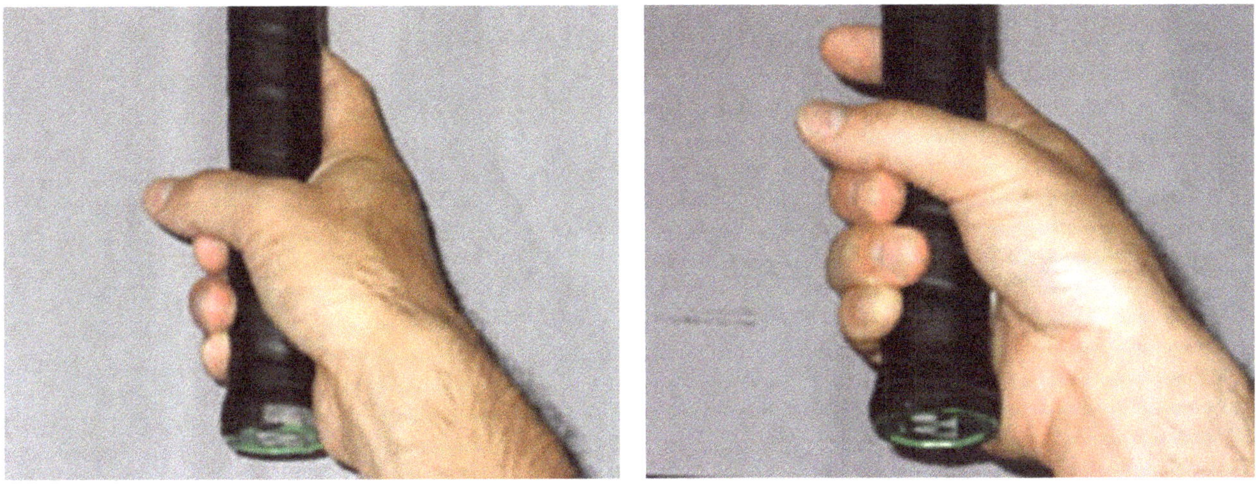

(a) (b)

FIGURE 4: (a) Eastern and (b) western grip style.

locations have been reported previously, including injuries affecting athletes in rowers with a fourth metacarpal stress fracture caused by awl gripping [10] and in a softball pitcher with a fifth metacarpal stress fracture caused by curveball pitching [11].

Stress fractures should be suspected in patients with a recent increase in physical activity or repeated excessive activities eliciting pain. There were no specific physical findings such as tenderness along the metacarpal bone in the dorsal hand or swelling. Plain radiographs usually show periosteal reaction, thickness of the cortex, and fracture lines; in early-onset cases, such abnormal signs are absent. Furthermore, these are relatively minor findings and may be easily overlooked. For early stress fracture diagnosis, MRI and bone scintigraphy are useful [12] as shown in the current case series.

Patients without apparent fracture lines in radiographs do not need external fixation, and temporarily suspending the maneuver related to the metacarpal stress fracture is sufficient. All patients in these cases returned to sports after tenderness and swelling along the metacarpal disappeared, callus on radiographs was confirmed, or bone marrow edema (high signal change) disappeared on MRI. None showed recurrence after return to sports activity.

In conclusion, we report a case series of metacarpal stress fractures and demonstrate that this condition is not as rare as previously reported. Metacarpal stress fractures are generally ignored since the clinical and radiological findings are mostly unclear. If an athlete experiences hand pain without acute onset during sports activities, especially in racket sports, the presence of a metacarpal stress fracture should be assessed by MRI.

## Abbreviations

A-P: Anteroposterior
CT: Computed tomography
FEA: Finite element analysis
MRI: Magnetic resonance imaging.

## Consent

We got the consent of all participants to publish or participate in this case report.

## Authors' Contributions

KN chiefly drafted the manuscript. YK revised the manuscript critically for important intellectual content and carried out the acquisition of data. DC revised the manuscript critically for important intellectual content. NS carried out the acquisition of data. SS carried out the acquisition of data. SN carried out the acquisition of data. YI helped to revise the manuscript and conducted the final approval of the manuscript to be submitted. All authors have read and approved the current manuscript.

## Acknowledgments

We would like to thank Editage (https://www.editage.jp) for English language editing.

## References

[1] S. Orava, J. Puranen, and L. Ala-Ketola, "Stress fractures caused by physical exercise," *Acta Orthopaedica Scandinavica*, vol. 49, no. 1, pp. 19–27, 1978.

[2] J. Iwamoto and T. Takeda, "Stress fractures in athletes: review of 196 cases," *Journal of Orthopaedic Science*, vol. 8, no. 3, pp. 273–278, 2003.

[3] K. Muramatsu and R. Kuriyama, "Stress fracture at the base of second metacarpal in a soft tennis player," *Clinical Journal of Sport Medicine*, vol. 15, no. 4, pp. 279-280, 2005.

[4] D. V. Knudson, "Factors affecting force loading on the hand in the tennis forehand," *The Journal of Sports Medicine and Physical Fitness*, vol. 31, no. 4, pp. 527–531, 1991.

[5] Y. Murakami, "Stress fracture of the metacarpal in an adolescent tennis player," *The American Journal of Sports Medicine*, vol. 16, no. 4, pp. 419-420, 1988.

[6] A. Bespalchuk, K. Okada, J. Nishida, S. Takahashi, Y. Shimada, and E. Itoi, "Stress fracture of the second metacarpal bone," *Skeletal Radiology*, vol. 33, no. 9, pp. 537–540, 2004.

[7] K. Fukuda, H. Fujioka, I. Fujita et al., "Stress fracture of the second metacarpal bone in a badminton player," *The Kobe Journal of Medical Sciences*, vol. 54, no. 3, pp. E159–E162, 2008.

[8] R. Balius, C. Pedret, A. Estruch, G. Hernández, Á. Ruiz-Cotorro, and J. Mota, "Stress fractures of the metacarpal bones in adolescent tennis players: a case series," *The American Journal of Sports Medicine*, vol. 38, no. 6, pp. 1215–1220, 2010.

[9] K. N. Waninger and J. A. Lomnardo, "Stress fracture of index metacarpal in an adolescent tennis player," *Clinical Journal of Sport Medicine*, vol. 5, no. 1, pp. 63–67, 1995.

[10] E. M. Parsons, J. P. Goldblatt, and J. C. Richmond, "Metacarpal stress fracture in an intercollegiate rower: case report," *The American Journal of Sports Medicine*, vol. 33, no. 2, pp. 293-294, 2005.

[11] A. D. Jowett and P. D. Brukner, "Fifth metacarpal stress fracture in a female softball pitcher," *Clinical Journal of Sport Medicine*, vol. 7, no. 3, pp. 220-221, 1997.

[12] Y. Ishibashi, Y. Okamura, H. Otsuka, K. Nishizawa, T. Sasaki, and S. Toh, "Comparison of scintigraphy and magnetic resonance imaging for stress injuries of bone," *Clinical Journal of Sport Medicine*, vol. 12, no. 2, pp. 79–84, 2002.

# 28

# Bilateral Reverse Total Shoulder Arthroplasty with Soft Tissue Release for Bilateral Posterior Fracture Dislocation after Status Epilepticus

George El Rassi,[1] Nabil Dib,[1] Joseph Maalouly,[1] Rita Moukarzel,[2] and Dany Aouad[1]

[1]Department of Orthopedic Surgery and Traumatology, Saint Georges University Medical Center, Balamand University, P.O. Box 166378, Achrafieh, Beirut 1100 2807, Lebanon

[2]Medical School, Lebanese American University Medical Center, Lebanese American University, P.O. Box 13-5053, Chouran, Beirut 1102 2801, Lebanon

Correspondence should be addressed to Dany Aouad; dany_aouad@hotmail.com

Academic Editor: Hiroshi Takahashi

Proximal humerus fracture is a common orthopedic presentation, with bimodal age distribution. On the other hand, bilateral proximal humerus fracture dislocation is a rarely reported pathology, especially when it is not the result of direct trauma. We present a case of a 71-year-old female patient found to have simultaneous bilateral 4-part proximal humerus fractures following status epilepticus treated surgically with bilateral reverse shoulder arthroplasty with constraint and soft tissue release. In a patient with recurrent status epilepticus episodes, the combination of constrained reverse shoulder arthroplasty and the extensive soft tissue release should decrease the rate of failure and dislocation dramatically. We conclude, after reviewing the literature, that there is no straightforward algorithm for treating such patients and that a clear classification should take into account both bone quality and patient comorbidities which has yet to be developed.

## 1. Introduction

Proximal humerus fractures constitute a fair proportion of worldwide reported fracture cases, with a 5-8% frequency [1] (incidence: 82 per 100,000 per year [2]). A bimodal distribution may be described. Indeed, while they mostly occur due to high-energy traumas, convulsions, and electrocutions in young patients, less energy is needed for their induction in osteoporotic older patients. Furthermore, the glenoid and acromial parameters can have an effect on concomitant rotator cuff tear incidence [3, 4]. The Neer classification stratifies proximal humerus fractures into 2-, 3-, and 4-part fractures [5, 6]. Also, bilateral cases are much less commonly recorded when compared to unilateral proximal humerus fractures, representing approximately 1% of the observed cases [7]. Furthermore, bilateral posterior fracture dislocation is even rarer with only 2 cases reported in the literature [8, 9]. In a previous article, the authors contributed [10] to discussing a rarely reported scenario whereby an elderly woman presented with bilateral proximal humerus fractures and was treated with bilateral open reduction and internal fixation with a plate and screws, with good outcomes upon follow-ups. Furthermore, a recent case report [11] describes bilateral reverse shoulder arthroplasty as the surgical management of a patient presenting with trauma-induced bilateral proximal humerus fractures. In this article, we present a case of simultaneous bilateral 4-part proximal humerus fractures in an elderly woman with status epilepticus treated surgically with bilateral reverse shoulder arthroplasty.

## 2. Case Report

This is the case of a 71-year-old female patient with history of bilateral carotid arteries stenosis status post left endarterectomy. Her surgery was complicated with a partial seizure postop and was discharged on antiepileptic medications. Two days after discharge, the patient was brought to the emergency department with status epilepticus. She was found

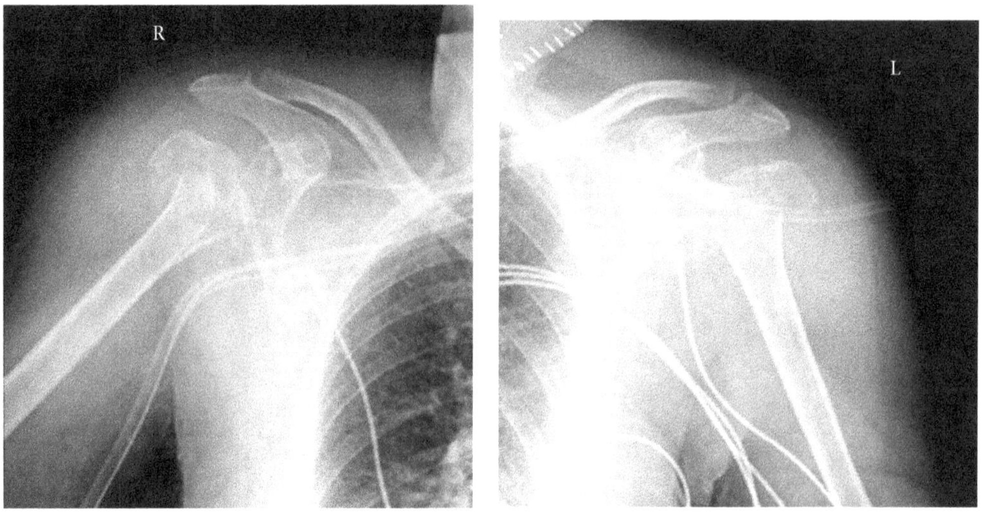


(a) (b)

Figure 1: (a) X-ray radiograph of the right shoulder showing a comminuted proximal humerus fracture. (b) X-ray radiograph of the left shoulder showing a comminuted proximal humerus fracture.

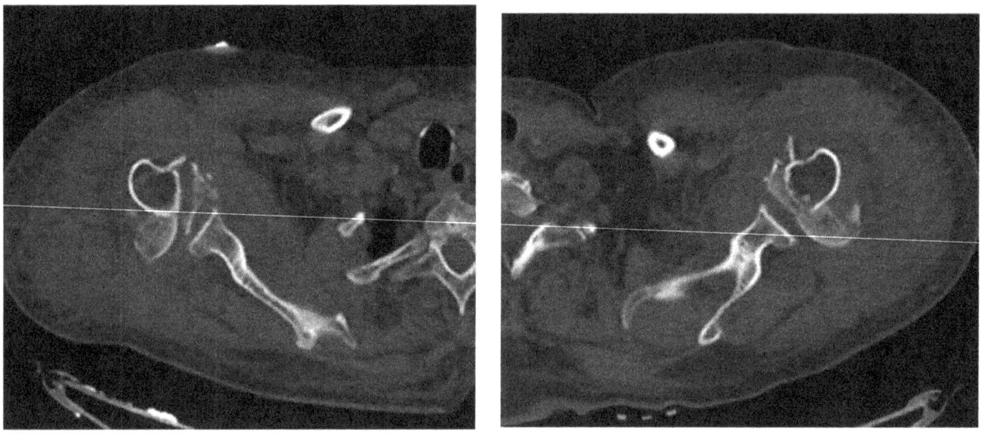

(a) (b)

Figure 2: (a) CT of the right shoulder showing a comminuted displaced fracture of the proximal humerus. (b) CT of the left shoulder showing a comminuted displaced fracture of the proximal humerus.

to have simultaneous bilateral proximal humerus fracture dislocations on radiographs (Figure 1) and CT scans (Figure 2).

She was treated with bilateral reverse total shoulder arthroplasty (Figure 3).

Using the deltopectoral approach, dissection down to the glenohumeral joint and identification of the biceps with subsequent tenotomy and suture tagging are performed. Also, the greater and lesser tuberosities were identified and a suture was passed in each one for reconstruction over the prosthesis. Excision of the humeral head followed by preparation of the glenoid was conducted. Then, glenoid base and glenosphere were placed. In addition, soft tissue was done, including release of the proximal fibers of the pectoralis major, followed by preparation of the humerus and insertion of a cemented stem in neutral rotation with removal of cement excess. In addition, the lesser tuberosity was reattached to the humeral component more medialized than the native joint, leading to less tension and subscapularis muscle pull to decrease future possible seizure-induced posterior dislocations. Finally, bone grafting of the proximal humerus was done and a constrained cup was placed to prevent dislocations as well as to reconstruct the tuberosities over the prosthesis. The same technique was used for the contralateral side simultaneously, with a total operative time of four hours. Shoulders were immobilized for six weeks with initiation of physical therapy program at two weeks postoperatively, increasing intensity progressively. Follow-up radiographs showed no failure or displacement of the prosthesis despite two episodes of partial seizures. Satisfactory results were observed after six months as for the Penn shoulder score [12], and the patient received 55/100 for the left shoulder and 60/100 for the right one.

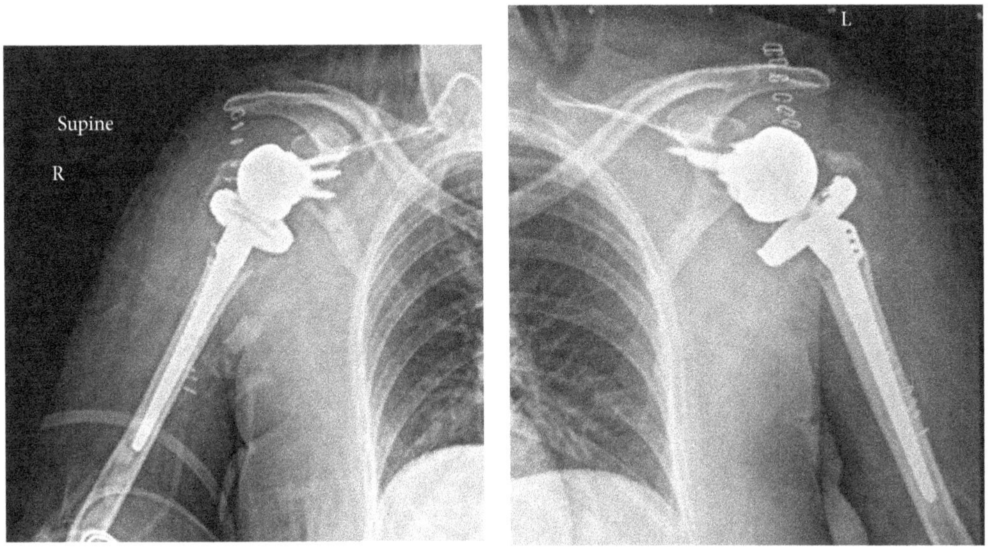


(a) (b)

FIGURE 3: (a) Postoperative X-ray radiograph of the right shoulder showing reverse shoulder arthroplasty. (b) Postoperative X-ray radiograph of the left shoulder showing reverse shoulder arthroplasty.

## 3. Discussion

As is the case in symmetrical structures in the human body, the treatment of bilateral, simultaneous fractures in the proximal humerus is identical to the modalities used to treat a unilateral fracture, as long as they both are identical in nature and grade of their injury. It thus ensues that nonoperative treatment, minimally invasive methods, hemiarthroplasty, reverse shoulder arthroplasty, and ORIF were all possible, acceptable treatment plans when dealing with this case. A large literature review released in 2015 [13] and comparing 4500 patients showed that attributes slightly improved functional outcomes to patients treated with ORIF, though with significantly higher revision rates. Secondly, an article published in 2019 [14] dealing with 425 cases including three modalities (ORIF, reverse shoulder arthroplasty, and hemiarthroplasty) concludes that ORIF and reverse shoulder arthroplasty confer the same postoperative range of motion when used to treat proximal humerus fractures. However, patients treated with ORIF had a higher rate of reoperation when compared to the group treated via RSA. In yet another article published in 2020 [15], concerning the surgical treatment of complex proximal humerus fractures in elderly patients and including 60 patients, it is concluded that complications rates (30% vs. 10%) and revision rates (20% vs. 3%) were significantly more severe in patients treated with ORIF. It thus may be asserted that RSA is the more predictable surgical management option between the two, even though both have been shown to be efficacious treatments for proximal humerus fractures.

The typical position of the shoulder during a convulsion is adduction, internal rotation, and flexion. The humeral head is forced superiorly and posteriorly over the glenoid cavity. Further convulsions cause the humeral head to be impinged against the glenoid rim resulting in a complex proximal humerus fracture [8].

In addition, a literature review published in 2004 [16] entails a 4-fold increase in the occurrence of humerus fractures in seizure- or epilepsy-prone patients, mostly in patients older than 45. Furthermore, the same review links bilateral proximal humerus fractures as indicative of seizure-related events, witnessed or otherwise, mainly derived from strong muscular contractions causing internal rotation and adduction of the shoulder joints and subsequently more commonly found in men due to stronger musculature [16].

Moreover, in a recent multicenter randomized controlled trial of 124 elderly patients, reverse shoulder prosthesis was superior to open reduction and internal fixation in terms of outcomes [17]. Also, certain authors recommend reverse shoulder arthroplasty in elderly patients above 70 years of age, when reduction is not possible. The reported outcomes are satisfactory in these selected patients [18].

And in this case, in a patient with recurrent status epilepticus episodes, the combination of constrained reverse shoulder arthroplasty and the extensive soft tissue release, with a main focus on the shoulder adductors and internal rotators, should decrease the rate of failure and dislocation dramatically.

## 4. Conclusion

Conclusively, we finish by underlining the fact that a clear classification taking into account both bone quality and patient comorbidities has yet to be developed for the management of status epilepticus-induced posterior shoulder fracture dislocations. Fractures behave in different patterns according to patient age, underlying medicosurgical problems and traumatic patterns. More randomized control trials are needed so as to determine the precise guidelines which may be used in determining specifically appropriate surgical management for various types of fractures especially posterior fracture dislocations in a seizure-prone individual, with emphasis on the importance of the soft tissue procedure to decrease rates of recurrence.

## Consent

Full consent from the patient was obtained for publishing this article and images.

## References


[1] R. E. Rodriguez-Corlay, R. Velutini-Becker, and L. D. Aguilar-Alcalá, "Conservative treatment for bilateral displaced proximal humerus head fracture," *Cureus*, vol. 8, no. 6, article e657, 2016.

[2] A. P. Launonen, V. Lepola, A. Saranko, T. Flinkkilä, M. Laitinen, and V. M. Mattila, "Epidemiology of proximal humerus fractures," *Archives of Osteoporosis*, vol. 10, no. 1, p. 209, 2015.

[3] J. Maalouly, A. Tawk, D. Aouad et al., "Association of acromial morphological parameters and rotator cuff tears, and evaluation of the influence of age and gender on the parameters and impact on cuff tears: a study on a Middle Eastern population," *Asia-Pacific journal of sports medicine, arthroscopy, rehabilitation and technology*, vol. 20, pp. 17–23, 2020.

[4] J. Maalouly, A. Tawk, D. Aouad et al., "Is there an association between glenoid parameters and rotator cuff tears and the influence of gender: a retrospective study on a Middle Eastern population," *International Journal of Surgery Case Reports*, vol. 68, pp. 74–82, 2020.

[5] J. A. Baron, J. A. Barrett, and M. R. Karagas, "The epidemiology of peripheral fractures," *Bone*, vol. 18, no. 3, pp. S209–S213, 1996.

[6] C. M. Court-Brown, A. Garg, and M. M. McQueen, "The epidemiology of proximal humeral fractures," *Acta Orthopaedica Scandinavica*, vol. 72, no. 4, pp. 365–371, 2009.

[7] M. D. Gurzì, D. De Meo, M. Pugliese, L. Di Giorgio, P. Persiani, and C. Villani, "Bilateral posterior fracture-dislocation of the shoulder after epileptic seizure," *Trauma case reports*, vol. 13, pp. 35–41, 2018.

[8] J. L. Shaw, "Bilateral posterior fracture-dislocation of the shoulder and other trauma caused by convulsive seizures," *The Journal of Bone and Joint Surgery*, vol. 53, no. 7, pp. 1437–1440, 1971.

[9] K. M. Din and B. F. Meggitt, "Bilateral four-part fractures with posterior dislocation of the shoulder. A case report," *The Journal of Bone and Joint Surgery British volume*, vol. 65-B, no. 2, pp. 176–178, 1983.

[10] J. Maalouly, D. Aouad, N. Dib, A. Tawk, and G. El Rassi, "Simultaneous ORIF for bilateral comminuted proximal humerus fractures: case report in an elderly patient," *International Journal of Surgery Case Reports*, vol. 65, pp. 193–196, 2019.

[11] L. Ceri, N. Mondanelli, R. Sangaletti, V. Bottai, F. Muratori, and S. Giannotti, "Simultaneous bilateral reverse shoulder arthroplasty for bilateral four-part fracture of the proximal humerus in an elderly patient: a case report," *Trauma case reports*, vol. 23, p. 100242, 2019.

[12] B. G. Leggin, L. A. Michener, M. A. Shaffer, S. K. Brenneman, J. P. Iannotti, and G. R. Williams Jr., "The Penn shoulder score: reliability and validity," *The Journal of Orthopaedic and Sports Physical Therapy*, vol. 36, no. 3, pp. 138–151, 2006.

[13] A. K. Gupta, J. D. Harris, B. J. Erickson et al., "Surgical management of complex proximal humerus fractures-a systematic review of 92 studies including 4500 patients," *Journal of Orthopaedic Trauma*, vol. 29, no. 1, pp. 54–59, 2015.

[14] B. I. Yahuaca, P. Simon, K. N. Christmas et al., "Acute surgical management of proximal humerus fractures: ORIF vs. hemiarthroplasty vs. reverse shoulder arthroplasty," *Journal of Shoulder and Elbow Surgery*, vol. 29, no. 7, pp. S32–S40, 2020.

[15] A. Klug, J. Harth, R. Hoffmann, and Y. Gramlich, "Surgical treatment of complex proximal humeral fractures in elderly patients: a matched-pair analysis of angular-stable plating vs. reverse shoulder arthroplasty," *Journal of Shoulder and Elbow Surgery*, vol. 29, no. 9, pp. 1796–1803, 2020.

[16] R. H. Mattson and B. E. Gidal, "Fractures, epilepsy, and antiepileptic drugs," *Epilepsy & behavior: E&B*, vol. 5, Suppl 2, pp. 36–S40, 2004.

[17] A. N. Fraser, J. Bjørdal, T. M. Wagle et al., "Reverse shoulder arthroplasty is superior to plate fixation at 2 years for displaced proximal humeral fractures in the elderly," *The Journal of Bone and Joint Surgery*, vol. 102, no. 6, pp. 477–485, 2020.

[18] S. J. Stanbury and I. Voloshin, "Reverse shoulder arthroplasty for acute proximal humeral fractures in the geriatric patient: a review of the literature," *Geriatric orthopaedic surgery & rehabilitation*, vol. 2, no. 5-6, pp. 181–186, 2011.

# 29

# Distal Radius Salter-Harris III Transitional Fracture in an Adolescent Male

**Adam Kurland,[1] Brian Batko,[1] Jeremy Hreha,[1] and Ashley Ignatiuk[2]**

[1]*Department of Orthopaedic Surgery, Rutgers New Jersey Medical School, New Jersey, USA*
[2]*Department of Surgery, Plastic & Reconstructive Surgery Division, Rutgers New Jersey Medical School, New Jersey, USA*

Correspondence should be addressed to Adam Kurland; amk355@njms.rutgers.edu

Academic Editor: Wan Ismail Faisham

In contrast to the well-described Tillaux fracture of the distal tibia, transitional fractures of the distal radius are exceedingly rare and have yet to be well described. Thus far, their presence in the literature has been limited to case reports and a singular series. None have involved a Salter-Harris III fracture pattern. We present the case of a 16-year-old male who sustained a Salter-Harris III transitional fracture of the distal radius with an associated ulnar styloid avulsion fracture secondary to a fall that was treated nonoperatively. Similar to the Tillaux fracture, examination of the distal radius transitional fracture should include computed tomography scan to better illustrate the pattern of injury and guide treatment.

## 1. Introduction

Transitional fractures are intra-articular fractures that occur during the process of physeal fusion in adolescents. It is estimated that up to 20% of physeal fractures in adolescents are transitional fractures [1]. They are most frequently found at the distal tibia [2], and the physiology of the closure of this physis is well understood [3–5]. Fractures of the distal radius are the most common pediatric fracture [6]; however, transitional fractures at this location are rare, and the physiology of the physeal closure of the distal radius has been only minimally elucidated [7]. Only one study has investigated this physeal closure using sequential MRIs and found that mineralization of this physis begins centroradially then ulnarly and progresses in a counterclockwise direction with completion at the peripheral dorsoradial area [7]. Their data also indicate that the process takes less than a year to complete, which suggests why this fracture pattern may be so uncommon [7].

To date, there have been few reports involving transitional fractures at the distal radius. A limited number of case reports and a case series involve triplane fractures of the distal radius but none yet that describe a Salter-Harris III fracture pattern [8–11]. We thus present this case of a 16-year-old male with a transitional, Salter-Harris III fracture of the dorsal ulnar corner of the distal radius.

## 2. Case Report

A 16-year-old right hand dominant Hispanic male presented to the emergency department complaining of left wrist pain after falling off of a bicycle onto an outstretched hand one day prior. On examination, the patient's skin was intact, and he had minor swelling from the midforearm to the hand. He was tender over the distal radius and ulnar styloid. No distal radioulnar joint instability was identified on exam when compared to the contralateral wrist. Motor strength was normal for his hand intrinsic muscles, but wrist flexion and extension were limited secondary to pain. Sensation was intact to light touch over the volar and dorsal aspects of the hand in median, ulnar, and radial nerve distributions. He had a palpable radial pulse and brisk capillary refill at all digits.

Plain radiographs of the left wrist showed a minimally displaced ulnar styloid avulsion fracture and a Salter-Harris III fracture of the distal radius involving only the dorsal ulnar corner which progressed from the dorsoulnar end of the distal radial epiphysis in the sagittal plane proximally into

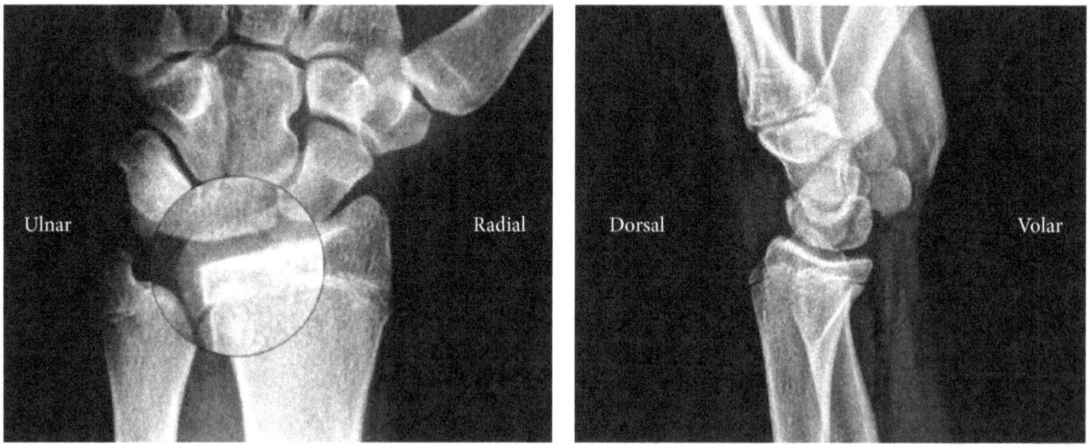


Figure 1: Plain PA and lateral radiographs of the left wrist demonstrating intra-articular fracture at dorsoulnar lip of the radius.

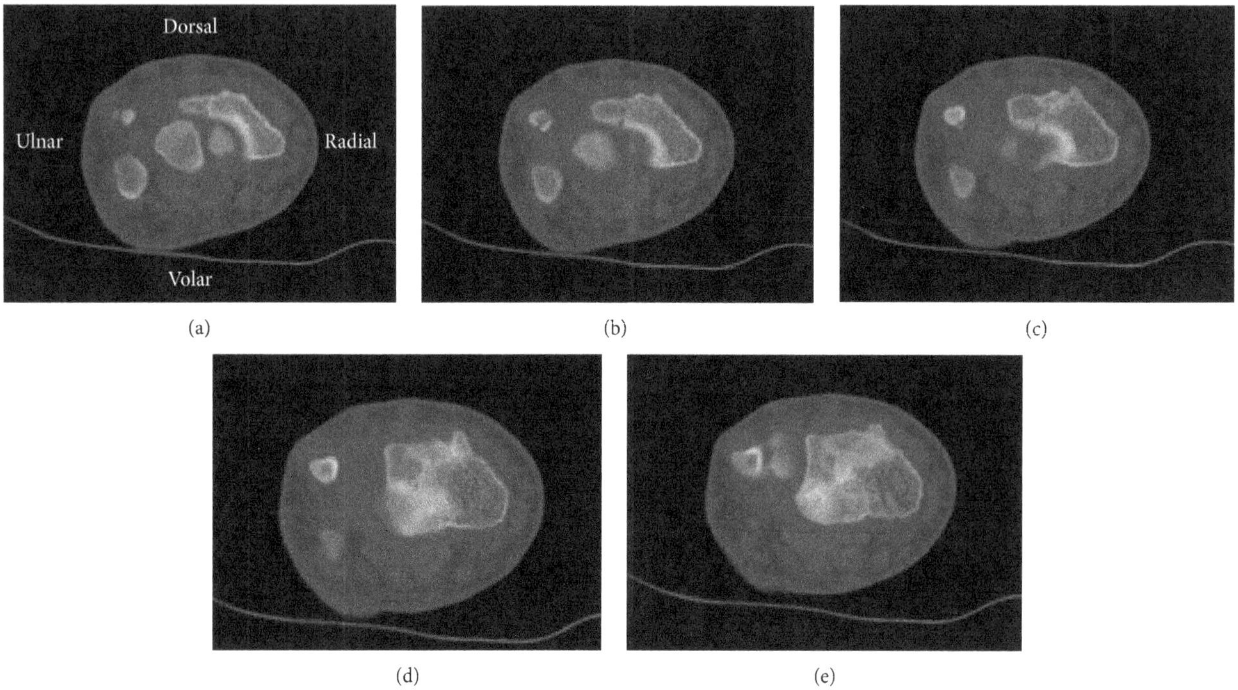


Figure 2: Sequential axial CT views (proximal to distal) demonstrating intra-articular extent of the fracture through the dorsal rim of the radial physis. (d) Shows the radial epiphysis fully in view, revealing the most volar extent of the fracture line dorsal to the volar ulnar rim.

the physis separating the dorsal and volar ulnar rims and extending ulnarly through the physis and into the distal radial ulnar joint (Figure 1). There was no articular step-off. Also visible was the predominantly closed physeal plate and mild negative ulnar variance. The patient was placed in a well-padded sugar-tong splint and made nonweight bearing to his left upper extremity.

The patient was transitioned to a short arm cast at 1.5 weeks with repeat radiographs demonstrating maintained articular alignment and with no distal radioulnar joint instability. A CT scan was attempted at this time but due to patient scheduling conflicts could not be obtained. At 4 weeks after the initial presentation, the cast was removed. The patient had improved range of motion but with only subtle pain and remained tender to palpation at the wrist. CT scan obtained 6 weeks postinjury showed an intra-articular distal radius fracture along the dorsal rim of the radius that had largely healed, while the physis of the distal radius was shown to be narrowed and largely fused (Figures 2–4). He was placed in a volar resting splint that could be removed for gentle range of motion exercises. By his latest follow-up visit at 3 months postinjury, the patient had returned to his normal activities of daily living. He was nontender at the wrist and had full wrist flexion and extension, as well as painless radial and ulnar deviation. Due to restrictions from COVID-19, the patient only had a telehealth visit, and thus, no radiographic imaging is available demonstrating a fully healed fracture.

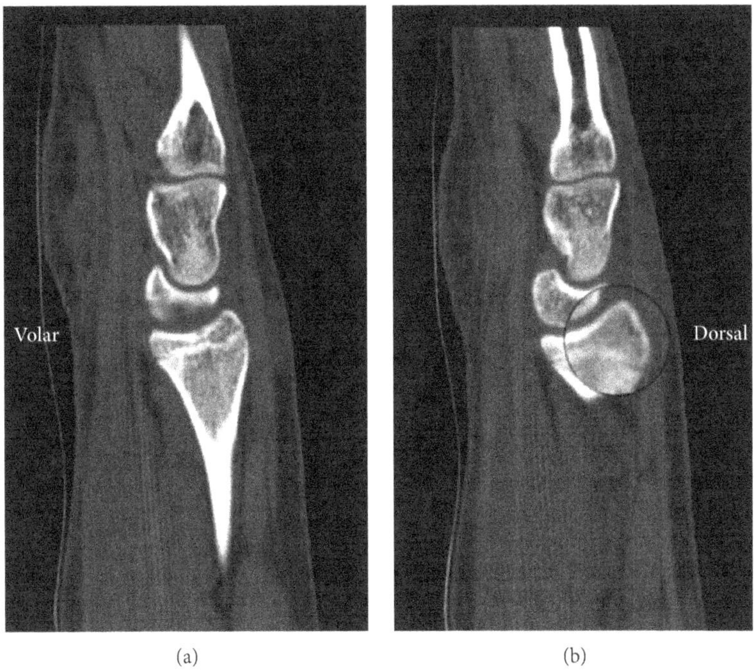


FIGURE 3: Sagittal CT view showing intra-articular extent of the fracture through the dorsal rim of the radius with interval healing.

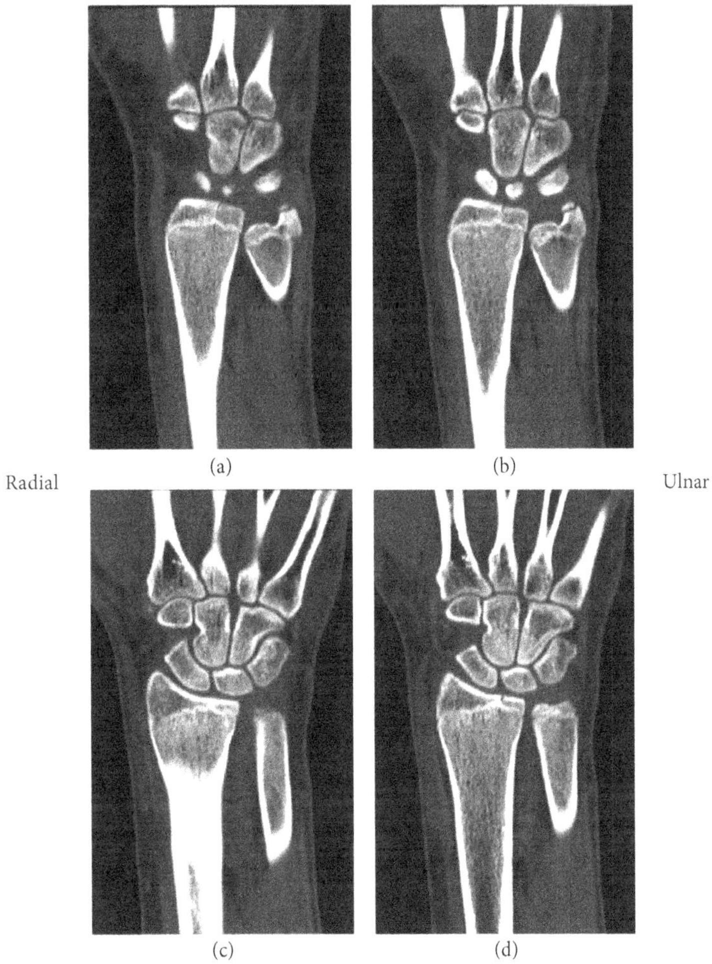


FIGURE 4: Coronal CT view showing location of fracture at dorsal rim with interval healing and narrowed and fusing radial physis.

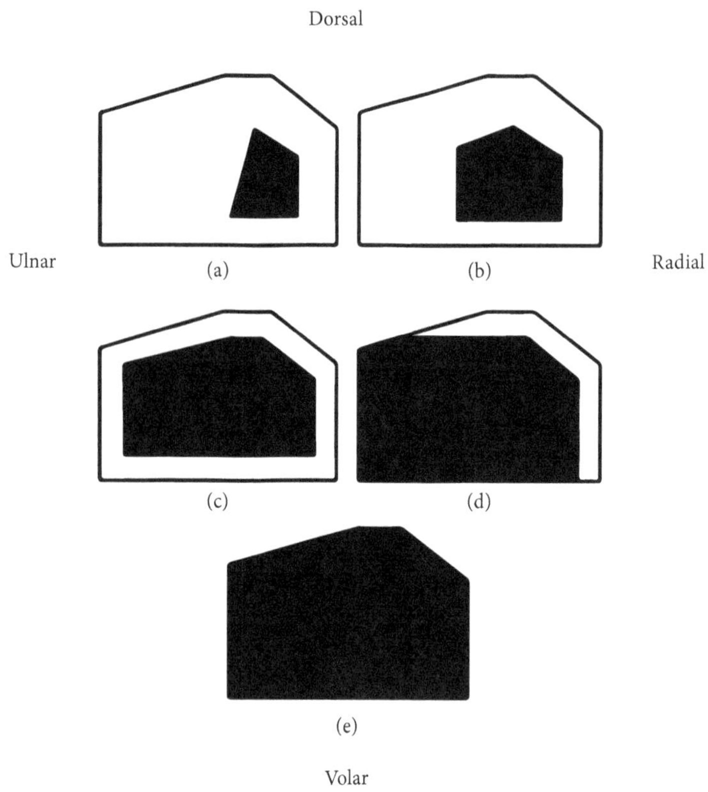


FIGURE 5: Sequence of fusion of the distal radial physis as identified by Kraus et al. [7]. Reprinted with permission.

## 3. Discussion

In contrast to Tillaux fractures of the distal tibia, transitional fractures of the distal radius are exceedingly rare and have yet to be well described. The physeal closure process of the distal radius takes less than a year to complete [7], as opposed to approximately 18 months in the distal tibia [1], which suggests why this fracture pattern may be so rare. Typically, if the dorsal and volar ulnar rims fragment, they do so concurrently as two distinct pieces. Rarely, one fractures while the other remains intact. The fracture presented in our case involves only the dorsal ulnar corner and traverses the dorsoulnar rim of the patient's physis, which is consistent with the region of the physis that is last to fuse [7] (Figure 5). As such, it is likely the progression of fusion that is responsible for our patient's unusual fracture pattern.

Treatment of transitional fractures of the distal radius should be managed similar to other adolescent transitional fractures. We recommend obtaining a CT scan to better define fracture displacement as this will dictate treatment. Similar to transitional fractures of the distal tibia, we suggest nonoperative management of intra-articular fractures with < 2 mm of displacement. If displaced, reduction and screw fixation is recommended. Closed reduction with k-wire fragment manipulation can be attempted; however, if displacement remains, open reduction is necessary. A dorsal approach to the distal radius is recommended to adequately visualize the fracture. Screw fixation across the physis can be performed with minimal deformity risk as patients are near the end of growth and physeal function.

In conclusion, transitional fractures of the distal radius are exceedingly rare and occur due to the physiology of physeal closure described by Kraus et al. [7]. To our knowledge, we are the first to present a case of Salter-Harris III transitional fracture of the distal radius. Treatment of these fractures should be managed similar to other adolescent transitional fractures. Greater than 2 mm of displacement seen on CT scan warrants operative fixation. Further study of Salter-Harris III fractures of the distal radius is needed to elucidate the long-term results of these fractures.

## References

[1] J. Kärrholm, "The triplane fracture: four years of follow-up of 21 cases and review of the literature," *Journal of Pediatric Orthopaedics. Part B*, vol. 6, no. 2, pp. 91–102, 1997.

[2] D. Schneidmueller, C. von Rüden, J. Friederichs, and V. Bühren, "Übergangsfraktur," *Der Unfallchirurg*, vol. 119, no. 6, pp. 517–526, 2016.

[3] L. von Laer, "Classification, diagnosis, and treatment of transitional fractures of the distal part of the tibia," *The Journal of Bone and Joint Surgery. American Volume*, vol. 67, no. 5, pp. 687–698, 1985.

[4] J. R. Cass and H. A. Peterson, "Salter-Harris type-IV injuries of the distal tibial epiphyseal growth plate, with emphasis on

those involving the medial malleolus," *The Journal of Bone and Joint Surgery. American Volume*, vol. 65, no. 8, pp. 1059–1070, 1983.

[5] J. C. Hoeffel, P. Lascombes, T. Poncelet et al., "Tillaux's fracture," *Journal de Radiologie*, vol. 70, no. 3, pp. 213–217, 1989.

[6] J. C. Cheng and W. Y. Shen, "Limb fracture pattern in different pediatric age groups: a study of 3,350 children," *Journal of Orthopaedic Trauma*, vol. 7, no. 1, pp. 15–22, 1993.

[7] R. Kraus, J. Reyers, V. Alt, R. Schnettler, and L. A. R. S. D. Berthold, "Physiological closure of the physeal plate of the distal radius: an MRI analysis," *Clinical Anatomy*, vol. 24, no. 8, pp. 1010–1015, 2011.

[8] T. Rauer, H. Pape, J. G. Gamble, N.'. Vitale, S. Halvachizadeh, and F. Allemann, "Transitional fracture of the distal radius: a rare injury in adolescent athletes. *Case series and literature review*," *European Journal of Medical Research*, vol. 25, no. 1, 2020.

[9] S. García-Mata and A. Hidalgo-Ovejero, "Triplane fracture of the distal radius," *Journal of Pediatric Orthopaedics. Part B*, vol. 15, no. 4, pp. 298–301, 2006.

[10] A. A. Parkar, S. Marya, and S. Auplish, "Distal radius triplane fracture," *The Annals of The Royal College of Surgeons of England*, vol. 96, no. 8, pp. e6–e7, 2014.

[11] R. Kraus, G. Szalay, C. Meyer, O. Kilian, and R. Schnettler, "Die Distale Radiusfraktur - eine Torwartverletzung bei Kindern und Jugendlichen," *Sportverletz Sportschaden*, vol. 21, no. 4, pp. 177–179, 2007.

# 30

# Clinical and Biomechanical Outcomes of One-Stage Treatment of a Simultaneous Ipsilateral Patellar Tendon and ACL Tear Combined with a Tibial Plateau Fracture: A Case Study

**Petros Ismailidis,[1,2,3] Rolf Kernen,[4] Christian Egloff,[1] Corina Nüesch,[1,2,3] Annegret Mündermann,[1,2,3] and Sebastian Andreas Müller[1]**

[1]*Department of Orthopaedics and Traumatology, University Hospital Basel, Spitalstrasse 21, 4031 Basel, Switzerland*
[2]*Department of Biomedical Engineering, University of Basel, Gewerbestrasse 14, 4123 Allschwil, Switzerland*
[3]*Department of Clinical Research, University of Basel, Schanzenstrasse 55, 4056 Basel, Switzerland*
[4]*Clinic for Orthopedics "Claraortho", Claragraben 82 4058 Basel, Switzerland*

Correspondence should be addressed to Petros Ismailidis; petrosismailidis@gmail.com

Academic Editor: Zbigniew Gugala

Simultaneous ipsilateral patellar tendon (PT) and anterior cruciate ligament (ACL) tear is a rare injury. Associated meniscal and ligamentous injuries are common but frequently initially missed. In contrast, to date, there is no report of associated fractures. We report on a 40-year-old female Caucasian patient presenting with a ski injury resulting in simultaneous ipsilateral patellar tendon and ACL tear combined with a tibia plateau fracture and a medial and lateral meniscus lesion. ORIF of the tibia as well as one-stage primary reconstruction of the PT and ACL and suturing of the menisci was conducted. The final follow-up was 2 years postoperatively. Lower extremity kinematic, kinetic, and muscle activity measurements were conducted. Although the clinical result was excellent, altered joint kinematics went along with large side-to-side difference in hip and knee joint moments during midstance and terminal stance. During weight acceptance, vastus medialis and hamstring muscles showed greater relative activity in the injured than the uninjured side. This case demonstrates the possibility of excellent early and midterm results with a one-stage approach and suitable rehabilitation scheme. Biomechanical measurements could further help evaluate the outcome of the treatments and implications for the development of potential secondary damage.

## 1. Introduction

Simultaneous ipsilateral patellar tendon (PT) and anterior cruciate ligament (ACL) tear is a rare injury. A systematic review in 2018 identified 28 cases in 17 published reports in the English literature [1]. Associated meniscal and ligamentous injuries are common but frequently initially missed [1]. In contrast, to date, there is no report of associated fractures. Moreover, there are no established treatment algorithms: open and arthroscopic approaches, as well as one- or two-stage approaches, have been described [2]. In our study, we report on a patellar tendon and ACL tear combined with a tibia plateau fracture in a middle age physically active female patient.

## 2. Case Report

Written patient consent was received and archived. A 40-year-old patient without any preexisting injury or morbidity suffered a knee injury while skiing. The exact injury mechanism was not clear; however, the patient described no direct impact and recalls a twisting injury. The patient initially presented herself to a local health center. The X-rays revealed a fracture of the tibia. Both the PT and the ACL rupture were initially overlooked. The patient was referred to our institution for the definitive treatment. On presentation at our institution, there was a large knee effusion with a palpable infrapatellar gap. Straight leg raise was impossible. X-ray analysis (Figure 1) revealed—in addition to the

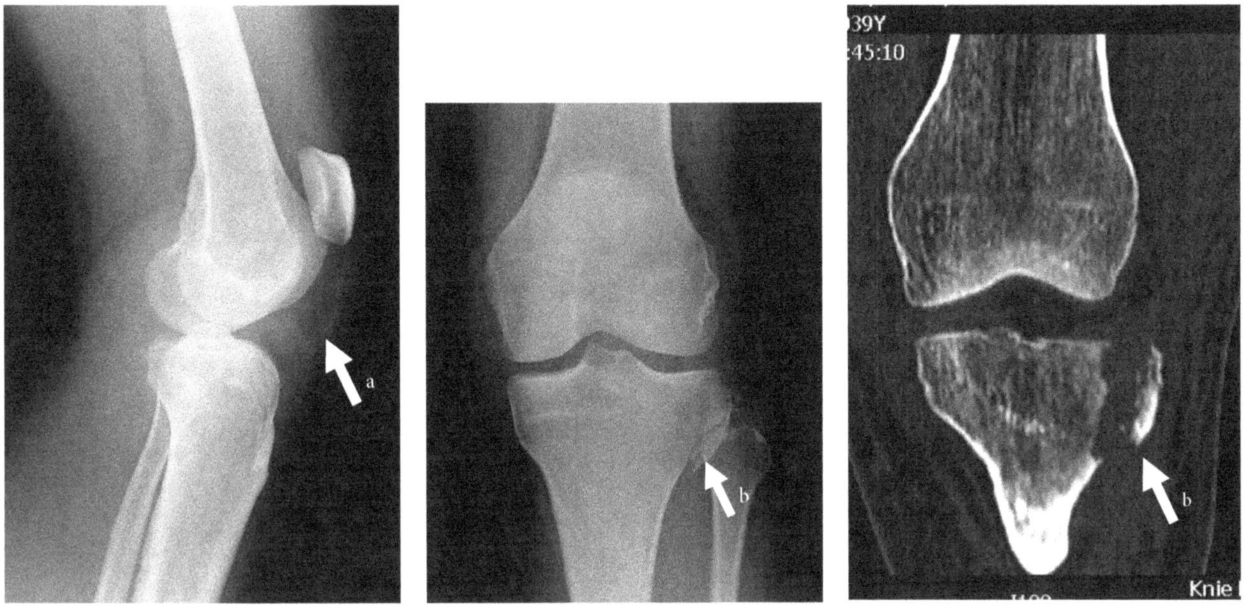


(a) (b) (c)

FIGURE 1: Preoperative X-rays: anterior-posterior (a), lateral (b), and coronal (c) view CT. Note the patella alta with a Caton Deschamps index of 1.5 (A) as an indirect sign of the PT rupture, as well as tibial plateau fracture (B).

lateral tibial plateau fracture—a patella alta (Caton Deschamps index [3] of 1.5) and raised the suspicion of a PT injury. Specific ACL tests were not reliable because of the large effusion and pain, which did not allow manipulation required for the tests. The CT scan (Figure 1) allowed the further evaluation of the tibial plateau fracture (Schatzker type 1 [4]) and the proximal migration of the patella and confirmed the diagnosis of PT rupture. The patient was scheduled for surgery on the following day with the diagnosis of a tibial plateau fracture and PT rupture. No MRI was conducted.

The operation was performed through an anterior midline incision. The diagnosis of a full thickness PT tear was confirmed, and a complete proximal tear of the ACL as well as a bucket handle injury of both menisci was diagnosed (Figure 2(a)). We decided to immediately suture both menisci and to perform a primary repair of the ACL and PT. Furthermore, there were chondral lesion Grades I-II [5] at both femoral condyles that were not addressed surgically.

The tibial plateau fracture was reduced and fixed with a lateral 4.5 mm T-Plate (Figures 2 and 3). The plate was manually contoured to best fit the tibia anatomy, the proximal screws were partially threaded to achieve interfragmentary compression, and the rest of the screws were normal cortex screws. The ACL was ruptured on the femoral side (Sherman type 1 [6]). The tibial stump was anchored 5 mm Mersilene Tape (Ethicon, Somerville, NJ) whip stitches and then passed through a femoral tunnel at the femoral origin of the ACL and secured on the femoral side with a 3.5 mm screw used as a suture post. The menisci were sutured with horizontal inside-out mattress stitches using number 2-0 Mersilene (Ethicon, Somerville, NJ) sutures. Finally, the PT was repaired using number 2 Vicryl whip stitches and secured with a McLaughlin cerclage with a 1.5 mm wire (Figures 2 and 3).

The knee was protected in a mobile brace for 6 weeks. The patient was mobilized with protected weight bearing of 15 kg for 6 weeks; the allowed range of motion (ROM) was restricted to 30° of flexion and gradually increased in increments of 30° every 2 weeks. The early physiotherapy focused on gradually regaining ROM including contiguous passive motion and quadriceps function with closed chain exercises. Stationary cycling and proprioceptive exercises were initiated 4 months posttrauma. Running was initiated at 6 months.

The postoperative follow-up showed no complications. The patient had a ROM of 90-0-0° 6 weeks after surgery. There was no breakage of the cerclage. Three months postoperatively, the cerclage was removed and a diagnostic arthroscopy was performed. The arthroscopy showed complete healing of the ACL and both menisci (Figure 4). The return to daily activities was uncomplicated already 6 months postoperatively. One year postoperatively, the lateral tibia plate was removed. A control arthroscopy was recommended. This would allow us to inspect the menisci and ACL reconstruction as well as perform a notchplasty in case of an intraoperatively ascertained ACL impingement. The arthroscopy was not performed because of the lack of cost coverage by the health insurance company and additionally because the patient was fully satisfied with the result and wanted to limit the intervention to the implant removal only.

The final follow-up was 2 years postoperatively: the IKDC Score was 90, the Lysholm Score 94, and the ROM 145-5-0° (contralateral ROM 150-0-10°). Isokinetic knee flexor and extensor strength tests were performed at 60°/s and 240°/s using an isokinetic dynamometer (Biodex System 4 Pro: Biodex Medical Systems, Shirley, NY, USA). At 240°/s, knee flexor strength was 5.0% higher and knee extensor strength and work were 20% and 22% lower, respectively, in the injured leg than in the contralateral leg. At 60°/s, knee

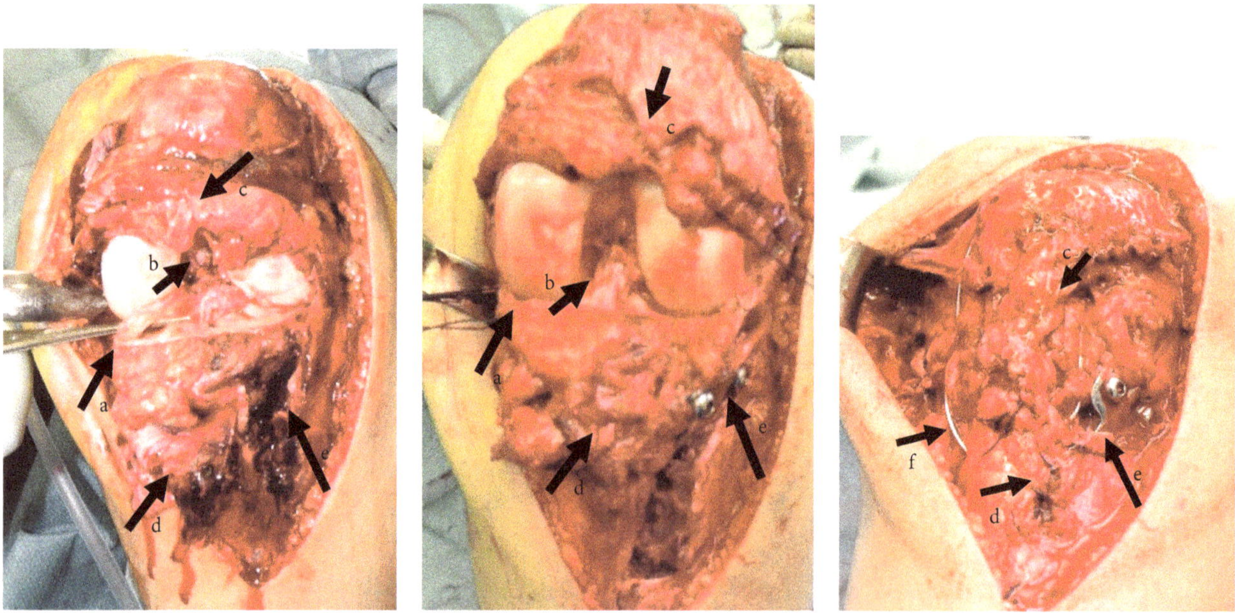


(a) (b) (c)

FIGURE 2: Intraoperative photos after the exposure of the joint (a); after the ORIF of the tibia, ACL reconstruction, and meniscus suturing (b); and after the PT repair (c). Note on the figures: (A) bucket handle tear of the medial meniscus before and after suturing, (B) absence of the ACL in the notch, the tibial stump of the ACL, and the reconstructed ACL, (C) the proximal and (D) distal stump of the PT before and after reconstruction, (E) the tibial plateau fracture before and after ORIF, and (F) the McLaughlin wire.

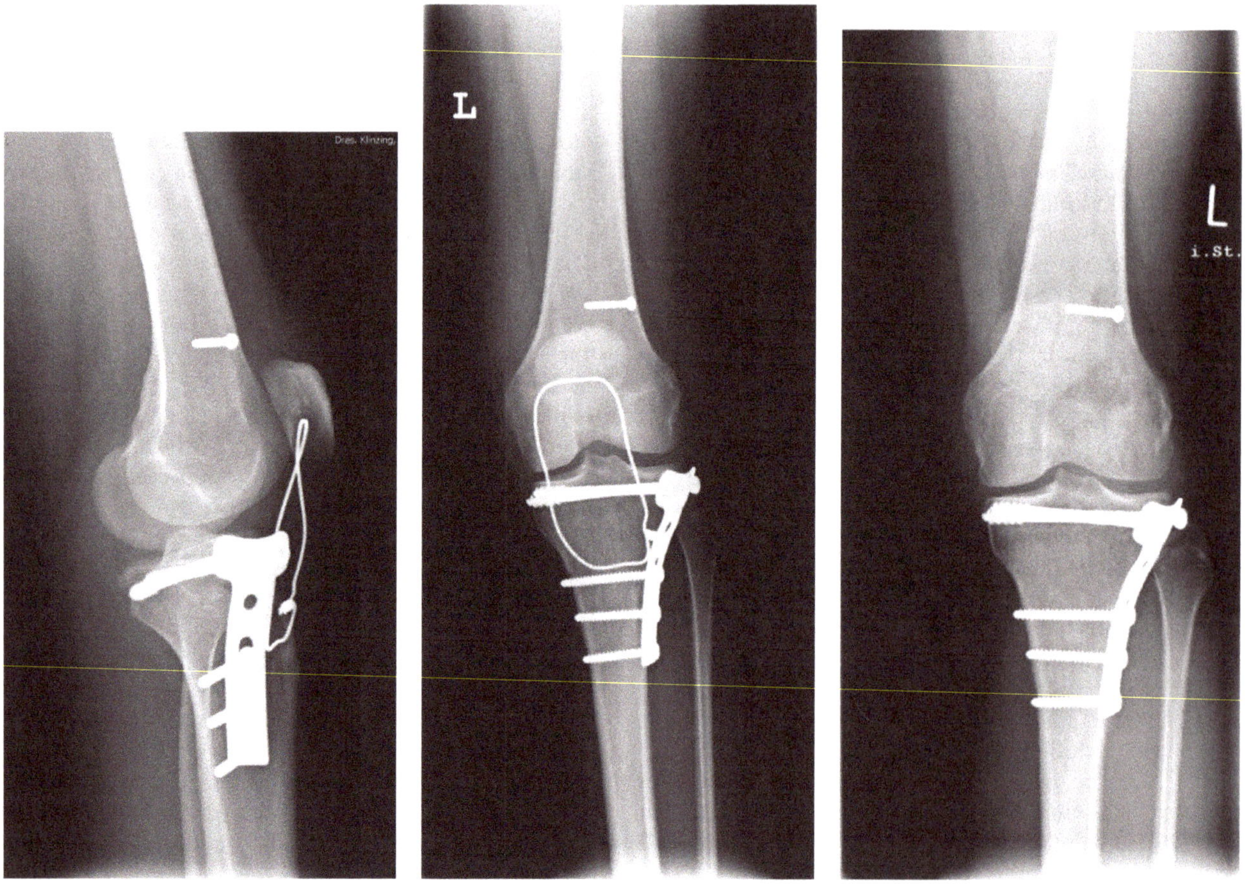


(a) (b) (c)

FIGURE 3: Radiographic result after the operation (a, b) and after the removal of the McLaughlin wire (c).

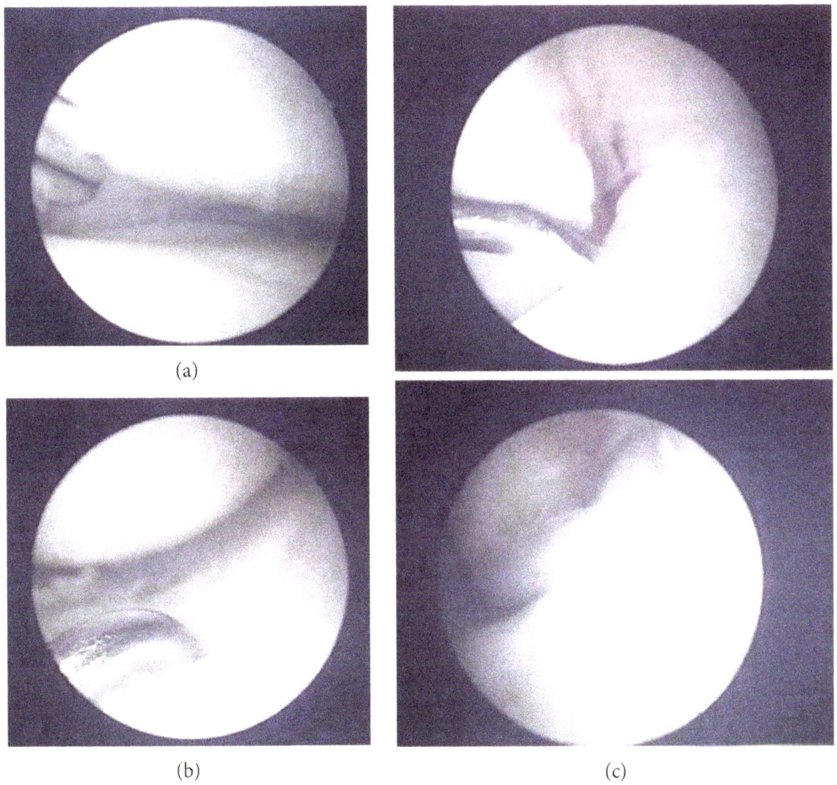

FIGURE 4: Arthroscopic views of the medial (a) and lateral (b) meniscus and the ACL (c) 3 months postoperatively. The ACL and both menisci were healed.

flexor strength was 5% higher and knee extensor strength and work were 7% and 8% lower, respectively, with a clear delay in force production of the knee extensors in the injured leg compared to the contralateral leg.

Lower extremity kinematic and kinetic data and muscle activity were collected during overground walking at 1.7 ± 0.1 m/s using an 8-camera motion analysis system (Vicon, Oxford, UK; sampling rate: 120 Hz), two force plates (Kistler, Winterthur, Switzerland; sampling rate: 2400 Hz), and a 12-channel surface electromyography (EMG) system (myon AG, Schwarzenberg, Switzerland, sampling rate 2400 Hz). Throughout the gait cycle, both the hip and the knee were in more flexed positions on the injured than the uninjured side (Figure 5). The injured knee presented a 6° extension deficit during terminal stance and a 16° higher flexion throughout swing. This altered joint kinematics went along with large side-to-side difference in hip and knee joint moments during midstance and terminal stance (Figure 5). During this interval, knee extension moments were 65% lower and hip extension moments were 89% higher in the injured than the uninjured side despite similar vertical ground reaction forces in both sides. From terminal stance through swing, the ankle on the injured side was approximately 6° more dorsiflexed than that on the uninjured side. In midstance, the gastrocnemius medialis muscle was less activated and the ankle dorsiflexion moment was 6% smaller on the injured side than the uninjured side (Figure 6). The tibialis anterior and vastus lateralis muscles showed similar activities on both sides throughout the gait cycle. During weight acceptance, vastus medialis and hamstring muscles showed greater relative activity in the injured than the uninjured side. During early swing, relative hamstring muscle activity was lower in the injured than uninjured side.

## 3. Discussion

Simultaneous ipsilateral PT and ACL tear is a rare injury with only very few studies reporting on this injury, the largest of which reports on 6 patients [7]. Hence, there is no clear evidence on the optimal diagnostic procedures, treatment, or expected outcomes. However, the existing literature reported a few interesting findings.

*3.1. Associated Injuries.* With the exception of two reported cases [7, 8], combined PT and ACL tears always occurred with associated ligamentous or meniscal injuries. While only one case reported a knee dislocation on the initial X-rays [9], a dislocation and spontaneous reduction before the consultation could be possible in our case as in all other cases reporting on PT and ACL injury. Rupture of the medial collateral ligament (MCL) was the most frequent (66.0%) ligament injury, and 69.0% of patients had an injury in either one or both menisci [1]. In contrast, to date, there is no report of associated fractures. PT and ACL rupture or the associated injuries are commonly missed at initial clinical and radiological diagnostics and only diagnosed intraoperatively. Cumulatively, in 43.3% of the reported cases, the ACL or the PT rupture was initially missed [1]. While in these studies, X-rays of the knee in two planes were the standard diagnostic procedure; preoperative CT or MRI was not conducted

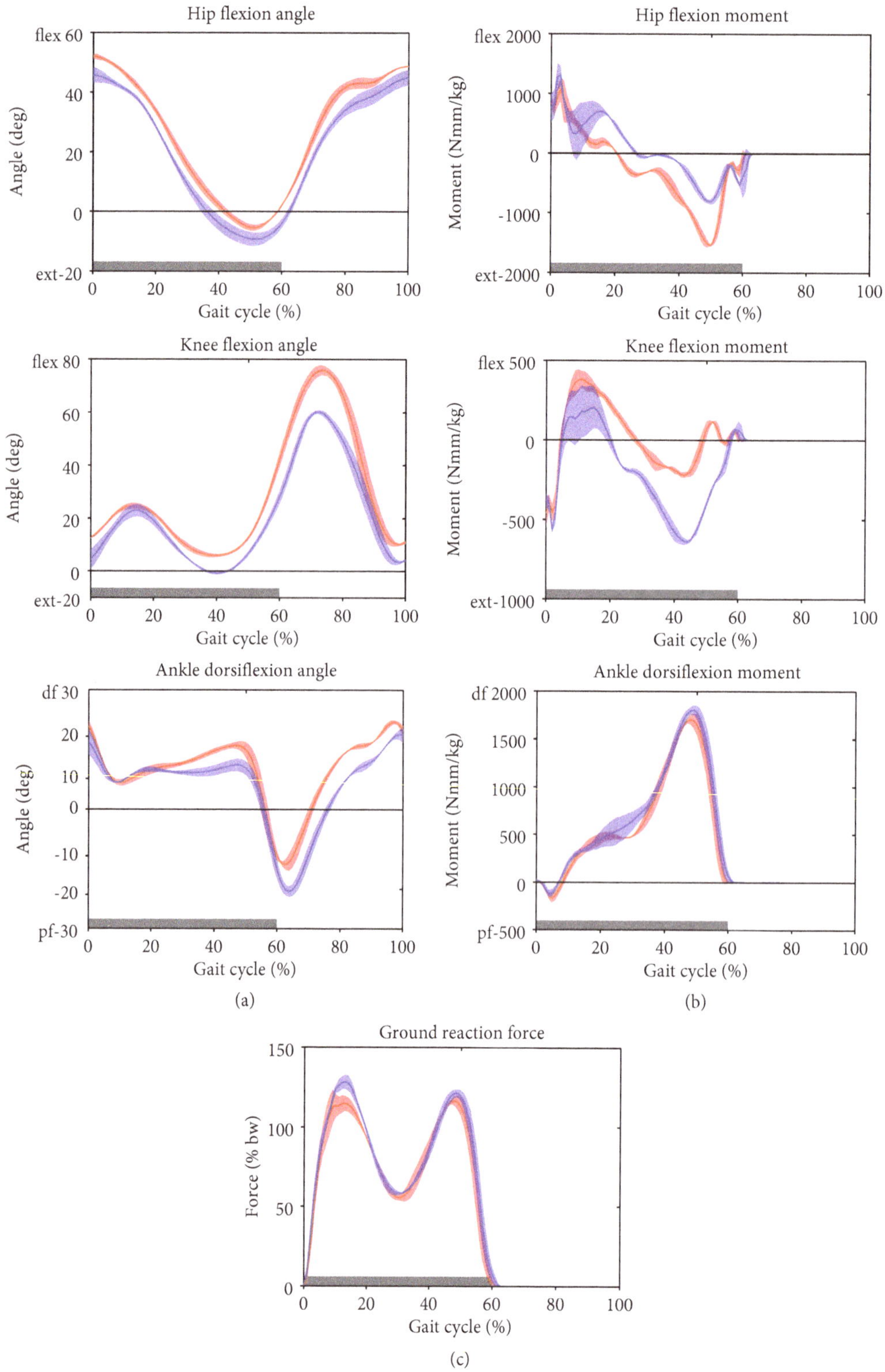


FIGURE 5: Joint angles (a) and resultant external joint moments (b) in the sagittal plane and vertical ground reaction force (c) during walking. Gait data was normalized to one gait cycle.

routinely. In our case, a part of the injury was also missed by the initial diagnostic procedures.

*3.2. Treatment Strategies.* Previously reported cases were treated with various treatment strategies. Apart from one case where the patient was presented with a delay of 2 months [8], the PT injury was always directly repaired, while in most reports (75%), the ACL was also addressed surgically. Of these, 50% were one-stage procedures (primary PT repair and ACL reconstruction), and the other 50% were two-stage

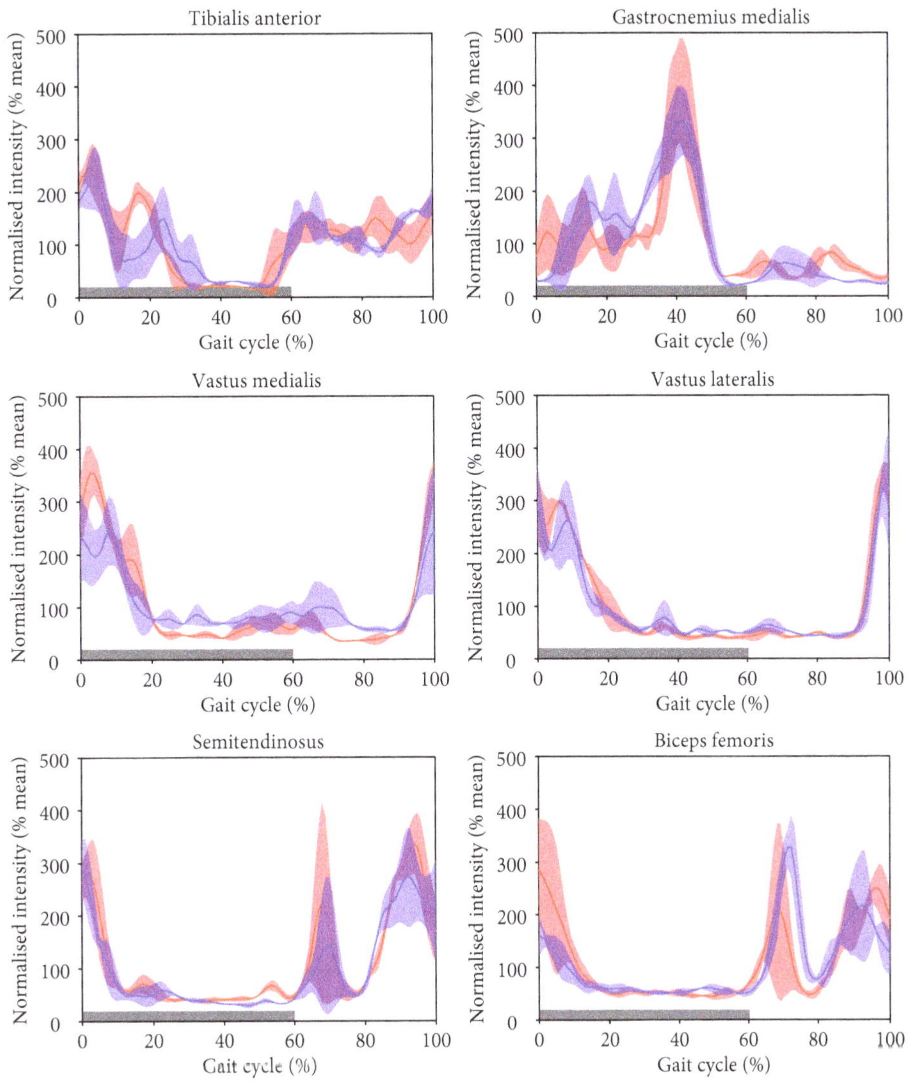


FIGURE 6: Relative muscle activity of selected lower extremity muscles during walking. Gait data was normalized to one gait cycle.

procedures (primary PT repair followed by ACL reconstruction) [1]. The rehabilitation scheme differed between reported cases: most authors prescribed some kind of ROM restriction similar to that commonly used after PT reconstructions and in contrast to the early ROM mobilization usually used after ACL reconstruction. The rehabilitation of the PT repair (restricted ROM) theoretically conflicts with that of the ACL (early ROM encouraged) leading some authors to the decision of waiting for the full rehabilitation of the PT injury before addressing the ACL. In our opinion and as demonstrated in this case, a combined scheme is feasible; the rehabilitation alone should be no reason to avoid a one-stage approach, especially if the ACL is avulsed proximally and amenable for a primary repair. Although no specific literature for combined ACL and PT injuries exists, current concepts of treating multiligament injuries in the knee also imply this principle: all injured structures should be reconstructed concurrently [10] so that an early postoperative knee ROM can be initiated in order to minimize the risk of postoperative stiffness.

Of the authors reporting an ACL reconstruction, 77% used an autograft while the rest used an allograft or a prosthetic ligament [7]. None of the surgeons reported on a direct reconstruction of the ACL. Some authors of previous reports preferred an arthroscopic ACL reconstruction and reported good results using this technique [7]. Arthroscopic ACL reconstruction with autograft or allograft is a standardized procedure with usually good results [11]. However, we believe that—because an open approach is necessary for the PT reconstruction—the ACL repair can be conducted directly through the same approach. In contrast to an autograft or allograft reconstruction, a direct repair seems like a risky option. Historically, direct repair of the ACL has been widely abandoned in favor of ACL reconstruction because of the unpredictable results and the high rates of failure. However, recently, interest on direct repair has increased again with animal and human studies providing promising results given careful patient selection [12]. In the presence of a proximal tear, a direct repair appears to be a good option sparing the need for an autograft and offering the advantages of preserving proprioception and better reconstructing knee kinematics above all with the addition of an internal reinforcing bracing device [12].

*3.3. Outcome.* Good outcomes were reported for one- and two-stage approaches and for all surgical methods including arthroscopic and open arthroscopic-assisted techniques as well as open surgery. In all but one reported cases [8], patients achieved full knee extension and knee flexion above 120°. The follow-up varied from 6 months to 4 years. However, specific orthopedic scores were documented in only less than half of the cases, and strength measurements were only performed in three studies [13–15]. Although return to daily activities and sport is expected after a surgical repair, most studies did not specify the time frame in which this was achieved [2]. Although postoperative complications such as patella baja, surgical site infection [7], complex regional pain syndrome and stiffness [8], persistent patellofemoral crepitus [16], and arthrofibrosis [17] were reported, these complications did not negatively influence the long-term result except in one case [8] in which the partial PT rupture was not addressed surgically. In two systematic reviews on this topic, no significant difference in the outcome between the one- and two-stage approaches was detected [1, 2]. However, one of these reviews reported a significantly higher complication rate in the one-stage approach [2].

*3.4. Gait and Functional Analysis.* None of the previous studies has reported on gait analysis or EMG measurements. In our case, the clinically assessed extension deficit of 5° was also portrayed in the kinematics. Hence, the extension of the injured side was reduced through the stance phase, resulting in a higher knee flexion moment (Figure 5). Through the lack of full knee extension, the activity of the vastus medialis and biceps femoris necessary to stabilize the leg through the initial foot contact of the stance phase was increased, resulting in increased relative muscle intensity (Figure 6). Less knee extension during the terminal stance was associated with lower knee extension moments during the terminal stance in the injured limb and higher than normal knee extension moments in the uninjured limb indicating an overload of the contralateral knee. This underlines the importance of increased ROM and particularly of achieving full extension by anatomical ACL reconstruction avoiding anterior graft impingement and by early rehabilitation. Moreover, these results illustrate the need of kinematic and kinetic analysis to fully understand the functional results of the injury and prevent long-term secondary changes not only in the affected limb but also in the contralateral limb. In our case, the extension deficit of only 5°—presumably caused by the injury and clinically judged as not important—appears to have a significant impact on the gait biomechanics of the patient.

Only three previous studies on ACL and PT rupture performed strength measurements [13–15]. For instance, Mariani et al. [14] reported on three cases evaluating isometric strength in extension at 90° knee flexion reporting a deficit compared to the contralateral limb of 21, 24, and 6%, respectively. Cucchi et al. [13] measured isometric strength in knee extension from a starting position with the knee and hip flexed 90° in two patients and reported a strength deficit compared to the contralateral limb of −15% and +20%, respectively. Pérez et al. [15] performed measurements using a manual manometer and reported identical power of quadriceps and hamstrings of the injured leg compared to the contralateral side on the last follow-up of 18 months postoperatively. In our study, we performed isokinetic measurements and measured an increase of 5% in maximum knee flexor strength and a reduction of 19.6% in maximum knee extensor strength. Clearly, gradual strengthening of the extensor muscles is an important goal of the rehabilitation. While the real impact of the injury on the reduction in muscle strength and the period needed to recover is difficult to assess from these individual reports, there was still a knee extensor strength deficit at the final follow-up in 5 of the 7 patients measured [13–15]. This observation is concurrent in our patient who had lower knee extensor strength in the injured side. However, a more flexed knee position requires greater muscle forces represented as greater knee flexion moments during the first half of the stance. The lower force production capacity of the knee extensor muscle in the injured leg explains the greater relative muscle activity of the extensor muscles observed in the first half of the stance. Strengthening knee extensors in the injured limb may not only normalize joint motion during gait but also shift loads (measured by the surrogate joint moment) towards normal values and hence positively affect the long-term outcome after this complex injury.

## 4. Conclusion

To the best of our knowledge, this is the first case reporting on a simultaneous ACL and PT injury combined with a tibial plateau fracture in a nondislocated knee.

Overall, this case adds to the existing knowledge regarding the treatment of simultaneous PT and ACL rupture and emphasizes the need for extensive diagnostic procedures to capture and diagnose possible concomitant injuries. Moreover, the surgeon should rule out additional injuries intraoperatively. This case further shows the potential of excellent early and midterm functional results with a one-stage approach and suitable rehabilitation scheme. Lastly, our results confirm the direct repair as a possible operative technique in cases with proximal rupture of the ACL. Clearly, there is a need for further reports to fully understand and optimally treat combined ACL and PT injuries. Biomechanical measurements could further help evaluate the outcome of the treatments and implications for the development of potential secondary damage.

## Abbreviations

ACL: Anterior cruciate ligament
PT: Patellar tendon
ORIF: Open reduction internal fixation.

## References

[1] A. H. Matthews, E. J. Fraser, and B. Parkinson, "Management of simultaneous patellar tendon and anterior cruciate ligament ruptures—a systematic review of available literature," *Journal of Orthopaedic Trauma*, vol. 32, no. 8, pp. e320–e326, 2018.

[2] C. Meheux, R. Jack II, P. McCulloch, D. Lintner, and J. Harris, "Surgical management of simultaneous anterior cruciate ligament and patellar tendon ruptures: a systematic review," *The Journal of Knee Surgery*, vol. 31, no. 9, pp. 875–883, 2018.

[3] J. Caton, G. Deschamps, P. Chambat, J. L. Lerat, and H. Dejour, "Patella infera. Apropos of 128 cases," *Revue de Chirurgie Orthopédique et Réparatrice de l'Appareil Moteur*, vol. 68, no. 5, pp. 317–325, 1982.

[4] J. Schatzker, R. McBroom, and D. Bruce, "The tibial plateau fracture: the Toronto experience 1968–1975," *Clinical Orthopaedics and Related Research*, vol. 138, pp. 94–104, 1979.

[5] C. Slattery and C. Y. Kweon, "Classifications in brief: outerbridge classification of chondral lesions," *Clinical Orthopaedics and Related Research*, vol. 476, no. 10, pp. 2101–2104, 2018.

[6] M. F. Sherman, L. Lieber, J. R. Bonamo, L. Podesta, and I. Reiter, "The long-term followup of primary anterior cruciate ligament repair. Defining a rationale for augmentation," *The American Journal of Sports Medicine*, vol. 19, no. 3, pp. 243–255, 1991.

[7] Y. Levakos, M. F. Sherman, K. D. Shelbourne, S. Trakru, and J. R. Bonamo, "Simultaneous rupture of the anterior cruciate ligament and the patellar tendon. Six case reports," *The American Journal of Sports Medicine*, vol. 24, no. 4, pp. 498–503, 1996.

[8] R. D. Wissman, N. Vonfischer, and K. Kempf, "Acute concomitant anterior cruciate ligament and patellar tendon tears in a non-dislocated knee," *Journal of Clinical Imaging Science*, vol. 2, p. 3, 2012.

[9] J. Brunkhorst and D. L. Johnson, "Multiligamentous knee injury concomitant with a patellar tendon rupture," *Orthopedics*, vol. 38, no. 1, pp. 45–48, 2015.

[10] K. H. Frosch, A. Preiss, S. Heider et al., "Primary ligament sutures as a treatment option of knee dislocations: a meta-analysis," *Knee Surgery, Sports Traumatology, Arthroscopy*, vol. 21, no. 7, pp. 1502–1509, 2013.

[11] K. L. Poehling-Monaghan, H. Salem, K. E. Ross et al., "Long-term outcomes in anterior cruciate ligament reconstruction: a systematic review of patellar tendon versus hamstring autografts," *Orthopaedic Journal of Sports Medicine*, vol. 5, no. 6, pp. 232596711770973–232596711770979, 2017.

[12] C. F. van Eck, O. Limpisvasti, and N. S. ElAttrache, "Is there a role for internal bracing and repair of the anterior cruciate ligament? A systematic literature review," *The American Journal of Sports Medicine*, vol. 46, no. 9, pp. 2291–2298, 2018.

[13] D. Cucchi, A. Aliprandi, E. Nocerino, and P. Randelli, "Early combined arthroscopic treatment for simultaneous ruptures of the patellar tendon and the anterior cruciate ligament leads to good radiological results and patient satisfaction," *Knee Surgery, Sports Traumatology, Arthroscopy*, vol. 26, no. 4, pp. 1164–1173, 2017.

[14] P. P. Mariani, G. Cerullo, and G. Iannella, "Simultaneous rupture of the patellar tendon and the anterior cruciate ligament: report of three cases," *The Journal of Knee Surgery*, vol. 26, Supplement 1, pp. S053–S057, 2013.

[15] J. Pérez, G. A. Novoa, A. Pierobon et al., "Postoperative rehabilitation of simultaneous rupture of anterior cruciate ligament and patellar ligament: a case report," *Physiotherapy Research International*, vol. 23, no. 4, article e1735, 2018.

[16] A. S. Chiang, S. S. Shin, L. M. Jazrawi, and D. J. Rose, "Simultaneous ipsilateral ruptures of the anterior cruciate ligament and patellar tendon: a case report," *Bulletin of the NYU Hospital for Joint Diseases*, vol. 62, pp. 134–136, 2005.

[17] L. A. Futch, W. P. Garth, G. J. Folsom, and W. K. Ogard, "Acute rupture of the anterior cruciate ligament and patellar tendon in a collegiate athlete," *Arthroscopy*, vol. 23, no. 1, pp. 112.e1–112.e4, 2007.

# 31

# Cystic Echinococcosis of the Ilium Treated with Curettage and Microwave Thermoablation Followed by Bone Cement Installation: A Novel Treatment Technique for a Rare Disease

**Kyriakos Papavasiliou**,[1] **Sousana Panagiotidou**,[1] **Panagiotis Kakoulidis**,[1] **Antonia Bintoudi**,[2] **Kostoula Arvaniti**,[3] and **Eleftherios Tsiridis**[1]

[1]*Academic Orthopaedic Department, Papageorgiou General Hospital, Aristotle University Medical School, Thessaloniki Ring Road, 56403 Nea Efkarpia, Greece*
[2]*Department of Radiology, Papageorgiou General Hospital, Thessaloniki Ring Road, 56403 Nea Efkarpia, Greece*
[3]*Intensive Care Unit, Infection Control and AMS Unit, Papageorgiou General Hospital, Thessaloniki Ring Road, 56403 Nea Efkarpia, Greece*

Correspondence should be addressed to Kyriakos Papavasiliou; papavasiliou.kyriakos@gmail.com

Academic Editor: Mark K. Lyons

Bone cystic echinococcosis (CE) is a rare condition requiring a high level of suspicion during primary diagnosis. Wide excision of the lesion is the gold standard of treatment, posing however extreme challenges in certain parts of the skeleton, since it may well be accompanied by increased morbidity. We report the case of a 35-year-old Caucasian female with iliac bone CE, referred to our department (a regional referral center for the treatment of patients with musculoskeletal tumors). The patient reported gradually increasing dull pain at the right iliac fossa and antalgic gait, with an onset of approximately 5 years before her referral. Bone CE diagnosis was established based on physical examination, imaging studies, and two subsequent CT-guided core needle biopsies, performed within a period of 3 months, of which the second was diagnostic. Following a musculoskeletal tumor multidisciplinary meeting, it was decided that the optional treatment was the surgical removal of the cyst. Aiming to minimize the morbidity accompanying a wide resection of the lesion, we performed extended curettage of the lesion through a typical iliac spine approach, followed by microwave ablation of the walls of the remaining bone cavity. The remaining iliac defect was treated with the installation of polymethyl methacrylate bone cement. The patient reported immediate remission of symptoms postoperatively and was able to return to everyday activities two weeks postoperatively. She began oral treatment with albendazole on the 7th postoperative day. She remained symptom-free for a period of 25 months, until she developed a seroma at the gluteal area, which was treated with simple drainage. On her latest follow-up six months later, she remained symptom-free and was able to perform all her previous activities. Microwave ablation may serve as a useful adjuvant modality when treating patients with bone CE, in order to prevent relapse of the disease.

## 1. Introduction

Cystic echinococcosis (CE) is a parasitic infection caused in humans by *Echinococcus granulosus* sensu lato [1]. It mainly affects the liver and the lungs, while occurrence at skeletal parts is rather rare [2]. The spine, pelvis, and femur are the most common locations of CE or hydatid cysts at the skeleton, with a reported incidence ranging from 0.5% to 4% of patients with CE [2]. Treatment of bone CE is challenging, since the radical excision of the parasite is a rather difficult task, even after the wide resection of a lesion [3]. As a result, the rate of recurrence following surgical treatment is rather high, reaching 48% of cases [4].

We present the case of an unusual location of bone CE at the ilium, treated with intralesional curettage and microwave ablation, followed by the installation of polymethyl

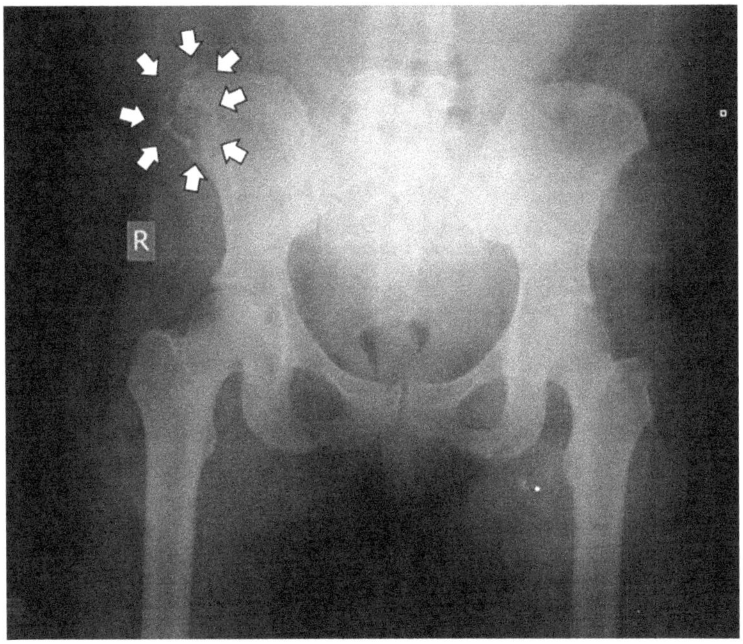


Figure 1: The initial standard anteroposterior radiograph of the patient's pelvis, depicting a lytic lesion (white arrows) at the iliac crest of the right ilium.

methacrylate (PMMA) bone cement into the remaining cavity to prevent postoperative fracture and potential relapse of the lesion. To the best of our knowledge, this is the first case in the English literature, presenting this novel adjuvant treatment modality as a means of treatment for bone CE.

This case has been reported according to the SCARE 2018 criteria [5].

## 2. Case Presentation

A 35-year-old Caucasian female was referred to our department (a regional referral center for the treatment of patients with musculoskeletal tumors), complaining about ongoing pain at her right ilium and intermittent limping for the past 5 years. Symptoms were not initiated by trauma. The patient had been working in a food processing factory for approximately 13 years and was the owner of a dog for a couple of years. Her medical history revealed an echinococcal cyst of the liver diagnosed 3 years before her referral and during investigation for anemia. She was on a regular follow-up schedule by general surgeons.

Upon clinical examination, the patient had antalgic gait and reported local tenderness elicited on palpation at the right ilium. The passive hip range of motion was normal, and no leg length discrepancy was detected. Further investigation with a plain radiograph of the pelvis (Figure 1) and Magnetic Resonance Imaging (MRI) (Figure 2) performed upon her first visit revealed an atypical lytic lesion at the right ilium. Laboratory tests showed a mild increase of the Erythrocyte Sedimentation Rate (ESR) (26 mm/hr) and of the C-Reactive Protein (CRP) (1.07 ng/L, normal range < 0.5 ng/L ). The patient subsequently underwent a Computed Tomography- (CT-) guided core needle biopsy (Figure 3) with a pathology report negative for malignancy yet nondiagnostic. The patient was given instructions for crutch-assisted partial weight bearing and reevaluation. Three months later, a second MRI scan was performed (Figure 4) and showed further destruction of the right ilium crest, with the presence of extended osteolytic areas. A second CT-guided biopsy followed, and the pathology report was positive for bone CE of the ilium.

The patient next underwent full staging. A contrast-enhanced CT scan of the abdomen revealed a $6.4 \times 4.5 \times 3.3$ cm calcified cystic lesion (Figure 5). A CT scan of the pelvis depicted a large cystic lesion at the iliac spine with osseous destruction of the right iliac bone anatomy (Figure 6). Following a musculoskeletal tumor multidisciplinary meeting with the ad hoc presence of an infectiologist and a general surgeon, it was decided that the optional treatment ought to be the surgical removal of the cyst and this should precede any other treatment, mainly due to the patient's ambulatory problems. Due to the location of the bone CE at the iliac crest and its size, and in order to prevent the increased morbidity that would accompany a wide excision, it was decided to implement a complex three-stage novel treatment technique, described as follows.

*2.1. Surgical Technique.* Under epidural anesthesia and following standard antibiotic prophylaxis administration (cefoxitin 2 gr IV q8hr for 24 hrs), with the patient in the supine position, we performed a standard incision along the iliac crest. The subcutaneous fat and the fascia were next incised, giving direct access to the right ilium and to the cyst. We then performed careful and extended curettage of the bone CE (stage 1), taking careful preventive measures to avoid the contamination of the surrounding tissues with the cyst's liquid content (the operative area was meticulously covered with compresses immersed in 20% hypertonic

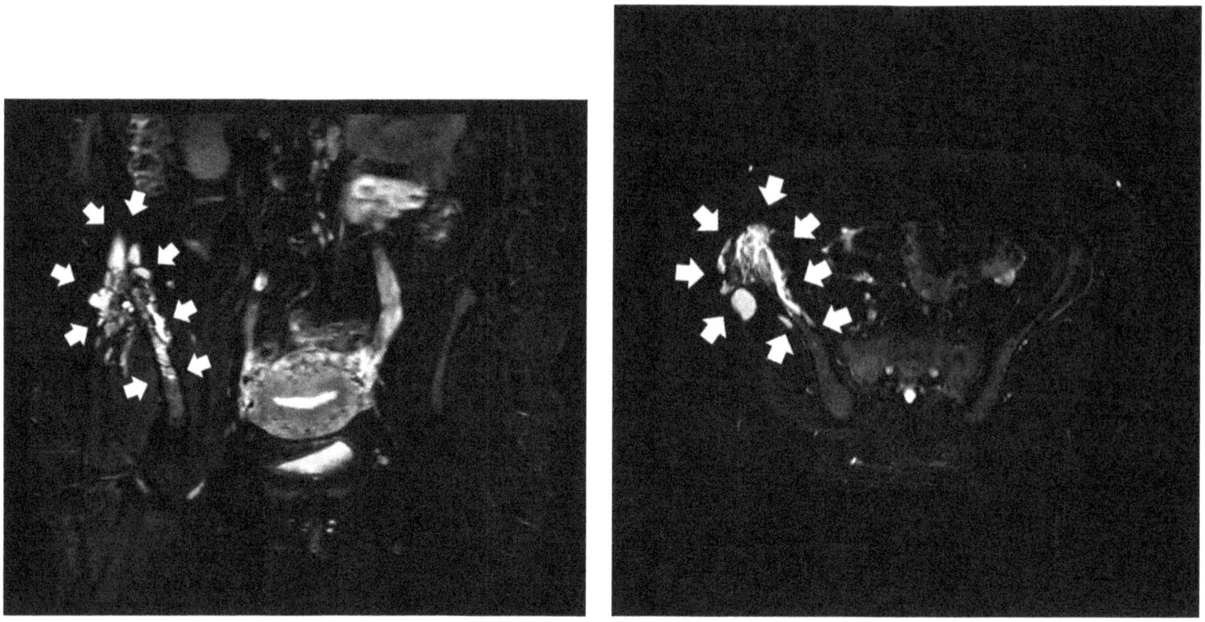

(a) (b)

FIGURE 2: The initial MRI scan of the patient's pelvis. Short TI Inversion Recovery-weighted image sequence (STIR) coronal (a) and axial (b) views. Both pictures demonstrate a lesion with extended bone edema and nonhomogenous appearance, originating from the area of interest along the right iliac crest, combined with extension to the adjacent soft tissue structures (white arrows).

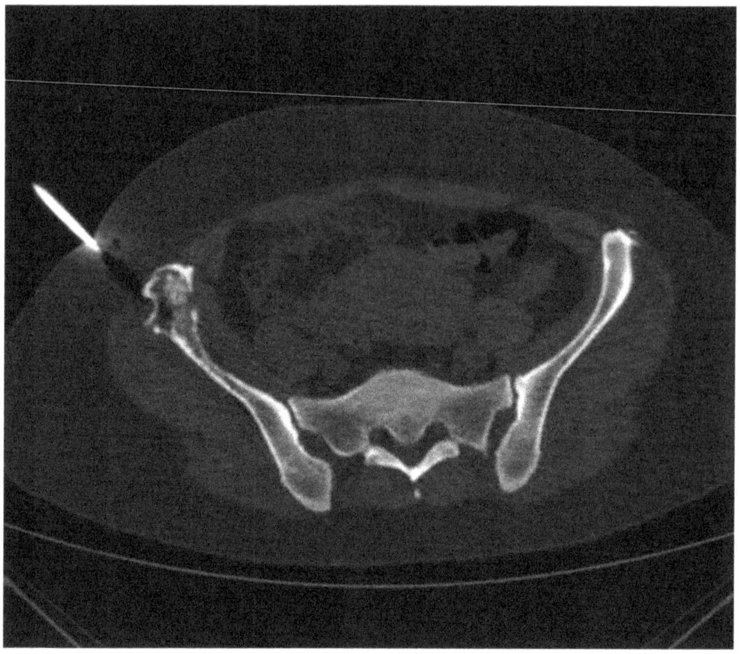

FIGURE 3: CT scan of the patient's pelvis (axial view) depicting the CT-guided core needle biopsy of the lesion at the right iliac crest.

saline). No viability of the parasite could be established in the products of the curettage, which nonetheless reconfirmed the diagnosis of bone CE. This was followed by the microwave thermoablation of the cyst's walls (stage 2), which was facilitated with the introduction to the bone cavity of an Amica™ (HS Hospital Service S.p.A., Rome, Italy) microwave thermoablation probe (16 gauge × 150 mm, combined with a mini choke and an internal water cooling system). The calculated total microwave output was 60 W at 2450 MHz, and the duration of the ablation was 6 min. The remaining bone cavity was filled with the installation of polymethyl methacrylate (PMMA) bone cement (stage 3) in order to prevent the potential development of a postoperative fracture and to prevent the potential relapse of the bone CE (Figure 7). The wound was closed in layers, and a simple vacuum drain was used.

The patient's postoperative course went uneventfully. The patient began crutch-assisted nonweight bearing

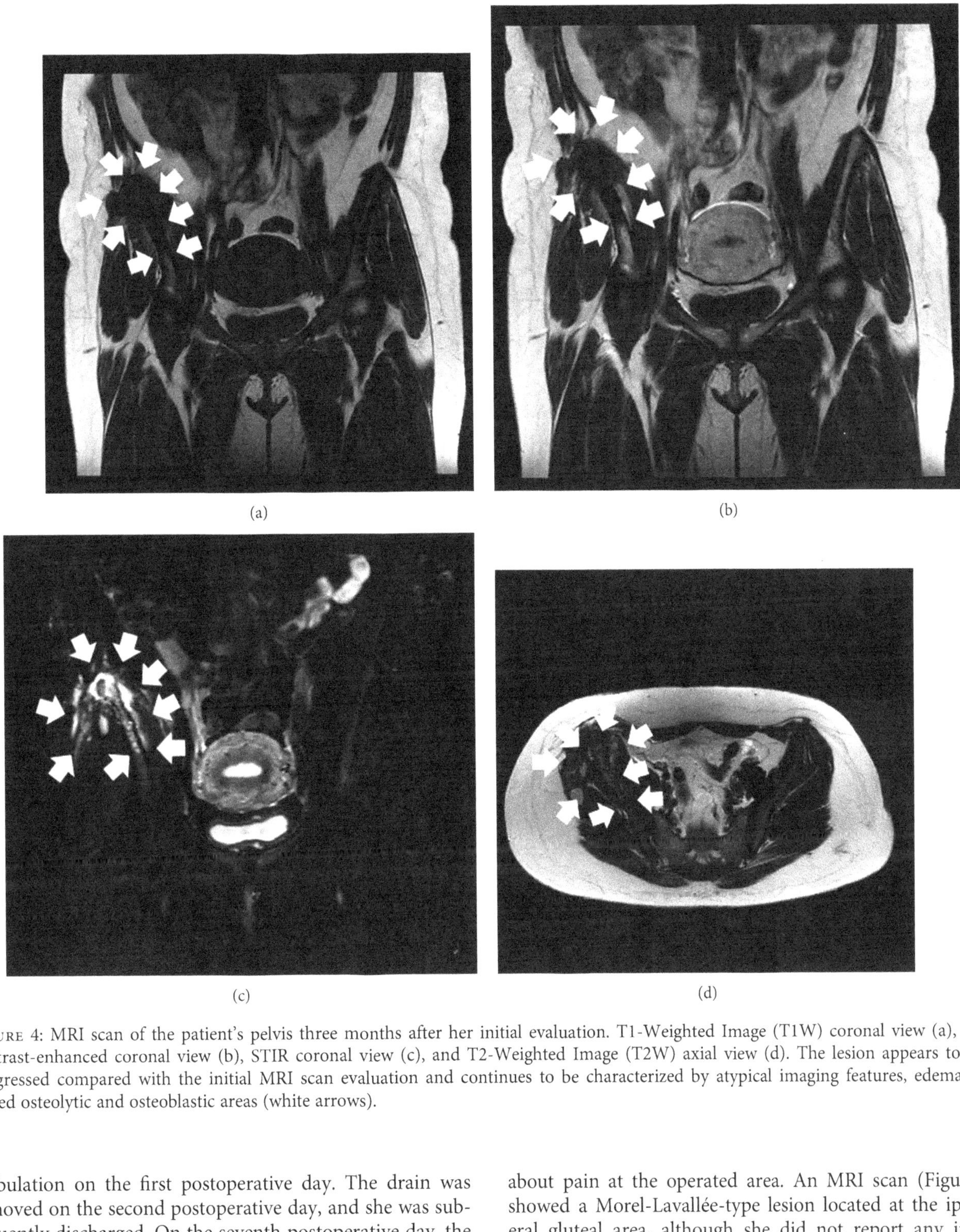

FIGURE 4: MRI scan of the patient's pelvis three months after her initial evaluation. T1-Weighted Image (T1W) coronal view (a), T1W contrast-enhanced coronal view (b), STIR coronal view (c), and T2-Weighted Image (T2W) axial view (d). The lesion appears to have progressed compared with the initial MRI scan evaluation and continues to be characterized by atypical imaging features, edema, and mixed osteolytic and osteoblastic areas (white arrows).

ambulation on the first postoperative day. The drain was removed on the second postoperative day, and she was subsequently discharged. On the seventh postoperative day, the patient commenced oral treatment with albendazole 400 mg q12hr. Crutch-assisted gradually increasing weight bearing ambulation begun at the second postoperative week. The patient was able to walk with no assistance at two months postoperatively, when she was also able to return to her usual everyday activities.

She remained symptom-free for almost 25 months following her operation, until she returned complaining about pain at the operated area. An MRI scan (Figure 8) showed a Morel-Lavallée-type lesion located at the ipsilateral gluteal area, although she did not report any injury whatsoever. The patient underwent uneventful CT-guided drainage of the seroma. Under local anesthesia and CT guidance, a 14-gauge catheter was inserted at the cystic lesion (Figure 9). Culture swabs obtained from the drained fluid came back negative for bone CE recurrence and/or microbial infection. The catheter remained in place for a period of 10 days, in order to facilitate the complete drainage of the cyst and to avoid its recurrence. While the

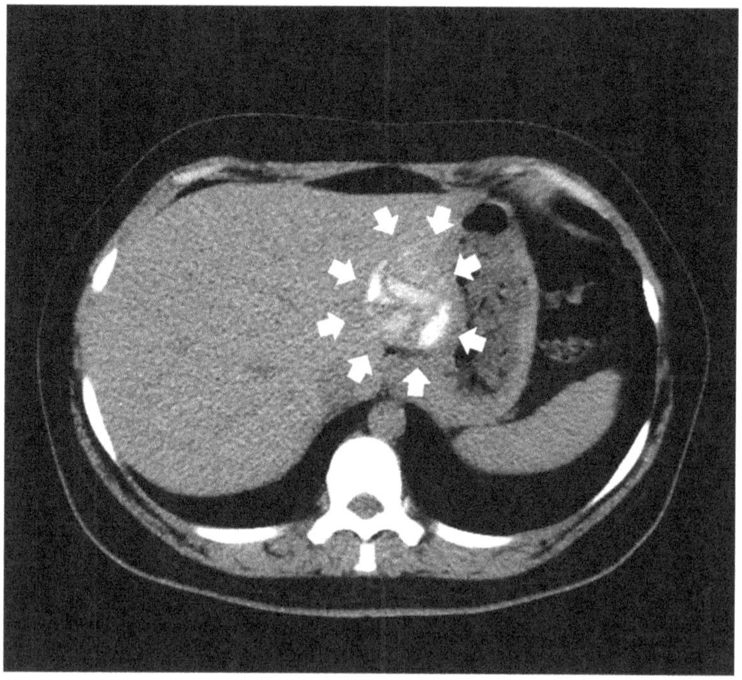

FIGURE 5: Contrast-enhanced CT scan of the abdomen (axial view) three months after the initial evaluation of the patient. Notice the existence of a single hydatid cyst with distinct calcified walls, arising from segment II of the left lobe of the liver (white arrows).

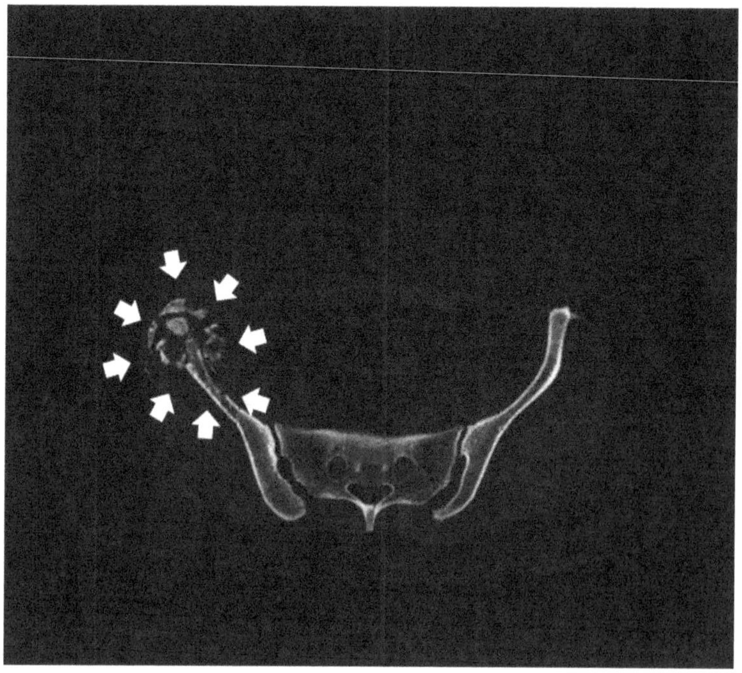

FIGURE 6: CT scan of the pelvis (axial view) of the patient three months after her initial evaluation. Notice the large cystic lesion at the iliac crest, with signs of the destruction of the ilium and areas of calcification (white arrows).

catheter was in place, the patient was under antibiotic prophylaxis (cefuroxime 500 mg PO q12hr) and fully ambulant. The catheter was removed uneventfully, and a subsequent CT scan confirmed the complete drainage of the cyst (Figure 10).

On her latest follow-up visit, at 31 months postoperatively (6 months following the seroma's drainage), the patient remains symptom-free, is still under oral antiparasitic therapy, has no signs of recurrence of the bone CE and of the seroma, and is scheduled to undergo hepatic surgery.

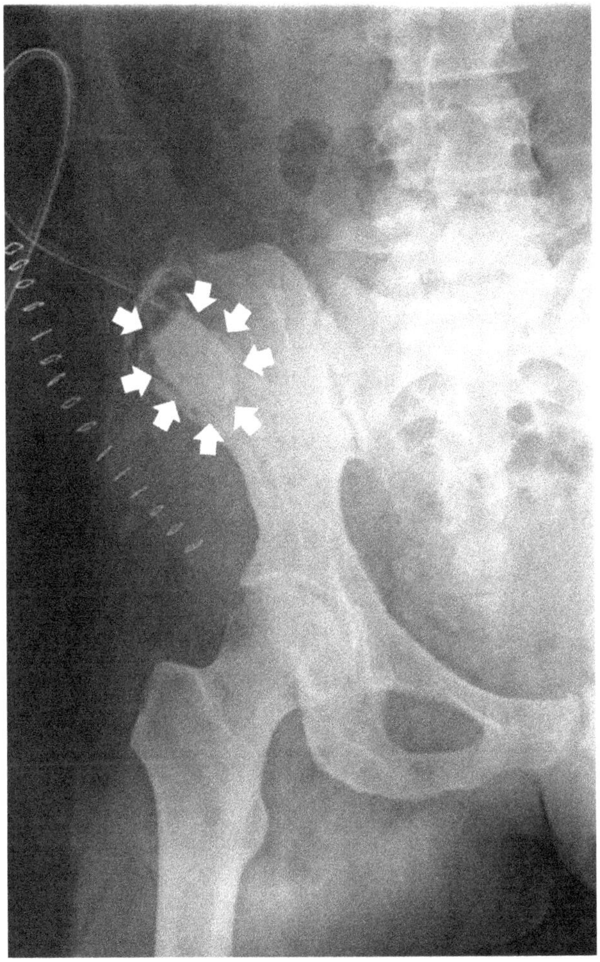

FIGURE 7: Immediate postoperative anteroposterior radiograph of the patient's hemipelvis, following the curettage of the cyst and the installation of PMMA at the remaining bone cavity (white arrows).

## 3. Discussion

Bone CE lesions are caused by the parasitic tapeworm *Echinococcus granulosus* [1, 2] and mainly occur in the trabecular bone, eventually extending to subcortical areas as the disease progresses [6]. They usually present with atypical imaging features and laboratory tests, hence posing a diagnostic problem and thus delaying treatment in early stages [6]. Differential diagnosis may include tumors and tumor-like lesions of the bone, tuberculosis, and fungal infections [7]. Echinococcal bone lesions may be unifocal or appear in multiple locations [2]. Most patients remain asymptomatic until the advanced stages of the disease, when symptoms like local pain and tenderness first appear [1]. Laboratory tests may reveal an elevated ESR, CRP concentration, and eosinophil count [8]. A positive antibody titer may also be helpful in the diagnosis [8].

The radiographic findings of bone CE are nonspecific [9]. Plain radiographs and CT scans may reveal a single or multiple osteolytic area(s), cortical thinning, calcification, and pathological fractures [9]. MRI scans are useful in order to accurately depict the extent of the disease and the potential extension to the adjacent soft tissues [9]. Bone CE can mimic tumors, simple cysts, and infections [8]. Further investigation with CT scans of the brain, lungs, and abdomen is essential while investigating a suspicious bony lesion of this type [10]. The bone biopsy and specimen culture are of utmost importance in the diagnosis of bone hydatid cysts [8, 11].

The gold standard when treating bone CE is the combination of surgical excision and antiparasitic therapy [3, 6]. There is a wide range of operative options, ranging from simple drainage or debridement to complete cyst excision, extensive bone removal, installation of bone grafts and PMMA, osteosynthesis, and arthroplasty [3]. The use of radiofrequency thermal ablation (RFA) as a treatment for hydatid cysts of the liver has been previously reported [12, 13]. The high temperature released in the cyst results in protein denaturation and further destruction of the germinal layer [14].

There are only a few cases of bone CE of the ilium reported in the literature, and they were treated with a variety of operative and nonoperative methods. Gdoura et al. reported a case located at the pelvis, which was treated with hemipelvectomy, followed by femoropubic and sacral arthrodesis [15]. In another case, the authors showed good results with the combination of antiparasitic therapy, wide excision, and the use of PMMA [16]. Emami et al. reported a case of an intraoperatively diagnosed bone CE which was treated with partial iliac wing excision, instead of the scheduled sequestrectomy [17]. Neelapala et al. presented a case treated with total hip arthroplasty and subtotal removal of the bone CE, which later necessitated a revision operation due to component loosening [18]. Akhan et al. treated a patient with a large bone CE of the ilium by implementing the nonoperative percutaneous modified catheterization technique (MoCaT). This was the first time that this technique was used in bone CE, and it was proven successful not only in dealing with the patient's condition but also in obliterating the need for an operation, which would probably have been accompanied by increased morbidity, due to the extension and the location of the lesion [19].

Bone CE presents with increased recurrence rates, especially when radical excision cannot be achieved [20]. In the hereby reported case, we decided to use microwave thermoablation and installation of PMMA, as adjuvant therapies to the extended curettage we implemented in order to avoid the morbidity associated with the wide excision of bone CE, which is usually used in these cases. Microwave thermoablation increases tissues' temperature locally and in an absolutely controllable manner, leading to the thermocauterization of a lesion. The use of PMMA as a primary or adjuvant treatment modality for benign [21] and malignant bone tumors [22] is also a well-established method of treatment. Furthermore, following the curettage of bone CE, the subsequent installation of PMMA in the remaining cavity (which is also associated with locally increased temperature) was also shown to be effective in preventing disease recurrence, due to the necrotizing impact exerted on the parasitic infection. Last but not least, PMMA is also used as a means of stabilization in order to prevent a pathological fracture [3].

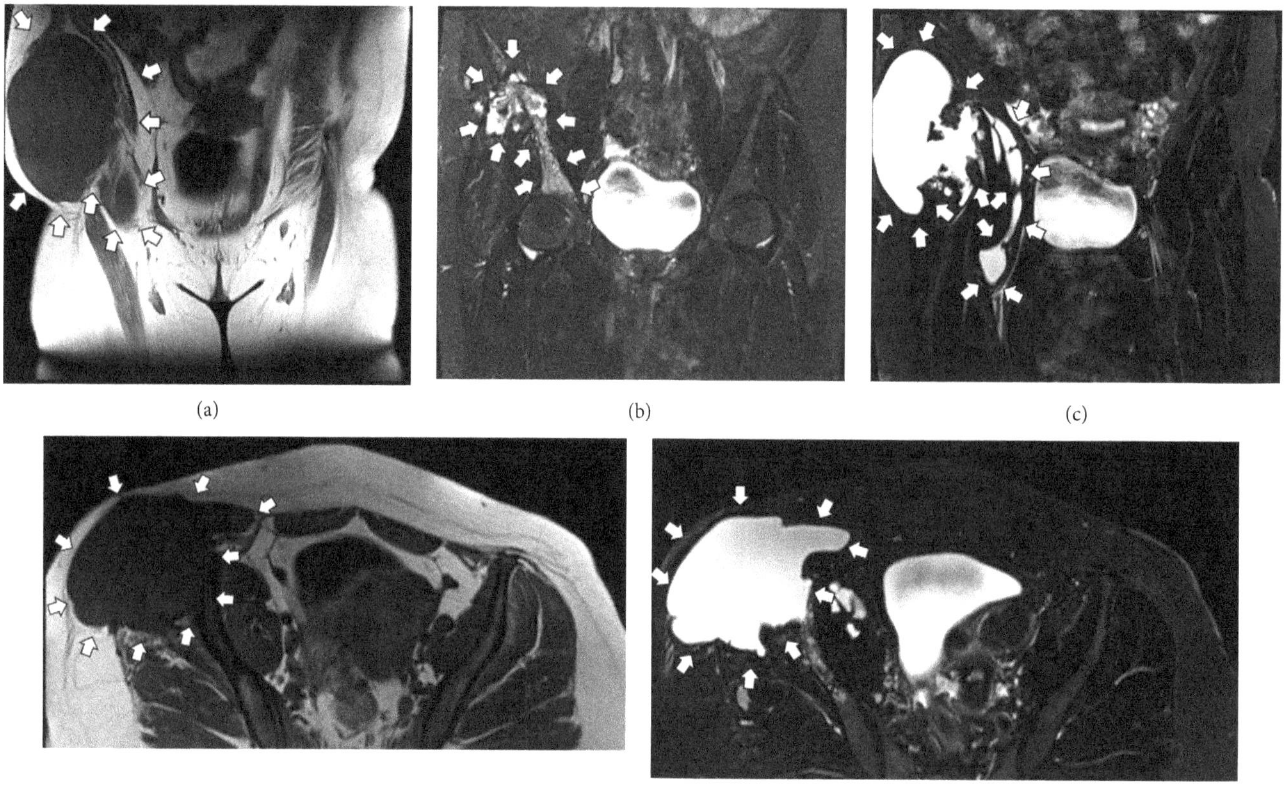

(a) (b) (c) (d) (e)

FIGURE 8: MRI scan of the patient's pelvis 25 months postoperatively. T1W coronal view (a), T2W coronal views (b, c), T1W axial view (d), and T2W axial view (e). Notice the extended Morel-Lavallée-type cystic lesion at the right gluteal area, with no sign of direct contact with the area where the cystic echinococcosis used to be at the iliac crest.

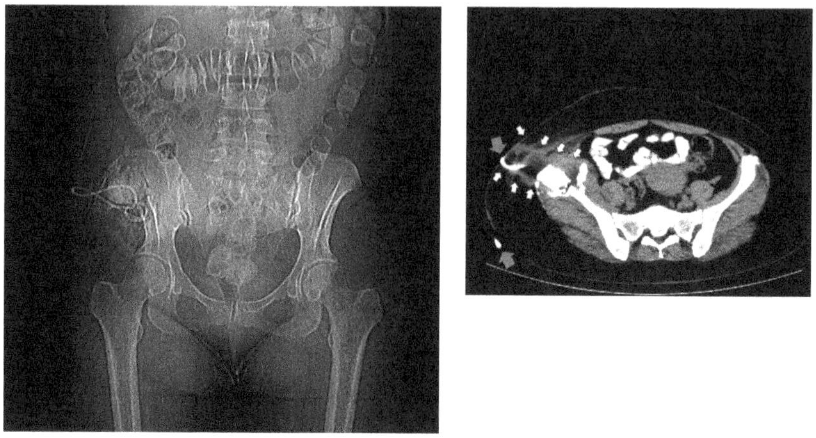

(a) (b)

FIGURE 9: CT scanogram of the patient's abdomen and pelvis (a) and CT scan (axial view) of the patient's pelvis (b) depicting the CT-guided insertion of the 14-gauge drainage catheter (gray arrows) into the Morel-Lavallée-type cystic lesion at the right gluteal area.

The combination of microwave thermoablation with the installation of PMMA seemed to have served well in order to avoid the recurrence of the bone CE. The development of a large seroma at the gluteal area 25 months postoperatively may be possibly attributed to the extended surgical approach implemented and to the preventive measures taken intraoperatively in order to prevent the contamination of the surrounding tissues, although this cause-and-effect model is neither certain nor verifiable. However, it cannot be related to the bone CE itself, since no recurrence could be established, and furthermore, it occurred after two years from its operative treatment.

To the best of our knowledge, this is the first case in the English literature, presenting this novel adjuvant treatment

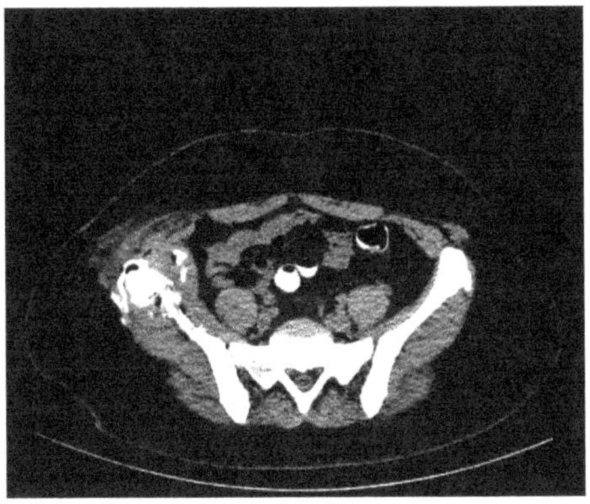

FIGURE 10: CT scan of the patient's pelvis (axial view) following the removal of the catheter that was used in order to drain the Morel-Lavallée-type cystic lesion at the right gluteal area, confirming the complete drainage of the cystic lesion.

modality as a means of treatment for bone CE. Although rare, bone CE may necessitate operative interventions accompanied by increased morbidity. The implementation of microwave thermoablation, along with other less invasive treatment modalities, may serve as a useful adjuvant technique, in order to increase the possibility of no recurrence, when less radical operative options are used.

## References


[1] S. Jain and P. Chopra, "Cystic echinococcosis of the pelvic bone with recurrences: a case report," *The Korean Journal of Parasitology*, vol. 49, no. 3, pp. 277–279, 2011.

[2] B. Monge-Maillo, M. Olmedo Samperio, J. A. Pérez-Molina et al., "Osseous cystic echinococcosis: a case series study at a referral unit in Spain," *PLoS Neglected Tropical Diseases*, vol. 13, no. 2, article e0007006, 2019.

[3] Q. Liang, H. Wen, A. Yunus, Z. Tian, F. Jiang, and X. Song, "Treatment experiences of pelvic bone hydatidosis," *International Journal of Infectious Diseases*, vol. 18, pp. 57–61, 2014.

[4] A. Neumayr, F. Tamarozzi, S. Goblirsch, J. Blum, and E. Brunetti, "Spinal cystic echinococcosis–a systematic analysis and review of the literature. Part 2. Treatment, follow-up and outcome," *PLoS Neglected Tropical Diseases*, vol. 7, no. 9, article e2458, 2013.

[5] R. A. Agha, M. R. Borrelli, R. Farwana et al., "The SCARE 2018 statement: Updating consensus Surgical CAse REport (SCARE) guidelines," *International Journal of Surgery*, vol. 60, pp. 132–136, 2018.

[6] H. O. Arik, M. Arican, N. K. Cetin, and U. Sarp, "Primary intraosseous hydatid cyst of femur," *Iranian Red Crescent Medical Journal*, vol. 17, no. 2, article e21070, 2015.

[7] M. Ciftdemir, A. Sezer, F. O. Puyan, C. Copuroglu, and M. Ozcan, "Hydatid disease of the femur with an extraosseous extent due to a former biopsy complicated by a pathological fracture," *Case Reports in Orthopedics*, vol. 2012, Article ID 169545, 4 pages, 2012.

[8] G. Toğral, Ş. M. Arıkan, T. Ekiz, A. F. Kekeç, and M. F. Ekşioğlu, "Musculoskeletal hydatid cysts resembling tumors: a report of five cases," *Orthopaedic Surgery*, vol. 8, no. 2, pp. 246–252, 2016.

[9] P. Polat, M. Kantarci, F. Alper, S. Suma, M. B. Koruyucu, and A. Okur, "Hydatid disease from head to toe," *Radiographics*, vol. 23, no. 2, pp. 475–494, 2003, quiz 536-7.

[10] J. Plant and S. Cannon, "Diagnostic work up and recognition of primary bone tumours: a review," *EFORT Open Reviews*, vol. 1, no. 6, pp. 247–253, 2016.

[11] S. E. Golzari and M. Sokouti, "Pericyst: the outermost layer of hydatid cyst," *World Journal of Gastroenterology*, vol. 20, no. 5, pp. 1377-1378, 2014.

[12] E. Brunetti and C. Filice, "Radiofrequency thermal ablation of echinococcal liver cysts," *Lancet*, vol. 358, no. 9291, p. 1464, 2001.

[13] C. Bastid, P. Ayela, and J. Sahel, "Traitement par radiofrequence d'un kyste hydatique hepatique complexe. À propos d'un cas," *Gastroentérologie Clinique et Biologique*, vol. 29, no. 2, pp. 191-192, 2005.

[14] E. Botsa, I. Thanou, I. Nikas, and L. Thanos, "Treatment of hepatic hydatid cyst in a 7-year-old boy using a new type of radiofrequency ablation electrode," *American Journal of Case Reports*, vol. 18, pp. 953–958, 2017.

[15] F. Gdoura, M. Trigui, W. Zribi et al., "Pelvic bone hydatidosis," *Orthopaedics & Traumatology: Surgery & Research*, vol. 96, no. 1, pp. 85–89, 2010.

[16] Y. Yildiz, K. Bayrakci, M. Altay, and Y. Saglik, "The use of polymethylmethacrylate in the management of hydatid disease of bone," *Journal of Bone and Joint Surgery. British Volume (London)*, vol. 83-B, no. 7, pp. 1005–1008, 2001.

[17] M. Emami, A. Vosoughi, I. Vadiee, S. Pakbaz, and S. Liaghat, "Primary hydatid disease of the ilium: a case report," *Iranian Red Crescent Medical Journal*, vol. 12, no. 2, pp. 190–194, 2010.

[18] V. S. Neelapala, C. R. Chandrasekar, and R. J. Grimer, "Revision hip replacement for recurrent hydatid disease of the pelvis: a case report and review of the literature," *Journal of Orthopaedic Surgery and Research*, vol. 5, no. 1, p. 17, 2010.

[19] O. Akhan, O. Yildiz, E. Unal, T. T. Ciftci, and D. Akinci, "Percutaneous treatment of bone hydatid cyst," *Cardiovascular and Interventional Radiology*, vol. 44, no. 7, pp. 1131–1134, 2021.

[20] A. Herrera and A. A. Martínez, "Extraspinal bone hydatidosis," *The Journal of Bone and Joint Surgery. American Volume*, vol. 85, no. 9, pp. 1790–1794, 2003.

[21] G. Koch, R. L. Cazzato, A. Gilkison, J. Caudrelier, J. Garnon, and A. Gangi, "Percutaneous treatments of benign bone tumors," *Semin Intervent Radiol.*, vol. 35, no. 4, pp. 324–332, 2018.

[22] K. Papavasiliou, K. Asteriadis, S. Panagiotidou, and E. Tsiridis, "Palliative surgical management of a metastatic lesion of the tibia with extension into the popliteal fossa using polytetrafluoroethylene felt and bone cement," *Case Reports in Orthopedics*, vol. 2020, Article ID 8845173, 8 pages, 2020.

# 32

# A 16-Year-Old Male with Thoracic Compression following Posterior Spinal Instrumentation and Fusion for Marfan-Associated Syndromic Scoliosis

**Mason Uvodich**[1] **Ross Barman**[2] **Adam Reitz**[3] **and Matthew Sexton**[2,4]

[1]*Mayo Clinic Department of Orthopaedic Surgery, USA*
[2]*Mayo Clinic Department of Anesthesiology and Perioperative Medicine, USA*
[3]*Kentucky College of Osteopathic Medicine, USA*
[4]*Department of Critical Care Medicine, USA*

Correspondence should be addressed to Mason Uvodich; uvodich.mason@mayo.edu

Academic Editor: Christian W. Müller

*Introduction.* Marfan syndrome is an autosomal dominant disorder caused by a mutation in the *FBN1* gene which affects connective tissue. The features of Marfan syndrome include many musculoskeletal abnormalities which require orthopaedic surgical intervention. Given the expansive phenotypic variations and comorbidities associated with Marfan syndrome, knowledge of perioperative risk factors and potential complications is essential. *Case.* In this case report, the authors describe a patient with Marfan syndrome who underwent spinal instrumentation and fusion from T3 to L4 for correction of syndromic scoliosis. The patient had a complicated perioperative course requiring significant fluid resuscitation and vasoactive medications to support blood pressure. He required intensive care unit level care for continued hemodynamic instability despite resuscitation in the postoperative period. Common causes of postoperative hypotension such as hypovolemic shock, sepsis, ongoing hemorrhage, and prolonged effects of anesthesia were diagnostically ruled out. Ultimately, the patient's refractory hypotension was determined to be from mechanical compression, both from prolonged intraoperative prone positioning exacerbated by pectus excavatum and from the surgically corrected spine decreasing the diameter of his thoracic cavity (as referenced by his postoperative Haller index). *Conclusion.* Mechanical compression of thoracic contents as a result of a worsening chest wall deformity can be a complication of spinal deformity correction.

## 1. Introduction

Marfan syndrome affects an estimated 1 in 10,000 people and is inherited in an autosomal dominant fashion. It is the result of a mutation in the extracellular matrix protein fibrillin-1 gene found on chromosome 15 which alters connective tissues [1]. Orthopaedic surgery is common in patients with Marfan syndrome because 60% will have scoliosis, and of those with scoliosis, an estimated 25% to 50% of patients will require surgical intervention for correction after failing conservative measures [2]. Marfan syndrome has a spectrum of manifestations that should be considered in the perioperative and ICU settings, such as predispositions to mitral valve prolapse, spontaneous pneumothorax, extreme scoliosis compressing other organs, sternal deformities, dilation of the ascending aorta, and aortic aneurysm. In the following case report, we present a unique case involving a pediatric patient with Marfan syndrome who presented to the ICU with refractory undifferentiated shock following posterior spinal instrumented fusion (PSIF) and deformity correction.

## 2. Case Description

A 16-year-old male with a past medical history of Marfan syndrome with severe pectus excavatum, significant scoliosis, and generalized anxiety disorder presented for PSIF from T3 to L4 to correct his scoliosis deformity. Preoperative evaluation demonstrated a left lumbar curve of 64 degrees and

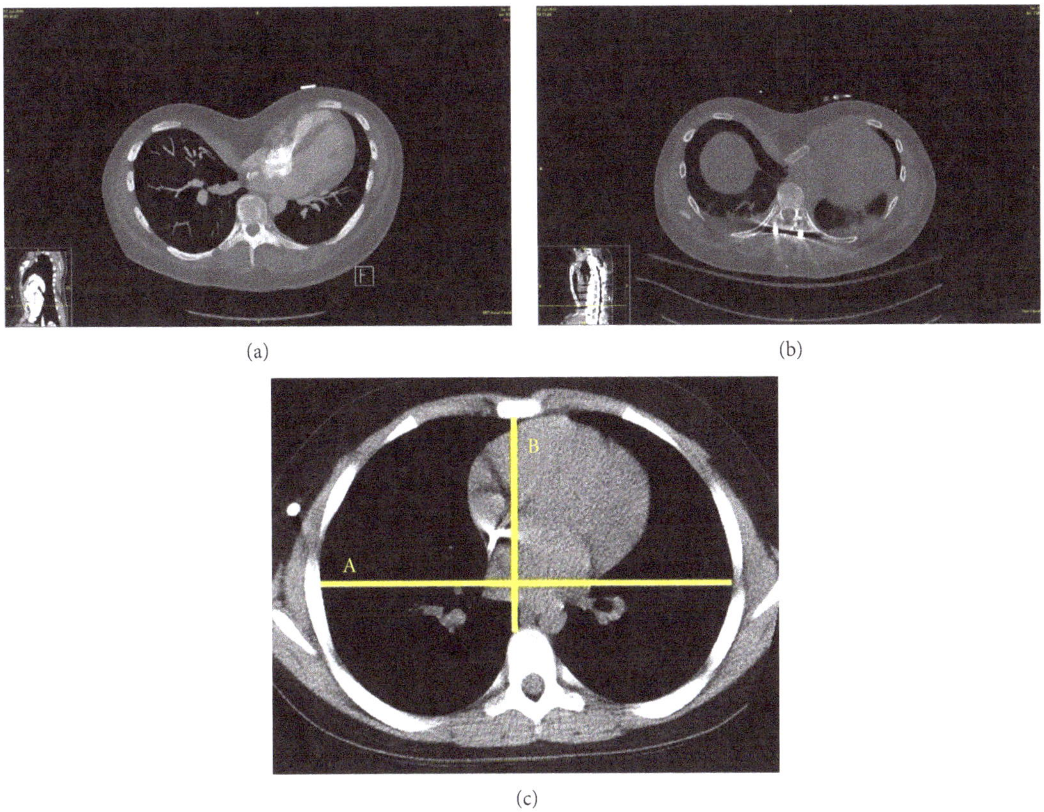


FIGURE 1: Comparison of preoperative and postoperative CT chest. Preoperative CT chest had a Haller index of 8.7. The anterior-posterior diameter minimum preoperatively was 3 cm (a). Postoperative CT chest had a Haller index of 11.3 (b). The anterior-posterior diameter minimum postoperatively was 2.3 cm. Example of a normal chest CT Haller index (c), with lines demonstrating measurements of the Haller index (ratio of A/B) [6].

lumbar kyphosis of 14 degrees. His curve corrected to 40 degrees with a fulcrum bend. Evaluation 1 year prior to the surgery revealed no cardiovascular abnormalities with a normal ejection fraction of 56%.

Induction of anesthesia and intubation were uncomplicated. His preprocedure vitals were stable and within a normal range. The patient was placed in a prone position. Due to the ongoing hemodynamic instability and need for abundant amounts of vasopressor support, the chest pads were repositioned which improved his hypotension for a time. The surgical aspects of the procedure proceeded uneventfully. The patient had transverse process pedicle hooks placed bilaterally at T3 and had navigated pedicle screws placed T4-L4. Facetectomies were performed at each level and a Cortrel-Dubousset derotation maneuver was performed to correct the scoliosis. Sequential distraction and compression was performed to correct the deformity in combination with in situ rod bending in both the coronal and the sagittal plane. Throughout the procedure, he had a significant vasopressor requirement. The patient received adequate crystalloid and colloid in addition to 4 units of fresh frozen plasma and approximately 600 cc of cell saver. The case lasted 10 hours and was complicated with 1.4 L of blood loss.

At the conclusion of the case, the patient was flipped supine and transferred to the postanesthesia care unit (PACU) intubated and on mechanical ventilator support in hopes to later extubate once his anesthetic dissipated. He was slow to emerge from anesthesia, and initial vital signs showed significant hypotension (systolic blood pressure 66 mmHg with a mean arterial pressure (MAP) of 54) and tachycardia into the 140s. The patient was started on phenylephrine and was transferred to the Surgical Intensive Care Unit (SICU) for ongoing management.

Over the next few hours, the patient became interactive and was extubated uneventfully; however, his hypotension continued despite phenylephrine which resulted in a transition to a norepinephrine infusion. His vitals continued to demonstrate a narrowed pulse pressure with hypotension and tachycardia, concerning for cardiac tamponade and/or active postsurgical bleeding. Laboratory investigations demonstrated a hemoglobin of 12.5 g/dL, international normalized ratio (INR) of 1.6, activated partial thromboplastin (APP) time of 30, and a fibrinogen of 155 mg/dL which improved to 187 mg/dL without intervention. He was given fluid boluses and continued on norepinephrine with minimal improvement. His initial postoperative labs were significant for a lactate of 3.6 mmol/L and a creatinine (Cr) of 0.8 mg/dL. His lactate peaked at 5.0 mmol/L. Given continued concern for myocardial depression, tamponade physiology, or active bleeding, he was assessed with an emergent formal bedside transthoracic echocardiogram and CT angiogram of the chest and abdomen. These demonstrated no active sources of bleeding, no pneumothoraces, and a relatively unfilled, hyperdynamic left ventricle with a postoperative Haller index that increased from 8.7 to 11.3 (Figure 1).

Over the next several hours, surveillance labs showed an evolving acute kidney injury and signs of global hypoperfusion as his lactate continued to rise. We suspected that his pectus excavatum had compromised his cardiac function by mechanical obstruction and that this compromise was exacerbated by significant intraoperative blood loss, fluid deficit, and residual effects of his anesthetic. Cardiothoracic surgery was consulted and gave consideration to immediate surgical intervention should the patient not improve with medical management. We utilized fluid boluses and vasopressor support over the course next 24 hours (Figure 2). He slowly improved hemodynamically. His acute kidney injury, lactate, and urine output improved, and he was ultimately transferred out of the ICU on postoperative day two without additional surgical intervention. Preoperative and postoperative radiographs demonstrating the spinal instrumentation and deformity correction are provided (Figure 3).

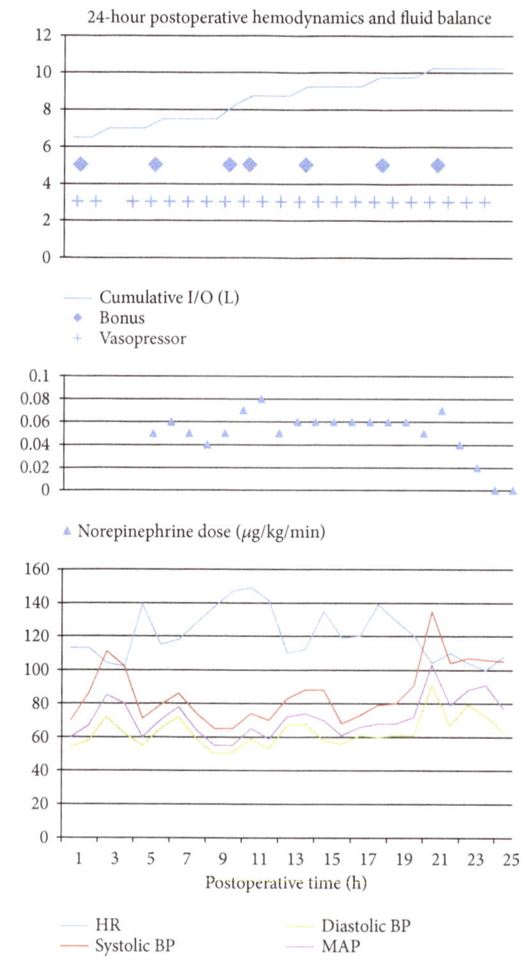


FIGURE 2: Postoperative hemodynamics and fluid balance data include measurements of blood pressure (BP) in millimeters of mercury (mmHg) and include systolic BP, diastolic BP, and mean arterial pressure (MAP). Heart rate (HR) is presented in beats per minute. Cumulative input and output (I/O) is for the patient's entire hospital course and is presented in liters (L). Starting at one hour postoperative, the patient was approximately 6 liters positive. Crystalloid and colloid boluses are designated under the same title "bolus," which is identified by diamonds in the graphs. Vasopressor refers to any vasopressive medication given in the postoperative period and is designated by crosses. Vasopressin and ephedrine were given in the early postoperative period followed by a transition to norepinephrine alone at approximately 4 hours postoperative. Norepinephrine was administered in micrograms per kilogram per minute (μg/kg/min) and was stopped approximately 23 hours postoperative.

## 3. Discussion

Adolescent scoliosis is classified as either idiopathic, neuromuscular, congenital, or syndromic. Marfan syndrome is a cause of syndromic scoliosis. The estimated prevalence of scoliosis in patients with Marfan syndrome varies but is greater than 30%, if not much higher [3]. Complication rates among patients with Marfan syndrome undergoing corrective procedures are typically higher than those among patients without Marfan syndrome [1, 4]. A retrospective review of a national registry found the most common complications to be pulmonary- or implant-related [4]. Kurucan et al. [4] also found that patients with Marfan syndrome did not have higher odds of cardiac complications compared to matched controls, although pediatric Marfan patients had a greater blood loss compared to controls. Perhaps the age or noncardiac surgery limits the cardiac complications in these patients, especially considering Marfan patients' known predisposition to aortic root and valvular pathology. In addition, there is limited literature describing intraoperative or postoperative sequelae of chest wall deformity particularly in scoliosis.

Intraoperative positioning is especially important for extended duration surgical procedures and likely played a role in our patient's refractory postoperative hypotension. While prone positioning has well-known complications of endotracheal tube displacement and ocular injury secondary to improper padding placement, abdominal compartment syndrome and reduced cardiac index are also frequently encountered in the postoperative course. Prone positioning during surgery affects the cardiac index by reducing stroke volume, and this risk is exacerbated by blood loss, intraoperative fluid shifts, and anatomic deformities that inherently obstruct cardiac output such as pectus excavatum or thoracic lordosis [5]. Mechanical obstruction is not relieved by vasopressors or fluid resuscitation; this is likely why our patient suffered from significant intraoperative hypotension.

Pectus excavatum is a deformity of the chest wall characterized by a posterior depression of the sternum and the adjacent costal cartilage. The deformity varies in depth by vertebral level [6]. The severity of pectus excavatum is graded via the Haller index which is the quotient of the transverse diameter of the chest wall divided by the smallest possible distance from the posterior aspect of the sternum to the anterior vertebral body [7]. A value > 3.5 is considered severe [8]. Our patient's Haller index was approximately 8.7 preoperatively which increased postoperatively to 11.3 (Figure 1). Without evidence of other causes for our patient's

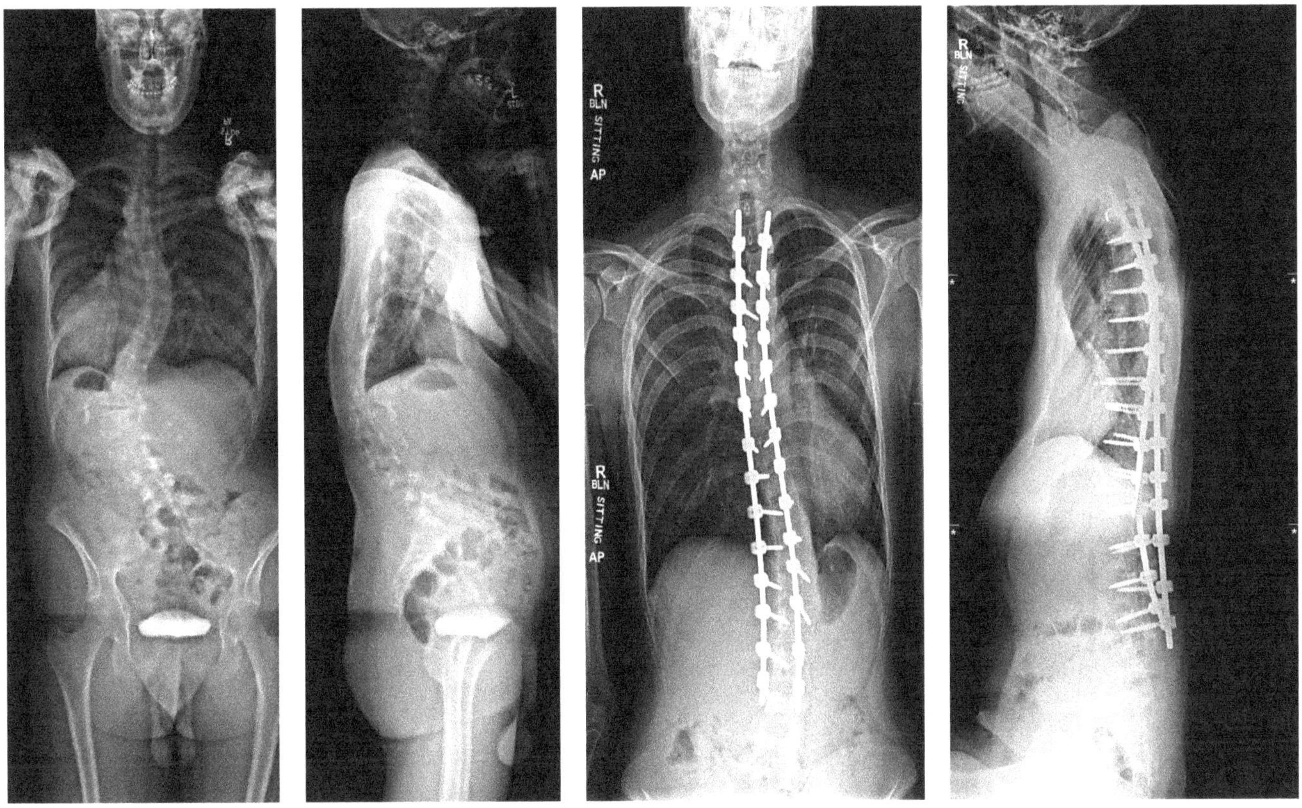


(a) (b) (c) (d)

Figure 3: Preoperative and postoperative radiographs. The top two images are the preoperative standing posterior-anterior (a) and lateral (b) plain radiographs of the entire spine. The bottom two images are six-month postoperative standing anterior-posterior (c) and lateral (d) plain radiographs of the spine.

hemodynamic instability, we considered this as the leading etiology in our patient.

Pectus excavatum is common in patients with Marfan syndrome (as well as carinatum) and occurs at a rate of approximately 30% [9]. There is a paucity of literature describing the effects of pectus excavatum on the perioperative complications of posterior spinal fusion in patients with Marfan syndrome. Overall, the rates of major complications in adolescent spine surgery for various etiologies are approximate at 3-20% [10, 11]. Main risk factors for major complications appear to be nonweight-bearing status, intraoperative blood loss, and preexisting pulmonary compromise [11]. Sternal compression of the heart with prone positioning has been reported to cause intraoperative hypotension [12]. A case report on a patient similar to ours who underwent elective surgical correction of his pectus excavatum following intolerance of prone positioning had a good outcome [13]. A recent study of 20 patients with pectus excavatum and scoliosis undergoing a corrective spine procedure within the thoracic spine had their pectus increase in severity in 11/20 patients [14]. Pectus excavatum has been shown to affect cardiac rotation and on occasion compress large vessels with prone positioning which is demonstrated in our patient's CT scan (Figure 1) [15, 16].

What is curious about our case is the prolonged hypotension after surgery. This initially suggested the more common causes of postoperative hypotension such as ongoing hemorrhage, fluid deficit secondary to blood loss or insensible losses, or myocardial stunning (from intraoperative positioning) [13, 17, 18]. However, upon further evaluation and based off of the patient's clinical course, we feel the patient's comorbid chest wall deformity, worsening Haller index, and prolonged prone positioning suggest an initial and continued mechanical compression of his thoracic contents that was made worse after his corrective surgery.

The effects of pectus excavatum on contributions to perioperative complications in Marfan patients are largely unstudied. Fortunately, our patient's hemodynamic instability improved with volume resuscitation and temporary vasoactive support, but one should also always consider additional causes within this patient population such as acute postoperative mechanical cardiac compression which warrants surgical evaluation.

## References

[1] B. J. Levy, J. F. Schulz, E. D. Fornari, and A. L. Wollowick, "Complications associated with surgical repair of syndromic scoliosis," *Scoliosis*, vol. 10, no. 1, p. 14, 2015.

[2] J. P. Gjolaj, P. D. Sponseller, S. A. Shah et al., "Spinal deformity correction in Marfan syndrome versus adolescent idiopathic scoliosis," *Spine (Phila Pa 1976)*, vol. 37, no. 18, pp. 1558–1565, 2012.

[3] M. di Silvestre, T. Greggi, S. Giacomini et al., "Surgical treatment for scoliosis in Marfan syndrome," *Spine (Phila Pa 1976)*, vol. 30, no. 20, pp. E597–E604, 2005.

[4] E. Kurucan, D. N. Bernstein, M. Ying et al., "Trends in spinal deformity surgery in Marfan syndrome," *The Spine Journal*, vol. 19, no. 12, pp. 1934–1940, 2019.

[5] M. M. Kwee, Y. H. Ho, and W. M. Rozen, "The prone position during surgery and its complications: a systematic review and evidence-based guidelines," *International Surgery*, vol. 100, no. 2, pp. 292–303, 2015.

[6] J. E. Archer, A. Gardner, F. Berryman, and P. Pynsent, "The measurement of the normal thorax using the Haller index methodology at multiple vertebral levels," *Journal of Anatomy*, vol. 229, no. 4, pp. 577–581, 2016.

[7] J. A. Haller Jr., S. S. Kramer, and S. A. Lietman, "Use of CT scans in selection of patients for pectus excavatum surgery: a preliminary report," *Journal of Pediatric Surgery*, vol. 22, no. 10, pp. 904–906, 1987.

[8] S. W. Daunt, J. H. Cohen, and S. F. Miller, "Age-related normal ranges for the Haller index in children," *Pediatric Radiology*, vol. 34, no. 4, pp. 326–330, 2004.

[9] F. De Maio, A. Fichera, V. De Luna, F. Mancini, and R. Caterini, "Orthopaedic aspects of Marfan syndrome: the experience of a referral center for diagnosis of rare diseases," *Advances in Orthopedics*, vol. 2016, Article ID 8275391, 6 pages, 2016.

[10] H. R. Weiss and D. Goodall, "Rate of complications in scoliosis surgery - a systematic review of the Pub Med literature," *Scoliosis*, vol. 3, no. 1, p. 9, 2008.

[11] B. J. Toll, A. F. Samdani, M. B. Janjua, S. Gandhi, J. M. Pahys, and S. W. Hwang, "Perioperative complications and risk factors in neuromuscular scoliosis surgery," *Journal of neurosurgery Pediatrics*, vol. 22, no. 2, pp. 207–213, 2018.

[12] D. Alexianu, E. T. Skolnick, A. C. Pinto et al., "Severe hypotension in the prone position in a child with neurofibromatosis, scoliosis and pectus excavatum presenting for posterior spinal fusion," *Anesthesia & Analgesia*, vol. 98, no. 2, pp. 334-335, 2004.

[13] B. T. Bafus, D. Chiravuri, M. E. van der Velde, B. I. Chu, R. Hirshl, and F. A. Farley, "Severe hypotension associated with the prone position in a child with scoliosis and pectus excavatum undergoing posterior spinal fusion," *Journal of Spinal Disorders & Techniques*, vol. 21, no. 6, pp. 451–454, 2008.

[14] R. Tauchi, N. Kawakami, T. Tsuji et al., "Evaluation of thoracic factors after scoliosis surgery in patients with both scoliosis and pectus excavatum," *European Spine Journal*, vol. 27, no. 2, pp. 381–387, 2018.

[15] Z. G. Chu, J. Q. Yu, Z. G. Yang, L. Q. Peng, H. L. Bai, and X. M. Li, "Correlation between sternal depression and cardiac rotation in pectus excavatum: evaluation with helical CT," *American Journal of Roentgenology*, vol. 195, no. 1, pp. W76–W80, 2010.

[16] J. M. Galas, M. E. van der Velde, S. D. Chiravuri, F. Farley, D. Parra, and G. J. Ensing, "Echocardiographic diagnosis of right ventricular inflow compression associated with pectus excavatum during spinal fusion in prone position," *Congenital Heart Disease*, vol. 4, no. 3, pp. 193–195, 2009.

[17] J. L. Nates, M. Nunnally, R. Kleinpell et al., "ICU admission, discharge, and triage guidelines: a framework to enhance clinical operations, development of institutional policies, and further research," *Critical Care Medicine*, vol. 44, no. 8, pp. 1553–1602, 2016.

[18] Y. Vaidya, S. M. Cavanaugh, and A. S. Dhamoon, *Myocardial stunning and hibernation*, StatPearls, Treasure Island (FL), 2019.

# 33

# Paediatric Posttraumatic Cyst-Like Lesions: A Report of Two Cases and Review of the Literature

**R. Jansen**,[1] **F. van Rooijen**,[1] **J. P. Toirkens**,[2] **A. T. Besselaar**,[1] **and J. J. Tolk**[1]

[1]*Máxima MC, Department of Orthopaedic Surgery and Trauma, P.O. Box 90052, 5600 PD Eindhoven, Netherlands*
[2]*Máxima MC, Department of Radiology, P.O. Box 90052, 5600 PD Eindhoven, Netherlands*

Correspondence should be addressed to J. J. Tolk; jaap.tolk@mmc.nl

Academic Editor: John Nyland

Posttraumatic cyst-like lesions are a rare finding after greenstick fractures in children. These asymptomatic, cystic lesions become radiologically apparent 2-4 months after the initial trauma. Conventional radiographs typically show nonexpansile, well-circumscribed lesions in the cortex, proximal to the fracture site. It is important to recognize them as benign to prevent unnecessary concern and additional imaging or invasive diagnostic procedures. No treatment is indicated, as they eventually resolve spontaneously in 1 to 3 years. The two cases of posttraumatic cyst-like lesions after paediatric forearm fractures are presented.

## 1. Introduction

Posttraumatic cyst-like lesions in children are quite a rare phenomenon with only approximately 30 cases reported in literature [1–5]. The cystic lesions are usually first spotted on conventional radiographs as nonexpansile, well-circumscribed lucent lesions in the cortex, no larger than 10 mm [4, 6]. In more than 80% of the cases, the lesions were located in the distal radius. They become radiologically apparent 2-4 months and occur most frequently after greenstick or torus fracture of the distal radius in children [1]. These are benign lesions and should not be confused with more aggressive or expansive lesions such as osteomyelitis or bone tumours [1–6]. It is therefore important to be informed about these benign posttraumatic bone cysts to prevent unnecessary further diagnostics or even invasive diagnostic methods.

## 2. Case

*2.1. Case 1.* A 4-year-old female presented with pain over the left wrist after a fall down the stairs. Clinical examination revealed tenderness over the distal radius and ulna with a limited range of motion. Initial X-rays showed a Salter-Harris type 2 fracture of the distal radius, with minimal dorsal displacement and a small line on the ulna suggestive for an ulnar fissure (Figures 1(a) and 1(b)).

She was treated conservatively with a below-elbow cast and regained a full range of motion after only two weeks of treatment. After six months follow-up, an X-ray was obtained to monitor potential growth disturbance. The images showed the fracture had healed completely and showed no signs of growth disturbance. However, it also revealed the three well-circumscribed lucent lesions in the cortex, proximal to the earlier fracture site (Figure 2). The cysts were asymptomatic with no signs of inflammation, osteolysis, or signs suggesting osteomyelitis and were therefore recognized as benign posttraumatic bone cysts. At one-year follow-up, no additional lesions or growth of the lesions was discovered. No further follow-up or investigation was deemed necessary.

*2.2. Case 2.* A 6-year-old girl presented with a painful and swollen left wrist after a fall. Clinical examination showed tenderness and soft tissue swelling over the distal radius with no limitations in range of motion. X-rays showed a distal forearm fracture with a Salter-Harris type 2 fracture of the distal radius and a greenstick fracture of the distal ulna (Figures 3(a) and 3(b)). She was treated conservatively with

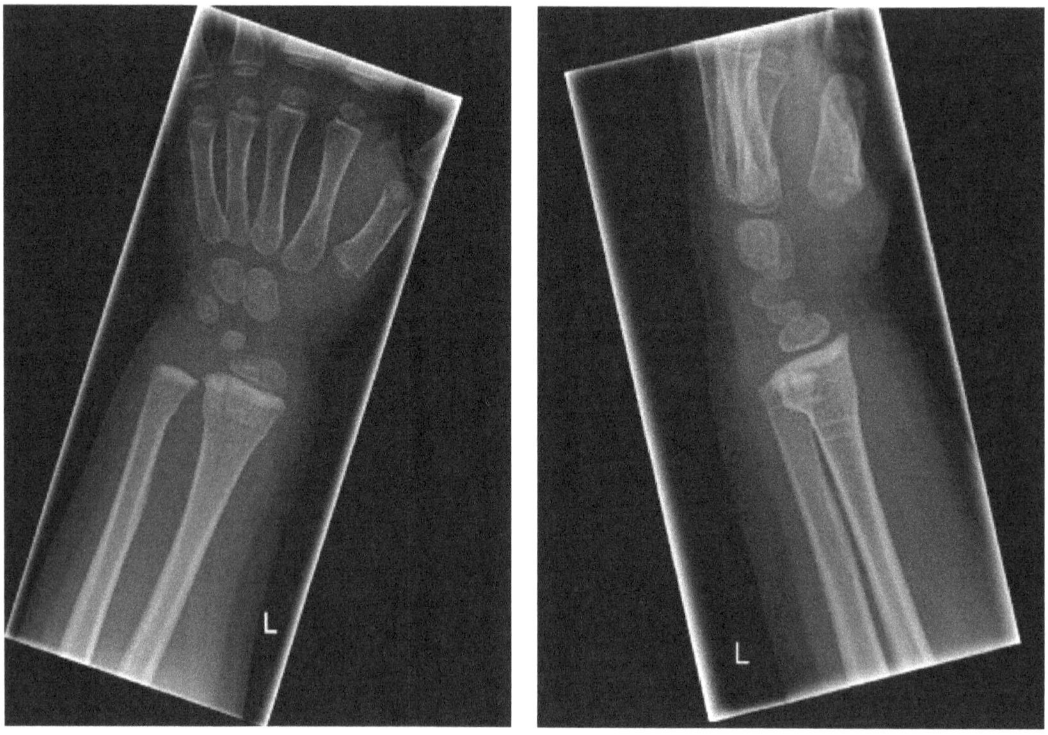

FIGURE 1: (a, b) Anteroposterior and lateral radiographs of the left wrist showing Salter-Harris type 2 fracture of the distal radius, with minimal dorsal displacement and a small line on the ulna suggestive for an ulnar fissure.

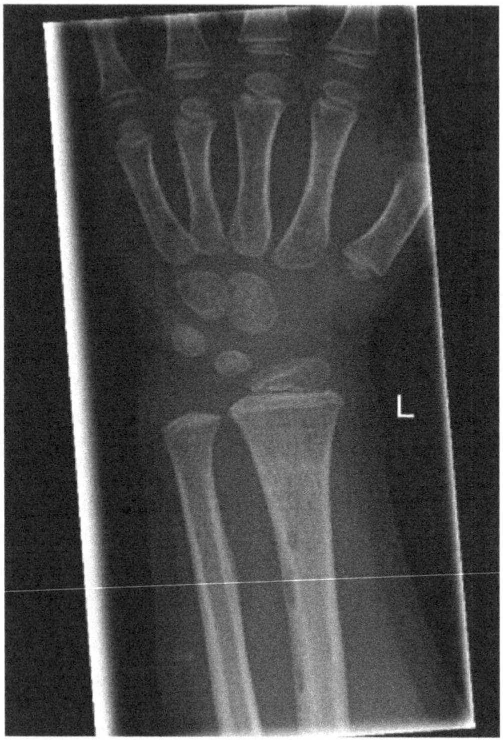

FIGURE 2: Anteroposterior radiograph showing complete consolidation and three well-circumscribed lucent lesions in the cortex, proximal to the previous fracture site.

a below-elbow cast for four weeks. At 4 weeks check-up, there was a good clinical recovery and X-rays showed a normal healing process.

After four months, she reported for follow-up with X-rays. The images not only showed consolidation of the fracture but also revealed two well-circumscribed lucent lesions in the cortex proximal to the previously fractured region (Figure 4(a)). The lesions were asymptomatic with no signs of inflammation, osteolysis, or osteomyelitis and were diagnosed as benign posttraumatic bone cysts.

She was seen for follow-up once more after six months at which point accompanying X-rays showed a decrease of the lucent lesions (Figure 4(b)). No further follow-up or investigation was required.

## 3. Discussion

Paediatric posttraumatic bone cysts are considered to be a quite rare phenomenon, with only around 30 cases reported in medical journals [1, 2, 7]. They appear in children ranging from 2 to 15 years old and can occur in single form or in multiple lesions. The exact prevalence is unknown; however, it is possible that they have a higher occurrence but remain underreported. Posttraumatic bone cysts usually appear a few months after an initial greenstick fracture [8]. This might add to underreporting, because treatment and radiographic follow-up will often have already ended by then for most children.

Regarding aetiology, the most widely accepted theory is that the lesions develop because of subperiosteal enclosure

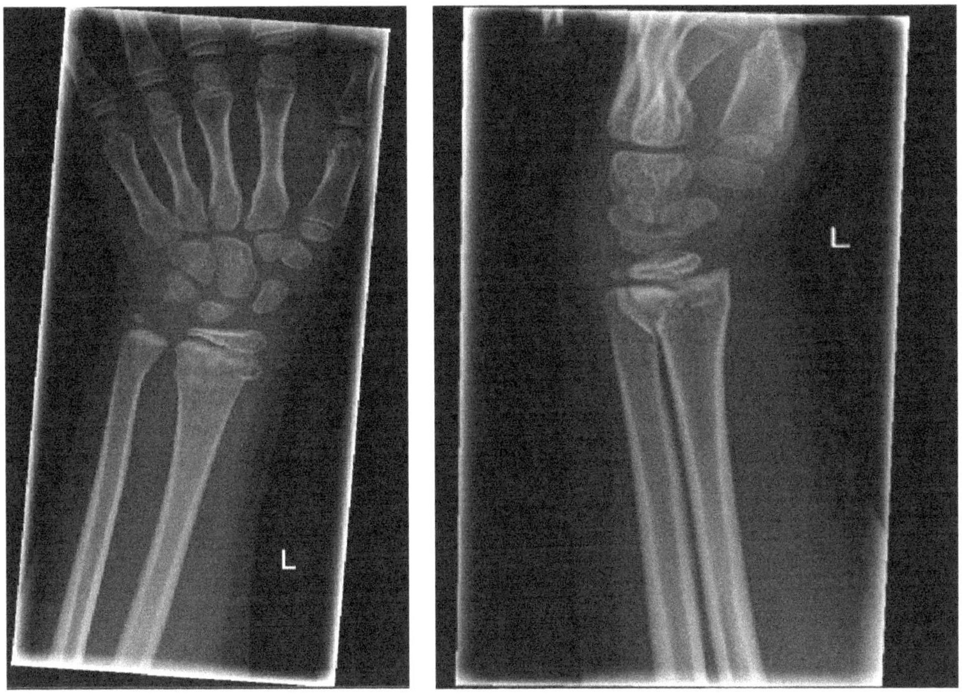

(a) (b)

FIGURE 3: (a, b) Anteroposterior and lateral radiographs of the left wrist distal forearm fracture showing a Salter-Harris type 2 fracture of the distal radius and a greenstick fracture of the distal ulna.

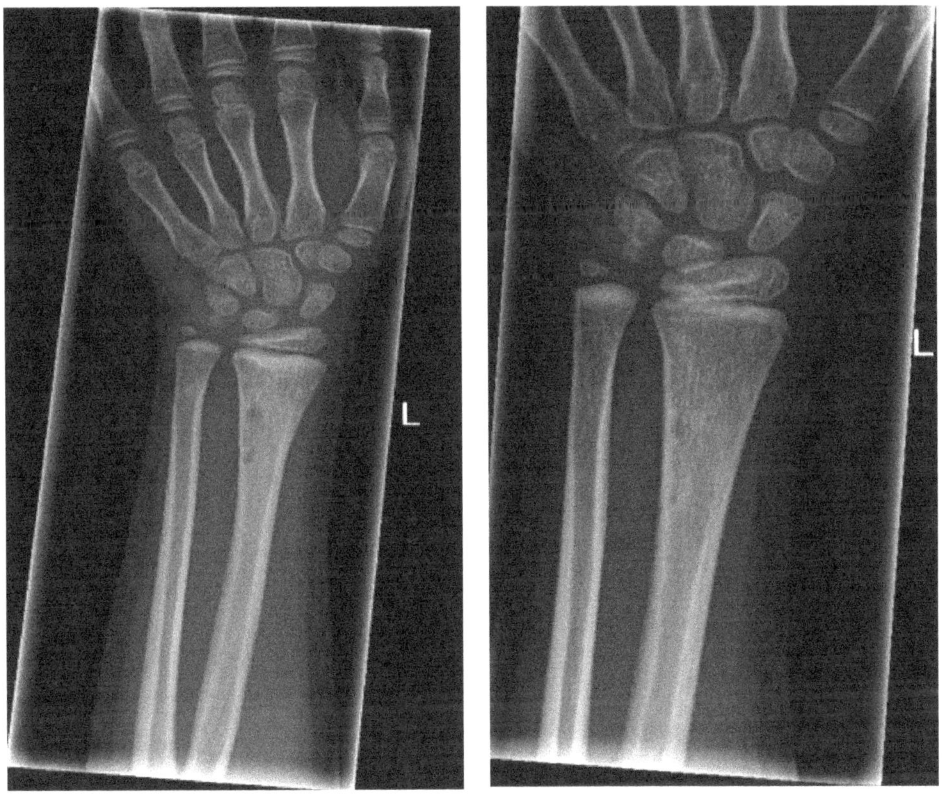

(a) (b)

FIGURE 4: (a) Radiograph showing complete bone healing of the fracture. Two well-circumscribed lucent lesions in the cortex proximal to the previously fractured region. (b) Radiograph showing the lucent lesions fading away.

of intramedullary fat after a fracture [1, 9–11]. Specifically in paediatric patients, the firm periosteum remains intact, allowing extravasated blood and fat derived from the fracture site to be encapsulated underneath. This theory was first suggested by Malghem et al. and supported by their analysis of the cysts on computed tomography (CT), which showed that the lesions seemed to consist of fatty content. They also stated that the lesions might actually appear much sooner after the trauma but initially remain concealed beneath the hematoma on early radiographs. After the hematoma clears up or becomes calcified, the lesions become apparent on radiographs [3].

The cysts are quite rare which is mainly caused by the fact that in order to arise there needs to be a sufficient trauma to cause a disruption of the cortex, while keeping the periosteum intact. In the cases presented, multiple cyst-like lesions are found. Cases of either single or multiple lesions have both been reported; this is probably related to the fracture pattern [1, 2, 7, 8]. The cysts are only reported in children, probably because their periosteum is thicker so it has a higher chance of staying intact during trauma.

While earlier reports mainly focused on imaging and further diagnostics, it is important to note that these benign cysts can easily be recognized on conventional X-rays. This is because of their occurrence after a fracture and their specific location in the cortex, proximal to the fracture. The typical radiological appearance is a radiolucency that is restricted to the cortical bone, having fatty radiodensity and appearing minimally aggressive. The lesions may be multiple or single and are rounded or oval in shape, nonexpansile, and usually less than 1 cm in diameter. Sequential radiographs show the lesions "migrating" away from the epiphyseal disc [4, 10]. Furthermore, these benign cysts eventually resolve spontaneously in 1-3 years, without interfering with the healing process of the fracture [6].

Regarding differential diagnosis, other diagnoses to be considered are simple bone cyst, aneurysmal bone cyst, eosinophilic granuloma, and osteomyelitis. Posttraumatic bone cysts are asymptomatic and are thus not accompanied by fever or pain. When either of these symptoms does occur, the diagnosis becomes less likely and further diagnostic methods are required. In the event of atypical clinical or radiographic presentation, additional imaging using magnetic resonance imaging (MRI) or CT is indicated.

On CT, the lesions can be observed as a fatty radiodensity, possibly accompanied by local thickening of cortical bone [8]. On MRI, the fatty content can be observed as round foci of increased signal intensity on T1-weighted images and intermediate signal intensity on T2-weighted images. Location corresponds to the cystic lesions on radiographs [3].

## 4. Conclusion

Posttraumatic cyst-like lesions are a rare finding after fractures in children. They typically present 2-4 months after the initial trauma as asymptomatic, nonexpansile, well-circumscribed lesions in the cortex. As no treatment is indicated, it is important to recognise them as benign to prevent unnecessary concern and additional diagnostic procedures.

## References

[1] G. Freire, R. Cruz, M. H. Valentim, T. G. Maerques, and P. D. Afonso, "Post-traumatic cyst-like lesion of cortical bone in children," *Skeletal Radiology*, vol. 48, no. 1, pp. 167–174, 2019.

[2] S. Houshian, N. W. Pedersen, T. Torfing, and N. Venkatram, "Post-traumatic cortical cysts in paediatric fractures: is it a concern for emergency doctors? A report of three cases," *European Journal of Emergency Medicine*, vol. 14, no. 6, pp. 365–367, 2007.

[3] N. G. Papadimitriou, J. Christophorides, T. A. Beslikas, E. G. Doulianaki, and A. G. Papadimitriou, "Post-traumatic cystic lesion following fracture of the radius," *Skeletal Radiology*, vol. 34, no. 7, pp. 411–414, 2005.

[4] J. C. Y. Beh and E. S. M. Hamouda, "Paediatric post-traumatic osseous cystic lesion following a distal radial fracture," *Journal of Radiology Case Reports*, vol. 10, no. 7, pp. 23–29, 2016.

[5] A. Asrian, M. Shahabpour, F. Tajdar, and H. de Boeck, "Post-traumatic cyst-like lesions of cortical bone in children," *Acta Orthopaedica Belgica*, vol. 76, no. 2, pp. 264–268, 2010.

[6] L. Pfister-Goedeke and M. Braune, "Cyst-like defects following fractures in children," *Pediatric Radiology*, vol. 11, no. 2, pp. 83–86, 1981.

[7] T. E. Moore, A. R. King, R. C. Travis, and B. C. Allen, "Post-traumatic cysts and cyst-like lesions of bone," *Skeletal Radiology*, vol. 18, no. 2, pp. 93–97, 1989.

[8] A. Courvoisier, E. Bourgeois, C. Durand, and J. Griffet, "Post-traumatic cyst-like lesion of the radius: a rare but benign lesion," *Diagnostic and Interventional Imaging*, vol. 95, no. 1, pp. 117–120, 2014.

[9] J. Malghem and B. Maldague, "Transient fatty cortical defects following fractures in children," *Skeletal Radiology*, vol. 15, no. 5, pp. 368–371, 1986.

[10] R. T. Roach, V. Cassar-Pullicino, and B. N. Summers, "Paediatric post-traumatic cortical defects of the distal radius," *Pediatric Radiology*, vol. 32, no. 5, pp. 333–339, 2002.

[11] C. D. Phillips and T. Keats, "The development of post-traumatic cystlike lesions in bone," *Skeletal Radiology*, vol. 15, no. 8, pp. 631–634, 1986.

34

# A Novel Approach to Augmenting Allograft Hamstring Anterior Cruciate Ligament Reconstructions Utilizing a Resorbable Type I Collagen Matrix with Platelet Rich Plasma

**Sean Mc Millan**,[1] **Danielle Thorn**,[2] **and Elizabeth Ford**[3]

[1]*Department of Orthopedics, Virtua Health System, 2103 Burlington-Mount Holly Rd, Burlington, NJ 08016, USA*
[2]*Department of Orthopedics, Virtua Health System, Burlington, NJ, USA*
[3]*Department of Orthopedics, Inspira Health System, Vineland, NJ, USA*

Correspondence should be addressed to Sean Mc Millan; mcmillansean@hotmail.com

Academic Editor: Athanassios Papanikolaou

*Background.* Anterior cruciate ligament reconstruction (ACLR) is one of the most common lower extremity orthopedic surgeries performed in the United States. Annually, between 100,000 and 200,000 ACL tears affect 1 in 3,000 people. The selection of autograft versus allograft for ACLR has been widely discussed in terms of risk of graft failure. Allograft reconstructions have been shown to have higher rerupture rates. One factor contributing to this risk is delayed biologic graft incorporation. *Methods.* A retrospective review was performed examining 14 patients who underwent an augmented quadruple-stranded hamstring allograft ACLR with a type I resorbable collagen matrix impregnated with platelet-rich plasma (PRP). *Results.* Within our clinical practice, the augmentation of quadruple-stranded hamstring allograft ACLR with a type I resorbable matrix impregnated with PRP has yielded good early clinical success at 2-year outcomes ($N = 14$). Zero ACLR failures have been reported to date in this series. *Conclusion.* This case series offers a novel approach for soft tissue allograft ACLR augmented with a type I collagen matrix impregnated with PRP. The authors theorize that this augmentation may improve biologic graft incorporation into the host bone tunnels.

## 1. Introduction

Anterior cruciate ligament reconstruction (ACLR) is one of the most common lower extremity orthopedic surgeries performed in the United States. The anterior cruciate ligament (ACL) is important for the stability of the knee, controlling against excessive motion. Furthermore, the ACL resists anterior tibial translation, while providing rotatory stability and proprioception. Annually, between 100,000 and 200,000 [1, 2], ACL tears affect 1 in 3,000 people in the general population at an estimated cost of $3 billion [3].

ACLR failure can be defined in a multitude of ways. Noyes and Barber-Westin defined ACLR failures requiring surgical correction as: a complete graft tear with >6 mm of anterior tibial displacement as compared to the healthy knee; a positive pivot shift test graded +2 or +3 compared to the healthy knee, with or without knee pain or inflammation, or subjective sensation of instability or functional limitations for daily life and/or sports activities [4]. Factors leading to ACLR failure include surgical technique, failed biology, and rehabilitation protocols.

Poor surgical technique has been identified as a risk of graft failure [5, 6]. More specifically, failure has been associated with mal-positioning of the graft in the femoral tunnel, resulting in increased graft load, abnormal knee kinematics, and/or instability of the knee joint [7]. Similarly, failure of biologic incorporation of the graft been correlated to ACL graft survivorship, specifically in the setting of allograft usage [5–7]. Benefits of autograft tissue for ACLR include decreased risk of tissue rejection, decreased procedural cost, and faster graft incorporation potential. Conversely, allograft tissue is favored in some instances due to decreased donor site morbidity, ease of surgical technique, decreased surgical time, and more predictable graft size [6]. Nevertheless, allograft ACLR has been associated with higher rates of graft failure compared to autograft tissue [8–13].

A primary reason for allograft ACLR failure has been attributed to a lack of biologic incorporation. Achieving biologic incorporation using allograft is a complex process that involves tissue integration, revascularization, and ultimately "ligamentization" into host tissue [14]. Delayed biologic incorporation of allograft tissue compared to autograft tissue has also been noted in the literature [14–17]. Scheffler et al. noted that allograft tissue incorporation was slower at both 6 weeks and 12 weeks compared to the incorporation of autograft tissue. This trend of "incorporation lag" continued out to 52 weeks. Various factors have been theorized as to the delayed incorporation, including allograft processing and purifications methods [14–19].

Consideration of the delicate balance between the attraction of allograft and the respect for biologic graft incorporation is a challenging dilemma for orthopedic surgeons. The introduction of ACLR scaffolds and biologic agents has been discussed to improve healing [20]. A systematic review by Andriolo et al. found a positive impact of platelet-rich plasma (PRP) in ACL graft ligamentization and inflammatory modulation. Additionally, acceleration of ACLR graft maturation and incorporation was seen [21–23]. The authors present a case series detailing a novel surgical approach to improve the outcomes of allograft ACLR utilizing a resorbable type I collagen matrix (TenoMend™) (Exactech, Gainesville, FL) soaked in PRP (Accelerate® PRP) (Exactech, Gainesville FL) (Figure 1). The resorbable type I collagen matrix is bovine-derived and is both chemically and mechanically machined. These unique properties provide a porous scaffold that enables acceptance of the PRP while permitting cellular incorporation between the graft and bone interface. Furthermore, the wrap acts to shelter the intra-articular portion of the graft from the negative effects of plasmin, thus allowing for the valuable nutrients to survive in the intra-articular environment [24, 25].

## 2. Materials and Methods

Institutional Board Review (IRB) approval at the lead authors' institution was obtained for this retrospective evaluation. A retrospective chart review from 2014 to 2016 was performed looking specifically at patients who underwent quadruple-stranded hamstring allograft ACLR with a type I collagen matrix augment impregnated with PRP. Hybrid grafts and autografts were excluded. All outcomes were extrapolated from this chart review. Outcomes were defined as a failure if there was an ACL graft retear or instability requiring revision ACLR. A total of 14 ACLR were identified within this time frame that met the above criteria. All patients underwent the following arthroscopic technique.

Routine diagnostic arthroscopy is performed, and confirmation of the ACL tear is noted. Next, two nonirradiated semitendinosus hamstring allografts are selected from the cadaver bank and thawed in a warm Bacitracin-infused saline bath. The allografts are measured and cut to equal lengths. Each end of the allograft is then whip-stitched. Next, the allografts are doubled over an adjustable button suture loop (Rigidloop Adjustable™) (MITEK, Raynham, MA) and tensioned to 20 pounds of force on a standard prep board for 20 minutes.

Whole blood (60 cc) is obtained from the patient at the time of surgery in a sterile fashion from the upper extremity. The blood is processed and separated using a gentle centrifugal technique (Accelerate® Autologous Platelet Concentrating System) (Exactech, Gainesville, FL). The PRP, or buffy coat layer, is collected at 6-10 ml of solution. The platelet-poor plasma (PPP) is also collected (10 cc) for later use in the procedure.

The collagen matrix is then cut to fit the semitendinosus graft and soaked in the PRP bath for a period of 5 minutes. Following this, the collagen wrap is placed around the hamstring allograft and sutured into place via a combination of 3-0 Vicryl interrupted and locking sutures (Figure 2). It should be noted that the collagen matrix is machined to come precurled, facilitating the ease of placement around the allograft tissue.

ACL tunnel preparation is then carried out in standard arthroscopic fashion via independent tunnel drilling consistent with an "anatomic" graft placement. The graft diameter had previously been sized at the conclusion of tensioning and prior to the application of the collagen graft. Typically, line-to-line drilling is undertaken; however, in instances where the graft is extremely snug in the sizer, the lead author elects to upsize by 0.5 mm for the tunnel drilling. On the tibial side, care is taken to preserve as much of the native ACL footprint as possible, allowing cellular migration from the native tissue across the graft and potentially leading to quicker ligamentization.

Upon completion of the tunnel preparation, the graft is carefully shuttled up through the tibial and femoral tunnels, and the adjustable button is flipped onto the lateral femoral cortex (Figure 3). The graft is secured into the tibial canal utilizing a screw and sheath technique within the four limbs of the graft under 20 pounds of manual tension. After checking the isometry and tension of the graft, attention is turned to the remaining PRP. Under a "dry scope technique," 3-4 ml of PRP is injected between the allograft tendons and the collagen wrap utilizing an 18-gauge spinal needle (Figure 4). The remaining PRP is then injected into the femoral and tibial tunnels. Finally, the previously harvested PPP is injected into the joint after the portals are closed. A standard soft tissue ACLR postoperative rehabilitation protocol is followed upon discharge.

## 3. Results

14 patients were identified to have undergone quadruple-stranded nonirradiated hamstring allograft ALCRs with a type I collagen wrap augmentation. The average age of the patients who underwent the procedure was 33 years of age (range 24-44). 0 out of 14 patients had reported rerupture at a minimum of 24 months postprocedure. None of the patients required further surgical intervention for instability. None of the patients had reported adverse events related to the surgical procedure. 1 of the 14 patients underwent repeat arthroscopy approximately 13

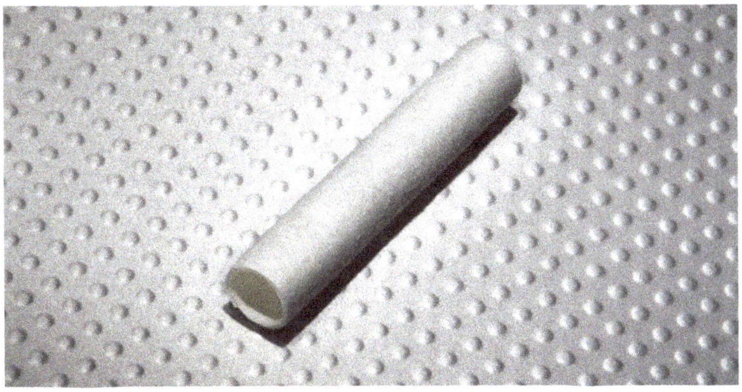

FIGURE 1: TenoMend™ comes as a machined pre-curled resorbable type I collagen. (Re-Printed with Permission from Exactech, Gainesville, FL).

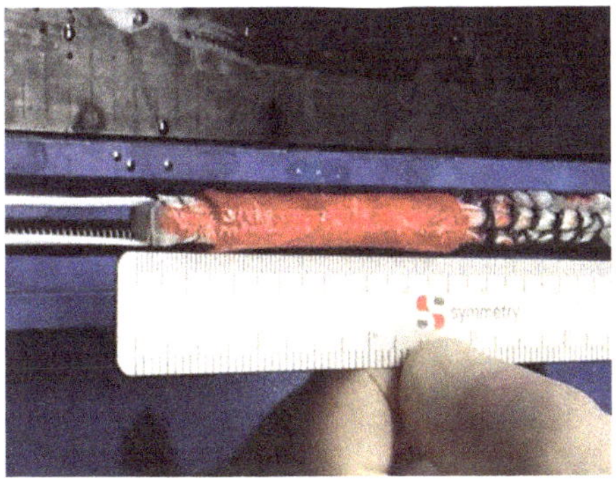

FIGURE 2: The soft tissue graft is tensioned on a standard prep board. The PRP-soaked TenoMend™ is sutured around the graft, ensuring coverage of the graft contained within the bone tunnels as well as the joint.

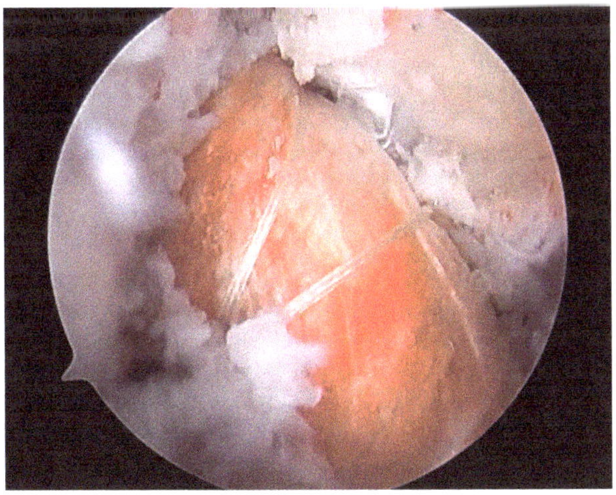

FIGURE 3: The graft has been secured into the femoral tunnel. The PRP-soaked collagen wrap maintains the biologic agent within the aqueous environment.

months postprocedure for a failed medial meniscus repair. The ACLR was noted to be intact at that time with signs of ligamentization.

## 4. Discussion

ACLR failure rates are a troubling problem for orthopedic surgeons, particularly in a younger or more athletic population. There is a disparity in the literature regarding the rate of ACLR failure rates [4, 6–12, 17, 19]. Contributing to the wide range of reported failure rates includes variation in graft choice, surgical technique, patient demographics, and the use of biologics as an augment. While each factor can have a certain measure of control placed upon them, it is nevertheless implicit upon the surgeon to explore all options that can optimize patient outcomes.

Several articles have discussed the risk of ACLR failure associated with allograft tissue [6–19]. A significant increase in ACLR failure has been shown in young patients who received allograft tissue in their reconstruction procedures [10–13, 19]. Kaeding et al., in a review of the data from the Multicenter Orthopaedic Outcomes Network (MOON) trials, found a four times higher ACLR graft failure rate when using allograft versus autograft in the population of 10–19 years. A meta-analysis of levels 2 and 3 studies, comparing primary patellar tendon autograft and allograft ACLRs, found approximately five times higher odds of graft rupture for patients who received allograft reconstructions [11]. Similarly, a meta-analysis of 20 studies by Prodromos et al. reported a 5% failure rate in autografts compared with a 14% failure rate in allografts ($P < 0.01$) [12]. Finally, a recent meta-analysis by Ellis et al. found allograft failure rates of 25.5% compared to 8.5% for bone-patella-bone autografts [13].

Delay in biologic graft incorporation has been of primary concern when considering allograft failures [19–21]. Rappé et al. found a 33% failure rate when using irradiated Achilles tendon allografts to a 2.4% failure rate when using nonirradiated Achilles tendon allografts [18]. The role of irradiation may weaken the integrity of the allograft tendon, predisposing it to tear in a highly active population. The advent of nonirradiated allografts has allowed for a decrease in the allograft failure rates; however, these numbers still exceed that of autograft ACLR

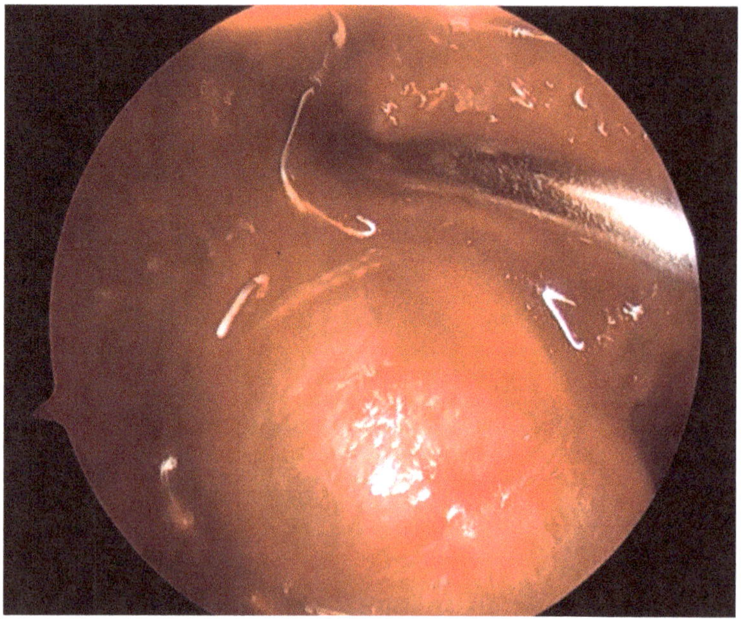

Figure 4: Under a dry environment, the remaining PRP is injected into the bone tunnels as well as within the collagen wrap.

outcomes [18]. Nonetheless, some surgeons or patients favor the use of allograft due to ease of procedure, availability without delay, decreased donor site morbidity, and decreased surgical time. Based upon this, the authors theorized that the addition of a porous type I collagen scaffold reconstituted with PRP could decrease the risk of failure by increasing the likelihood of biologic graft incorporation.

The concept of utilizing biologics as an augment for ACLR has gained popularity in recent years [19–23]. Fleissner et al. reported on 143 patients who underwent ACLR with autograft augmented with type I collagen matrix hydrated with PRP. In their series, the failure rate was 5% [19]. Of note, there was a 92% return to previous activity reported with return to play allowed, on average, at 22 weeks postprocedure. By way of comparison, Arden et al. noted in their ACLR group a return to preinjury sports participation of only 60% [26]. A second look arthroscopy on one ACLR for a separate injury demonstrated graft incorporation with neovascularization and ligamentization at 7 months postprocedure. Furthermore, Weiler et al. demonstrated that the adjunct of PRP on an ACLR can lead to advanced graft maturation and increased tensile strength [27]. Fleming et al. also found this to be true in their porcine model, further noting that biologic augmentation resulted in decreased ligament laxity [28].

The concept of utilizing type I collagen matrix, hydrated with a PRP clot to block plasmin from the healing environment, is a novel approach to a known hostile environment within the intra-articular knee joint. Murray et al. has done extensive work through their Bridge-Enhanced Anterior Cruciate Ligament Repair (BEAR) collagen scaffold research [29, 30]. The BEAR scaffold is applied to primary ACL repairs as opposed to ACLR. Nevertheless, one of the functions of the BEAR scaffold is to allow for and promote the formation of a protective fibrin clot between the native ACL and the remaining anatomic structures of the ACL within the knee joint. These authors note that one possible failure of previous work done on native ACL tear from healing is due to the failure of fibrin clot formation, which functions as a provisional scaffold within the ACL wound site. This deficiency is likely secondary to the ACL's location within the synovial cavity [2, 24, 25]. To circumvent this problem, collagen-platelet composites (CPCs) have been used as a substitute scaffolding material [25]. This scaffold simulates a fibrin clot, creating an environment conducive to healing within the gap between the torn ends of the ACL. Primary ACL repair is of particular interest because this treatment would avoid the morbidities associated with tissue harvest or allograft use, it would potentially retain the ligament insertion sites, and it could better preserve the proprioceptive nerves of the ACL.

This 14 patient case series on patients who underwent ACLR with a type I collagen augment impregnated with PRP demonstrated positive outcomes at of minimum 2 years postprocedure evaluation. The authors realize limitations exist. First, a small sample size is reported, and as such, this should be considered in the context of a case series. A second limitation is the lack of standardized laxity testing, such as KT-1000. Per standard postoperative protocol, the lead author does not routinely have this test performed on patients; however, chart review notes "negative Lachman" test at final follow-up on each of the 14 patients. Furthermore, there was the absence of subjective knee instability at the final follow-up. Anecdotally, the authors feel that there was less knee laxity in the patients who underwent the allograft ACLR with augmentation versus those who did not.

## 5. Conclusion

Improving patient outcomes in ACLR is a continuous journey for orthopedic surgeons. Many variables require contemplation by the treating surgeon when performing an ACLR. In situations where allograft tissue is to be used, steps should be taken to aid in the process of biologic graft incorporation. The authors feel that they present a compelling case series offering a novel approach to allograft ACLR utilizing a type I collagen wrap impregnated with PRP. Further investigation is warranted into this technique including a larger sample size, KT-1000 testing, and potentially tissue biopsy to evaluate for tissue viability.

## References

[1] M. D. Gordon and M. E. Steiner, "Anterior cruciate ligament injuries," in *Orthopaedic Knowledge Update Sports Medicine III*, J. G. Garrick, Ed., p. 169, American Academy of Orthopaedic Surgeons, Rosemont, 2004.

[2] V. Musahl and J. Karlsson, "Anterior cruciate ligament tear," *The New England Journal of Medicine*, vol. 380, no. 24, pp. 2341–2348, 2019.

[3] M. M. Herzog, S. W. Marshall, J. L. Lund, V. Pate, and J. T. Spang, "Cost of outpatient arthroscopic anterior cruciate ligament reconstruction among commercially insured patients in the United States, 2005-2013," *Orthopaedic Journal of Sports Medicine*, vol. 5, no. 1, 2017.

[4] F. R. Noyes and S. D. Barber-Westin, "Revision anterior cruciate surgery with use of bone-patellar tendon-bone autogenous grafts," *The Journal of Bone and Joint Surgery. American Volume*, vol. 83, no. 8, pp. 1131–1143, 2001.

[5] B. R. Bach and M. T. Provencher, *ACL Surgery: How to Get it Right the First Time and What to Do if it Fails*, SLACK, Thorofare, NJ, 2010.

[6] J. A. Morgan, D. Dahm, B. Levy, M. J. Stuart, and and the MARS Study Group, "Femoral tunnel malposition in ACL revision reconstruction," *The Journal of Knee Surgery*, vol. 25, no. 5, pp. 361–368, 2012.

[7] P. Di Benedetto, E. Di Benedetto, A. Fiocchi, A. Beltrame, and A. Causero, "Causes of failure of anterior cruciate ligament reconstruction and revision surgical strategies," *Knee Surgery & Related Research*, vol. 28, no. 4, pp. 319–324, 2016.

[8] K. P. Spindler, J. E. Kuhn, K. B. Freedman, C. E. Matthews, R. S. Dittus, and F. E. Harrell Jr., "Anterior cruciate ligament reconstruction autograft choice: bone-tendon-bone versus hamstring: does it really matter? A systematic review," *The American Journal of Sports Medicine*, vol. 32, no. 8, pp. 1986–1995, 2004.

[9] G. Samitier, A. I. Marcano, E. Alentorn-Geli, R. Cugat, K. W. Farmer, and M. W. Moser, "Failure of anterior cruciate ligament reconstruction," *Archives of bone and joint surgery*, vol. 3, no. 4, pp. 220–240, 2015.

[10] C. C. Kaeding, B. Aros, A. Pedroza et al., "Allograft versus autograft anterior cruciate ligament reconstruction: predictors of failure from a MOON prospective longitudinal cohort," *Sports Health: A Multidisciplinary Approach*, vol. 3, no. 1, pp. 73–81, 2011.

[11] A. J. Krych, J. D. Jackson, T. L. Hoskin, and D. L. Dahm, "A meta-analysis of patellar tendon autograft versus patellar tendon allograft in anterior cruciate ligament reconstruction," *Arthroscopy: The Journal of Arthroscopic & Related Surgery*, vol. 24, no. 3, pp. 292–298, 2008.

[12] C. Prodromos, B. Joyce, and K. Shi, "A meta-analysis of stability of autografts compared to allografts after anterior cruciate ligament reconstruction," *Knee Surgery, Sports Traumatology, Arthroscopy*, vol. 15, no. 7, pp. 851–856, 2007.

[13] A. I. Cruz Jr., J. J. Beck, M. D. Ellington et al., "Failure rates of autograft and allograft ACL reconstruction in patients 19 years of age and younger," *JBJS Open Access*, vol. 5, no. 4, 2020.

[14] J. Ménétrey, V. B. Duthon, T. Laumonier, and D. Fritschy, ""Biological failure" of the anterior cruciate ligament graft," *Knee Surgery, Sports Traumatology, Arthroscopy*, vol. 16, no. 3, pp. 224–231, 2008.

[15] J. L. Carey, W. R. Dunn, D. L. Dahm, S. L. Zeger, and K. P. Spindler, "A systematic review of anterior cruciate ligament reconstruction with autograft compared with allograft," *The Journal of Bone and Joint Surgery. American Volume*, vol. 91, no. 9, pp. 2242–2250, 2009.

[16] S. U. Scheffler, T. Schmidt, I. Gangéy, M. Dustmann, F. Unterhauser, and A. Weiler, "Fresh-frozen free-tendon allografts versus autografts in anterior cruciate ligament reconstruction: delayed remodeling and inferior mechanical function during long-term healing in sheep," *Arthroscopy*, vol. 24, no. 4, pp. 448–458, 2008.

[17] G. G. Poehling, W. W. Curl, C. A. Lee et al., "Analysis of outcomes of anterior cruciate ligament repair with 5-year follow-up: allograft versus autograft," *Arthroscopy*, vol. 21, no. 7, pp. 774–785, 2005.

[18] M. Rappé, M. Horodyski, K. Meister, and P. A. Indelicato, "Nonirradiated versus irradiated Achilles allograft: in vivo failure comparison," *The American Journal of Sports Medicine*, vol. 35, no. 10, pp. 1653–1658, 2007.

[19] A. S. Berdis, K. Veale, and P. R. Fleissner Jr., "Outcomes of anterior cruciate ligament reconstruction using biologic augmentation in patients 21 years of age and younger," *Arthroscopy: The Journal of Arthroscopic & Related Surgery*, vol. 35, no. 11, pp. 3107–3113, 2019.

[20] A. M. Looney, J. D. Leider, A. R. Horn, and B. M. Bodendorfer, "Bioaugmentation in the surgical treatment of anterior cruciate ligament injuries: a review of current concepts and emerging techniques," *SAGE Open Medicine*, vol. 8, 2020.

[21] L. Andriolo, B. di Matteo, E. Kon, G. Filardo, G. Venieri, and M. Marcacci, "PRP augmentation for ACL reconstruction," *BioMed Research International*, vol. 2015, Article ID 371746, 15 pages, 2015.

[22] P. Vavken, P. Sadoghi, and M. M. Murray, "The effect of platelet concentrates on graft maturation and graft-bone interface healing in anterior cruciate ligament reconstruction in human patients: a systematic review of controlled trials," *Arthroscopy: The Journal of Arthroscopic & Related Surgery*, vol. 27, no. 11, pp. 1573–1583, 2011.

[23] M. Vogrin, M. Rupreht, D. Dinevski et al., "Effects of a platelet gel on early graft revascularization after anterior cruciate ligament reconstruction: a prospective, randomized, double-blind, clinical trial," *European Surgical Research*, vol. 45, no. 2, pp. 77–85, 2010.

[24] A. Günther, P. Markart, M. Kalinowski, C. Ruppert, F. Grimminger, and W. Seeger, "Cleavage of surfactant-incorporating fibrin by different fibrinolytic agents. Kinetics of lysis and rescue of surface activity," *American Journal of Respiratory Cell and Molecular Biology*, vol. 21, no. 6, pp. 738–745, 1999.

[25] M. E. Kroon, M. L. van Schie, B. van der Vecht, V. W. van Hinsbergh, and P. Koolwijk, "Collagen type 1 retards tube formation by human microvascular endothelial cells in a fibrin matrix," *Angiogenesis*, vol. 5, no. 4, pp. 257–265, 2002.

[26] C. L. Ardern, K. E. Webster, N. F. Taylor, and J. A. Feller, "Return to sport following anterior cruciate ligament reconstruction surgery: a systematic review and meta-analysis of the state of play," *British Journal of Sports Medicine*, vol. 45, no. 7, pp. 596–606, 2011.

[27] A. Weiler, C. Förster, P. Hunt et al., "The influence of locally applied platelet-derived growth factor-BB on free tendon graft remodeling after anterior cruciate ligament reconstruction," *The American Journal of Sports Medicine*, vol. 32, no. 4, pp. 881–891, 2017.

[28] B. C. Fleming, K. P. Spindler, M. P. Palmer, E. M. Magarian, and M. M. Murray, "Collagen-platelet composites improve the biomechanical properties of healing anterior cruciate ligament grafts in a porcine model," *The American Journal of Sports Medicine*, vol. 37, no. 8, pp. 1554–1563, 2009.

[29] A. N. Mastrangelo, P. Vavken, B. C. Fleming, S. L. Harrison, and M. M. Murray, "Reduced platelet concentration does not harm PRP effectiveness for ACL repair in a porcine in vivo model," *Journal of Orthopaedic Research*, vol. 29, no. 7, pp. 1002–1007, 2011.

[30] M. M. Murray, L. A. Kalish, B. C. Fleming et al., "Bridge-Enhanced Anterior Cruciate Ligament Repair: Two-Year Results of a First-in-Human Study," *Orthopaedic journal of sports medicine*, vol. 7, no. 3, 2019.

# 35

# Tuberculous Arthritis of the Knee with Rice Body Formation: A Report of a Rare Case

**Truong Nguyen Khanh Hung,[1,2] Tran Binh Duong,[2] Tran Phuoc Binh,[2] Dao Thanh Tu,[2] Huynh Phuoc Hau,[2] Truong Trong Tin,[3] Cao Thi,[3] and Le Van Tuan[2]**

[1]*College of Medicine, Taipei Medical University, Taipei City, Taiwan*
[2]*Orthopedic and Trauma Department, ChoRay Hospital, Ho Chi Minh City, Vietnam*
[3]*Orthopedic and Rehabilitation Department, University of Medicine and Pharmacy at Ho Chi Minh City, Ho Chi Minh City, Vietnam*

Correspondence should be addressed to Truong Nguyen Khanh Hung; drhung.bvcr@gmail.com, Tran Binh Duong; trungduong45@yahoo.com, Tran Phuoc Binh; bstranphuocbinh@gmail.com, Dao Thanh Tu; dr.thanhtu@yahoo.com, Huynh Phuoc Hau; drhauhuynh86@gmail.com, Truong Trong Tin; drtruongtrongtin@yahoo.com.vn, Cao Thi; caothibacsi@ump.edu.vn, and Le Van Tuan; drlevantuan.cr@gmail.com

Academic Editor: Dimitrios S. Karataglis

In this report, we present the case of a 53-year-old man with rice body formation in the right knee caused by tuberculous arthritis (TB arthritis). The patient visited our hospital in January 2018 with a seven-month history of swelling and pain in the right knee. He had no previous history of tuberculosis, and the results of the routine laboratory tests were within normal limits; he also tested negative for rheumatoid factor. Magnetic resonance (MR) imaging revealed multiple rice bodies in the right knee, measuring 5-8 mm. He underwent an arthroscopic operation in the right knee in January 2018 and received antituberculosis polytherapy for 6 months. He was followed-up for more than 01 year. The patient regained good function of the operated knee with no evidence of recurrence during the last follow-up in February 2019. *Conclusion.* The biggest challenge in diagnosing tuberculosis arthritis is the consideration of its possibility in the differential diagnosis, not only in endemic countries where tuberculosis is frequent. A high level of suspicion for TB should be maintained for every infection of the knee joint, particularly in the case of intra-articular rice bodies.

## 1. Introduction

Tuberculosis (TB) is a common and endemic disease in developing countries [1]. Approximately 10.4 million patients develop active infections worldwide, resulting in almost 1.4 million deaths annually [2]. Although the majority of newly diagnosed cases have pulmonary TB, various organs, bones, and joints may also be affected. Skeletal TB in particular accounts for approximately 10% to 35% of extrapulmonary cases, and the knee is the third most frequently affected site after the spine and hip [3]. Rice body formation in the knee is inconsistent but common in tuberculous and rheumatoid arthritis (RA) or/and tuberculous synovitis. However, it is not commonly encountered by arthroscopic surgeons [4]. Intra-articular rice body formation can occur in chronic inflammatory diseases such as RA, TB arthritis, chronic fungal infections, synovial chondromatosis, pigmented villonodular synovitis, gout, or systemic lupus erythematosus (SLE) [4, 5]. We present the case of a patient requiring arthroscopy of the right knee for arthritis, without a history of pulmonary TB or RA.

This review is intended to report a recent clinical case of TB arthritis of the knee and highlight the need for high levels of suspicion to correctly diagnose TB arthritis. The current concepts of clinical and surgical therapies for this condition have also been discussed.

## 2. Case Presentation

A 53-year-old male driver suffering from knee pain was referred to our orthopedic department in January 2018. He provided a history of continuous and progressive right knee pain since the past 1 year without any constitutional symptoms. On physical examination, his knee was swollen with restricted motion (range of movement 0–100 degrees). Pain was elicited on lateral compression of the femoral condyle. The fluid collected twice during knee arthrocentesis was clear.

Radiographs of the chest and affected knee appeared normal. He had no previous history of tuberculosis, and the results of the routine laboratory tests were within normal limits; he also tested negative for rheumatoid factor. Examination of the blood revealed a white blood cell (WBC) count of 11.38 G/L, C-reactive protein (CRP) level of 5.0 mg/dL, erythrocyte sedimentation rate (ESR) of V1: 34 mm/h and V2: 71 mm/h, and a rheumatoid factor level of 18.6 IU/mL. MRI showed multiple rice bodies measuring 5-8 mm in both T1- and T2-weighted sequences (Figure 1). The patient underwent arthroscopic surgery (Figure 2).

The histopathologic exam revealed granulomatous inflammation with caseous necrosis, suggestive of TB (Figure 3). This is the gold standard to diagnose TB. The polymerase chain reaction (PCR) test for *Mycobacterium tuberculosis* DNA was positive.

The patient was treated with antituberculosis polytherapy that continued for 6 months; it consisted of rifampin, isoniazid, pyrazinamide, and ethambutol in the intensive phase (usually based on 4 drugs) lasting 2 months and isoniazid and ethambutol in the continuation phase (usually with 2 drugs administered) lasting 4 months (2HRZE/4HR). The patient was checked follow up 1 month, 3 months (Figure 4), 6 months and 1 year, respectively. At more than 1-year follow-up, the patient experienced relief from pain and swelling with knee movements ranging from 0 to 120 degrees (Figure 5(a)). The follow-up MRI showed no rice bodies in the T1- and T2-weighted sequences (Figure 5(b)).

The patient provided consent to publish his clinical data in this case report. There are no conflicts of interest to declare.

## 3. Discussion

Rice bodies are shiny white structures with variable sizes and shapes. The shapes may either be like teardrops and nodules or be angular and flake-like [6]. In 1980, Cheung et al. elucidated a theory of synovial origin for rice body formation, in which the synovium undergoes inflammation followed by tiny infarcts and peeling of the infarcted tissue [7]. Two years later, Popert et al. proposed a theory of origin in the synovial fluid, independent of the synovial elements [8]. Musculoskeletal TB may manifest without constitutional symptoms. Pulmonary involvement has been found in only one-third of musculoskeletal TB cases leading to delays in diagnosis [9]; laboratory parameters such as ESR do not have much diagnostic value [10]. Drew et al. suggested that the diagnosis of TB arthritis requires a thorough history emphasizing on relevant travel, a careful physical examination, and appropriate diagnostic testing. In their report, the time for delayed diagnosis was between 2 months and 10 years [11].

According to the global tuberculosis (TB) report, 2017, of the World Health Organization, Vietnam is one of the high-burden countries with 13593 cases of diagnosed TB in 2016 [12]. However, musculoskeletal TB may manifest without constitutional symptoms. It is therefore essential to consider TB in the differential diagnosis as it may easily be misdiagnosed, particularly in patients without a history of TB or specific symptoms. TB should be considered a possible offending infectious agent in cases of unexplained joint pain and swelling. Arthroscopy with antituberculosis polytherapy is an effective treatment, but more research and a long-term follow-up process are necessary to observe the patient effectively.

According to all the reports, the gold standard for diagnosing TB arthritis is synovial biopsy, with positive results in 80% of cases [13, 14]. The findings typical of TB arthritis include granulomas, lymphocytes, and giant cells with caseation. Treatment may involve the use of splints for a short time to decrease acute and chronic symptoms in specific cases of TB arthritis and to prevent deformation of infected joints [15–17]. Surgical procedures should be limited to joints with severe cartilage destruction, deformation of infected joints, large abscesses, and infections with multidrug-resistant or atypical mycobacteria [16, 18]. The main treatment is antituberculosis polytherapy (for 12-18 months) and active-assisted non-weight-bearing exercises of the relevant joints throughout the postoperative period. Operative interventions (synovectomy and debridement) are required when the patient is not responding after 4-5 months of antituberculosis polytherapy [19, 20].

## 4. Conclusion

TB is still an important global public health problem. TB arthritis accounts for approximately 1-3% of all cases of TB and 10-11% of extrapulmonary TB cases [20]. The biggest challenge in diagnosing tuberculosis arthritis is to consider the possibility in the differential diagnosis, not only in endemic countries where tuberculosis is frequent. A high level of suspicion should be maintained for TB in every infection of the knee joint, particularly in cases with intra-articular rice bodies [13, 14, 20]. An early diagnosis and specific and adequate treatment may improve the possibility of maintaining good joint function [15–17]. The main treatment is antituberculous polytherapy (for 12-18 months) and active-assisted non-weight-bearing exercises of the relevant joint throughout the postoperative period [19, 20]. A high level of suspicion for TB should be maintained for every infection of the knee joint, particularly in the case of intra-articular rice bodies.

## Consent

The informed consent was obtained from the patient next of kin for the publication of this report and any accompanying images.

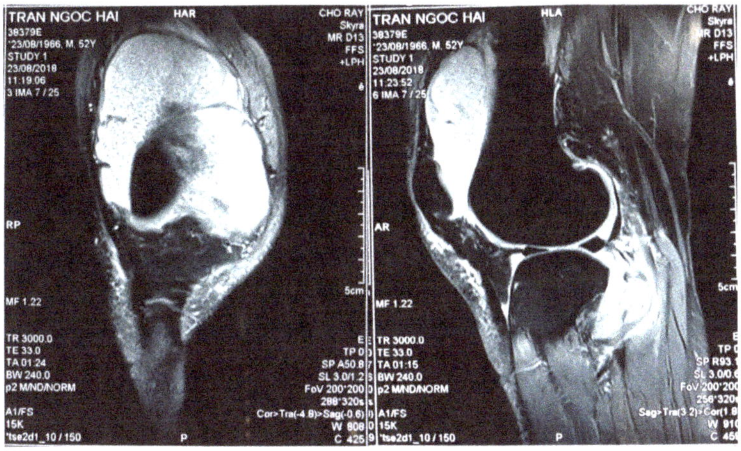


Figure 1: MRI showed multiple rice bodies.

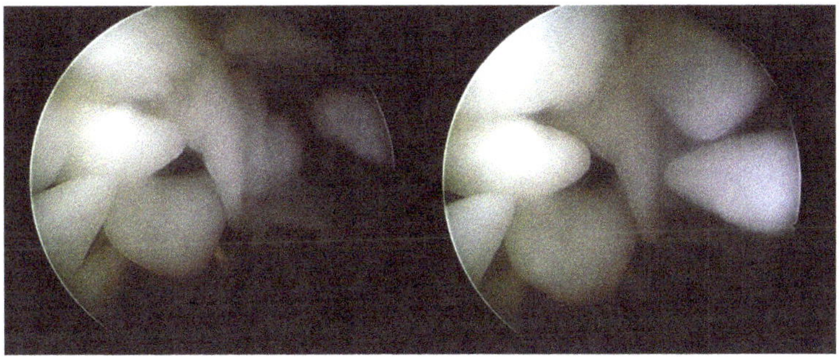

Figure 2: Rice bodies are seen during arthroscopy.

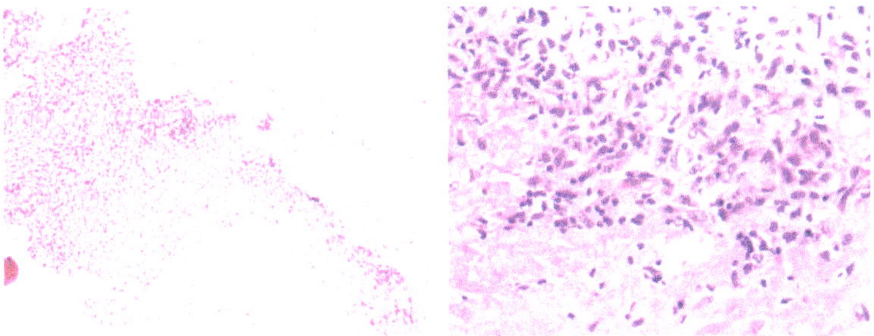

Figure 3: Synovial biopsy result.

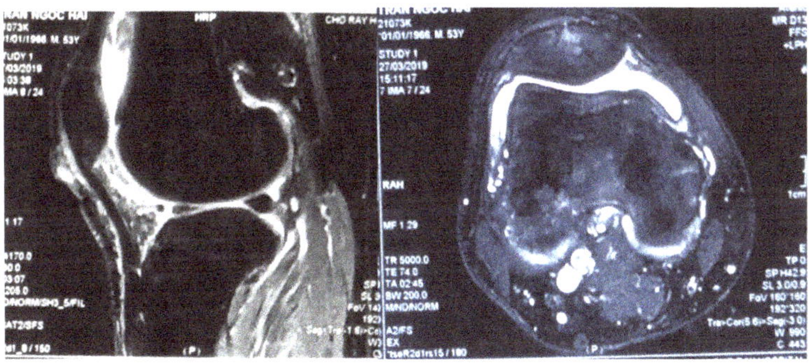

Figure 4: MRI after 3 months.

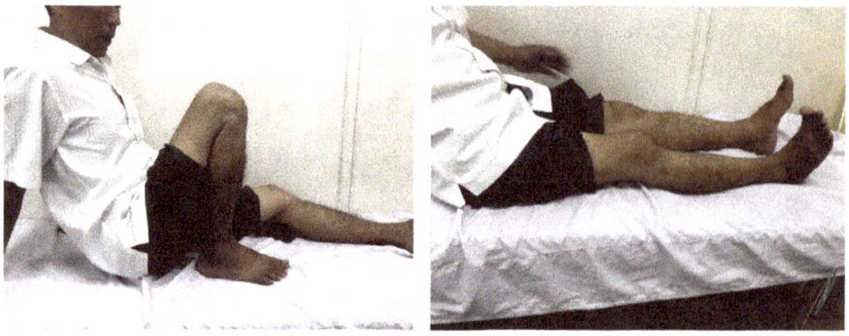

(a)

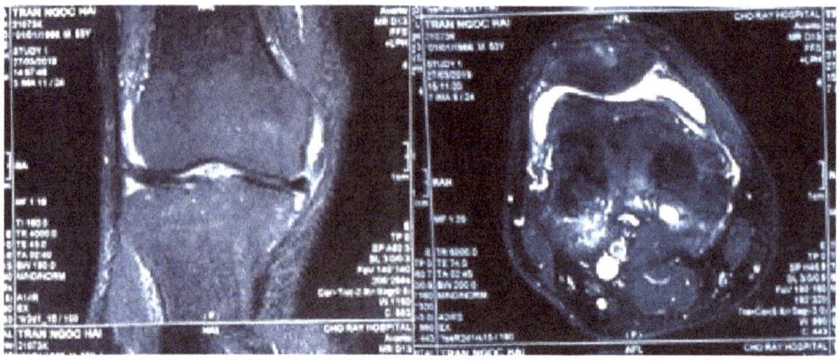

(b)

FIGURE 5: (a) The last follow-up, more than 1 year. (b) MRI of the last follow-up.

## Authors' Contributions

Hung drafted the manuscript. Duong, Hau, Binh, Tu, and Tin managed the case. Thi and Tuan revised the manuscript critically and the literature. They all read and approved the final manuscript.

## Acknowledgments

Truong Nguyen Khanh Hung is the submitting author and the first author. This research was carried out at the Orthopedic and Trauma Department, ChoRay Hospital, 201B Nguyen Chi Thanh Street, Ward 12, District 5, Ho Chi Minh City, Vietnam.

## References

[1] J. Amini, H. Poka, J. Kumbu et al., "The crisis of tuberculosis in Papua New Guinea-the role of older strategies for public health disease control," *Papua and New Guinea Medical Journal*, vol. 55, no. 1-4, pp. 1–4, 2012.

[2] WHO, "Global Tuberculosis Report 2016," June 2017, http://www.who.int/entity/tb/publications/global_report/gtbr2016_main_text.pdf?ua=1.

[3] H. M. Peto, R. H. Pratt, T. A. Harrington, P. A. LoBue, and L. R. Armstrong, "Epidemiology of extrapulmonary tuberculosis in the United States, 1993-2006," *Clinical Infectious Diseases*, vol. 49, no. 9, pp. 1350–1357, 2009.

[4] M. Tyllianakis, G. Kasimatis, S. Athanaselis, and M. Melachrinou, "Rice-body formation and tenosynovitis of the wrist: a case report," *Journal of Orthopaedic Surgery*, vol. 14, no. 2, pp. 208–211, 2006.

[5] S. Bayram, A. Erşen, M. Altan, and H. Durmaz, "Tuberculosis tenosynovitis with multiple rice bodies of the flexor tendons in the wrist: a case report," *International Journal of Surgery Case Reports*, vol. 27, pp. 129–132, 2016.

[6] J. R. Kichari and R. Bezooijen, "Flake-shaped rice bodies," *SA Journal of Radiology*, vol. 16, no. 4, pp. 140-141, 2012.

[7] H. S. Cheung, L. M. Ryan, F. Kozin, and D. J. McCarty, "Synovial origins of rice bodies in joint fluid," *Arthritis and Rheumatism*, vol. 23, no. 1, pp. 72–76, 1980.

[8] A. J. Popert, D. L. Scott, A. C. Wainwright, K. W. Walton, N. Williamson, and J. H. Chapman, "Frequency of occurrence, mode of development, and significance or rice bodies in rheumatoid joints," *Annals of the Rheumatic Diseases*, vol. 41, no. 2, pp. 109–117, 1982.

[9] C. Muangchan and S. Nilganuwong, "The study of clinical manifestation of osteoarticular tuberculosis in Siriraj Hospital, Thailand," *Journal of the Medical Association of Thailand*, vol. 92, Supplement 2, pp. 101–109, 2009.

[10] K. D. Vaughan, "Extraspinal osteoarticular tuberculosis; a forgotten entity?," *The West Indian Medical Journal*, vol. 54, p. 202, 2005.

[11] D. Triplett, E. Stewart, S. Mathew, B. R. Horne, and V. Prakash, "Delayed diagnosis of tuberculous arthritis of the

knee in an air force service member: case report and review of the literature," *Military Medicine*, vol. 181, no. 3, pp. e306–e309, 2016.

[12] WHO, "Global Tuberculosis Report 2017," August 2018, https://www.who.int/tb/publications/global_report/gtbr2017_main_text.pdf.

[13] S. Arthanari, S. Yusuf, and M. Nisar, "Tuberculosis of the knee complicating seronegative arthritis," *The Journal of Rheumatology*, vol. 35, no. 6, pp. 1227-1228, 2008.

[14] S. Lidder, K. Lang, M. Haroon, M. Shahidi, and M. El-Guindi, "Tuberculosis of the knee," *Orthopedic Reviews*, vol. 1, no. 1, article e24, 2009.

[15] M. M. Al-Qattan, A. Al-Namla, A. Al-Thunayan, and M. Al-Omawi, "Tuberculosis of the hand," *The Journal of Hand Surgery*, vol. 36, no. 8, pp. 1413–1421, 2011.

[16] S. H. Chen, C. H. Lee, T. Wong, and H. S. Feng, "Long-term retrospective analysis of surgical treatment for irretrievable tuberculosis of the ankle," *Foot & Ankle International*, vol. 34, no. 3, pp. 372–379, 2013.

[17] W. G. Dixon, K. L. Hyrich, K. D. Watson et al., "Drug-specific risk of tuberculosis in patients with rheumatoid arthritis treated with anti-TNF therapy: results from the British Society for Rheumatology Biologics Register (BSRBR)," *Annals of the Rheumatic Diseases*, vol. 69, no. 3, pp. 522–528, 2010.

[18] A. D. Bhargava, A. N. Malaviya, and A. Kumar, "Tuberculous rheumatism (Poncet's disease)- a case series," *The Indian Journal of Tuberculosis*, vol. 45, pp. 215–220, 1998.

[19] WHO, "Guidelines for treatment of drug-susceptible tuberculosis and patient care (2017 update)," April 2017, https://www.who.int/tb/publications/2017/dstb_guidance_2017/en/.

[20] C. Tseng, R. M. Huang, and K. T. Chen, "Tuberculosis arthritis: epidemiology, diagnosis, treatment," *Clinical Research on Foot & Ankle*, vol. 2, p. 131, 2014.

# 36

# Posterior Arthroscopic Treatment of a Massive Effusion in the Flexor Hallucis Longus Tendon Sheath Associated with Stenosing Tenosynovitis and Os Trigonum

**Ichiro Tonogai and Koichi Sairyo**

*Department of Orthopedics, Institute of Biomedical Science, Tokushima University Graduate School, 3-18-15 Kuramoto, Tokushima, Tokushima 770-8503, Japan*

Correspondence should be addressed to Ichiro Tonogai; i.tonogai@tokushima-u.ac.jp

Academic Editor: Akio Sakamoto

We report a rare case of massive accumulation of fluid in the flexor hallucis longus tendon sheath with stenosing tenosynovitis and os trigonum. A 34-year-old woman presented to our hospital with pain and swelling in the posteromedial aspect of the left ankle joint after an ankle sprain approximately 8 months earlier. There was tenderness at the posteromedial aspect of the ankle, and the pain worsened on dorsiflexion of the left great toe. Magnetic resonance imaging revealed massive accumulation of fluid around the flexor hallucis longus tendon. We removed the os trigonum, performed tenosynovectomy around the flexor hallucis longus, and released the flexor hallucis longus tendon via posterior arthroscopy using standard posterolateral and posteromedial portals. At 1 week postoperatively, the patient was asymptomatic and able to resume her daily activities. There has been no recurrence of the massive accumulation of fluid around the flexor hallucis longus tendon as of 1 year after the surgery. To our knowledge, this is a rare case report of extreme massive effusion in the flexor hallucis longus tendon sheath with stenosing tenosynovitis and os trigonum treated successfully by removal of the os trigonum, tenosynovectomy around the flexor hallucis longus, and release of the flexor hallucis longus tendon via posterior ankle arthroscopy.

## 1. Introduction

The flexor hallucis longus (FHL) tendon passes through a tendon sheath extending from the flexor retinaculum at the posterior talus through a fibroosseous tunnel along the medial calcaneus to the inferior aspect of the sustentaculum tali. The thick FHL tendon sheath lies just near the medial aspect of the talar process. If the os trigonum is present, it is usually entrapped and narrowed under the thick tendon sheath. Stenosing tenosynovitis of the FHL with involvement of the os trigonum has been reported as a major pathologic finding [1–4].

Effusion in the FHL tendon is often associated with stenosing tenosynovitis. Magnetic resonance imaging (MRI) is useful for assessing the degree of effusion and can confirm the diagnosis by the presence of excess fluid around the FHL in the region of the fibroosseous tunnel [5–7]. However, massive effusion around the FHL tendon is rare.

Here, we report on a patient who presented with massive effusion in the FHL tendon sheath with stenosing tenosynovitis involving an os trigonum, which was successfully treated by resection of the os trigonum, tenosynovectomy around the FHL, and release of the FHL tendon via posterior ankle arthroscopy. To our knowledge, this is a rare case report of extreme massive effusion around the FHL.

## 2. Case Report

A 34-year-old woman was referred to our department with an 8-month history of pain and swelling of the left ankle after sustaining an ankle sprain while descending a flight of stairs. She had no significant past medical history. Physical

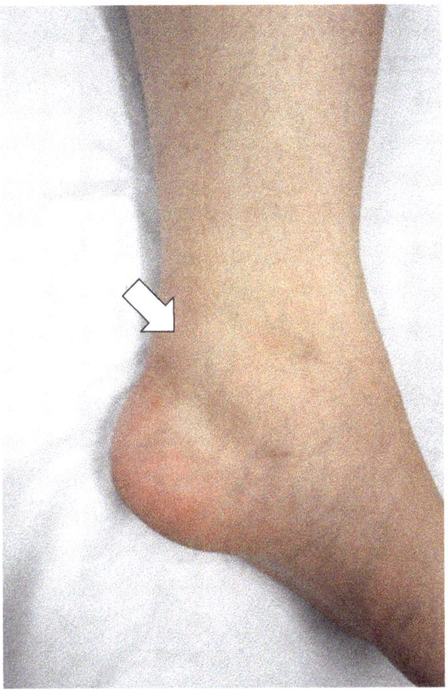

FIGURE 1: Preoperative photograph showing swelling of the posteromedial side of the left ankle (white arrow).

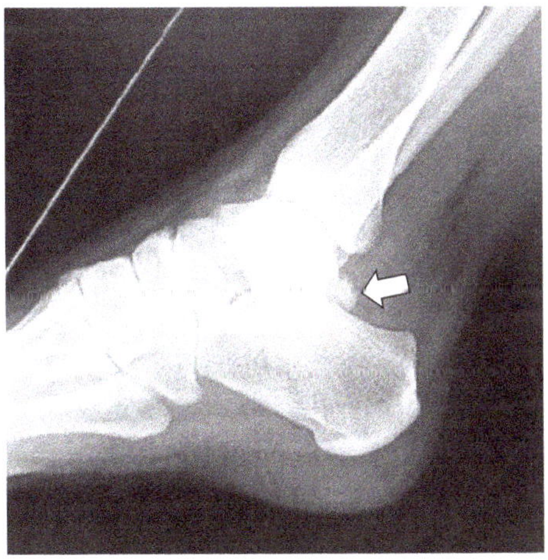

FIGURE 2: Lateral radiograph showing the os trigonum (arrow).

examination revealed swelling and tenderness on the medial side of the left ankle (Figure 1). There was slight limitation of range of motion at the ankle. The ankle pain worsened on dorsiflexion of the left great toe. No neurovascular deficit was noted. Her JSSF (Japanese Society for Surgery of the Foot) scale score was 69/100 (pain 20/40, function 39/50, and alignment 10/10). The patient rated her pain as 6/10 on a visual analogue scale (VAS). An os trigonum was visible on a weight-bearing lateral radiograph of the left ankle (Figure 2) and on a computed tomography (CT) scan (Figures 3(a) and 3(b)). MRI revealed massive effusion around the FHL tendon at a level proximal to the ankle joint posteriorly (Figures 4(a)–4(c)) and between the talar tubercles and the master knot of Henry (Figures 4(d)–4(f)). The preoperative diagnosis was massive effusion around the FHL with stenosing tenosynovitis and os trigonum. Initially, we injected a steroid and xylocaine into the posterior ankle space under ultrasound guidance. The pain decreased but returned within a few days and became persistent. Therefore, we proceeded to a surgical arthroscopic procedure.

The patient was positioned prone with a thigh tourniquet. Two portals were made 1 cm above the insertion of the Achilles tendon just medial and lateral to the tendon in line with the tip of the lateral malleolus, and then, we performed a posterior hindfoot endoscopy using the standard 2-portal technique described by van Dijk et al. [1]. The lateral portal was used mainly for visualization, and the medial one served as the working portal. A 4 mm 30-degree arthroscope was introduced through the portals and directed toward the second toe. The posterior aspect of the talus and os trigonum was then visualized (Figure 5(a)). The os trigonum was impinged between the posterior aspect of the talus and the calcaneus. The os trigonum on the posteromedial aspect of the talus was resected with a motorized shaver to visualize the entire FHL tendon sheath. The FHL was thick, and a fibroosseous tunnel was seen adherent to the tendon (Figure 5(b)). All fibrous tissues compressing the FHL were cut and removed with a motorized shaver. Next, the tendon was released (Figure 5(c)). Suction was performed along the FHL tendon toward a level proximal to the ankle joint posteriorly (Figure 5(d)) and anterior to the talar tubercles and the master knot of Henry (Figure 5(e)). There were no intraoperative complications.

After skin closure, a bulky dressing was placed without immobilization. The patient was encouraged to actively move the ankle and toes. Weight bearing was allowed after surgery as tolerated with return to normal daily activities after a week. The postoperative course was unremarkable. At the 1-year follow-up visit, the patient remained asymptomatic and MRI showed no recurrence of the fluid around the FHL (Figures 6(a)–6(d)). Her JSSF scale score had improved from 69/100 points to 100/100 points and her VAS score to 0/10.

The patient provided informed consent for the publication of this report.

## 3. Discussion

We have reported the case of a 34-year-old woman who presented with a massive effusion along the FHL tendon sheath with stenosing tenosynovitis and os trigonum. Although FHL tenosynovitis often occurs in the os trigonum syndrome, an extreme effusion along the FHL tendon is extremely rare.

The FHL is a secondary producer of torque at the ankle subtalar joint complex and hallux joints [8–10] but functions primarily as an active plantar flexor at the first metatarsophalangeal and hallux interphalangeal joints [11–13] and provides primary restraint to passive dorsiflexion at the first metatarsophalangeal joint [6, 7, 10, 14]. Given the finding by Hamilton and Chao that there is relative incongruity between the FHL and the fibroosseous tunnel when the foot is in extreme plantar flexion [7], it is possible that the FHL tendon was subjected to abnormal stresses in our patient

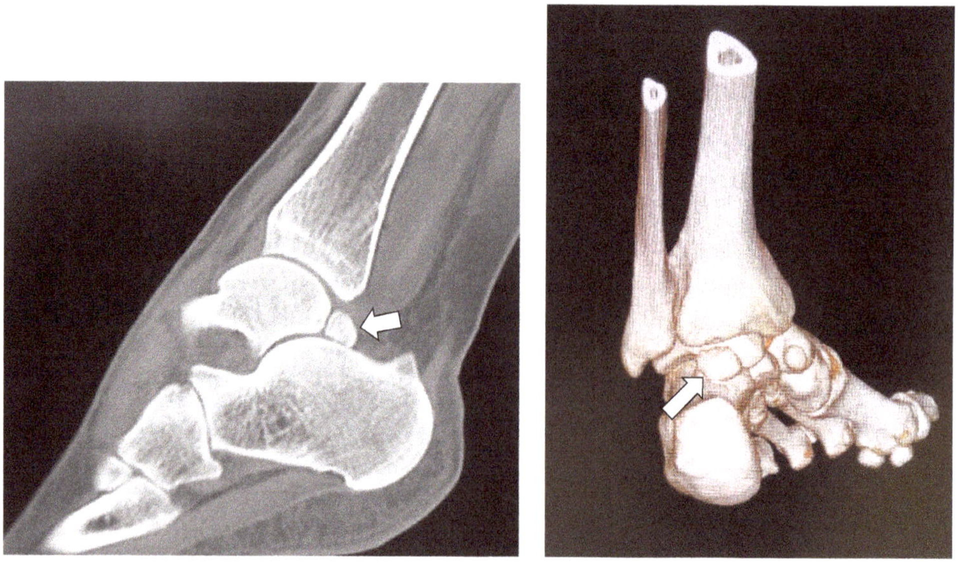

(a) (b)

Figure 3: Computed tomography images showing the os trigonum connected to the posterior aspect of the talus. (a) Plain image, sagittal view (arrow). (b) Three-dimensional image, posterior view (arrow).

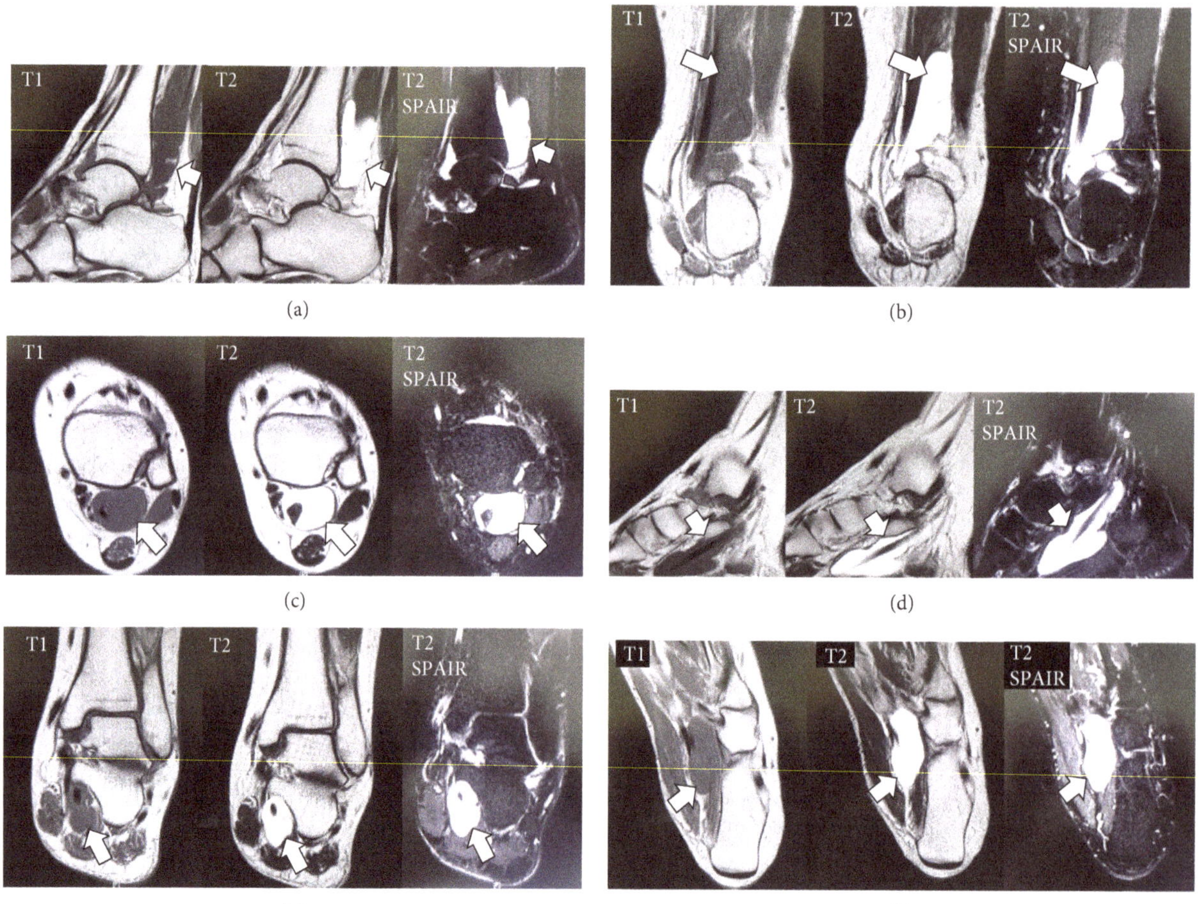


(a) (b) (c) (d) (e) (f)

Figure 4: T1-weighted, T2-weighted, and T2-spectral attenuated inversion recovery magnetic resonance images showing a massive effusion around the flexor hallucis longus (arrow) at a level proximal to the ankle joint posteriorly in the (a) sagittal, (b) coronal, and (c) axial planes and between the talar tubercles and the master knot of Henry in the (d) sagittal, (e) coronal, and (f) axial planes.

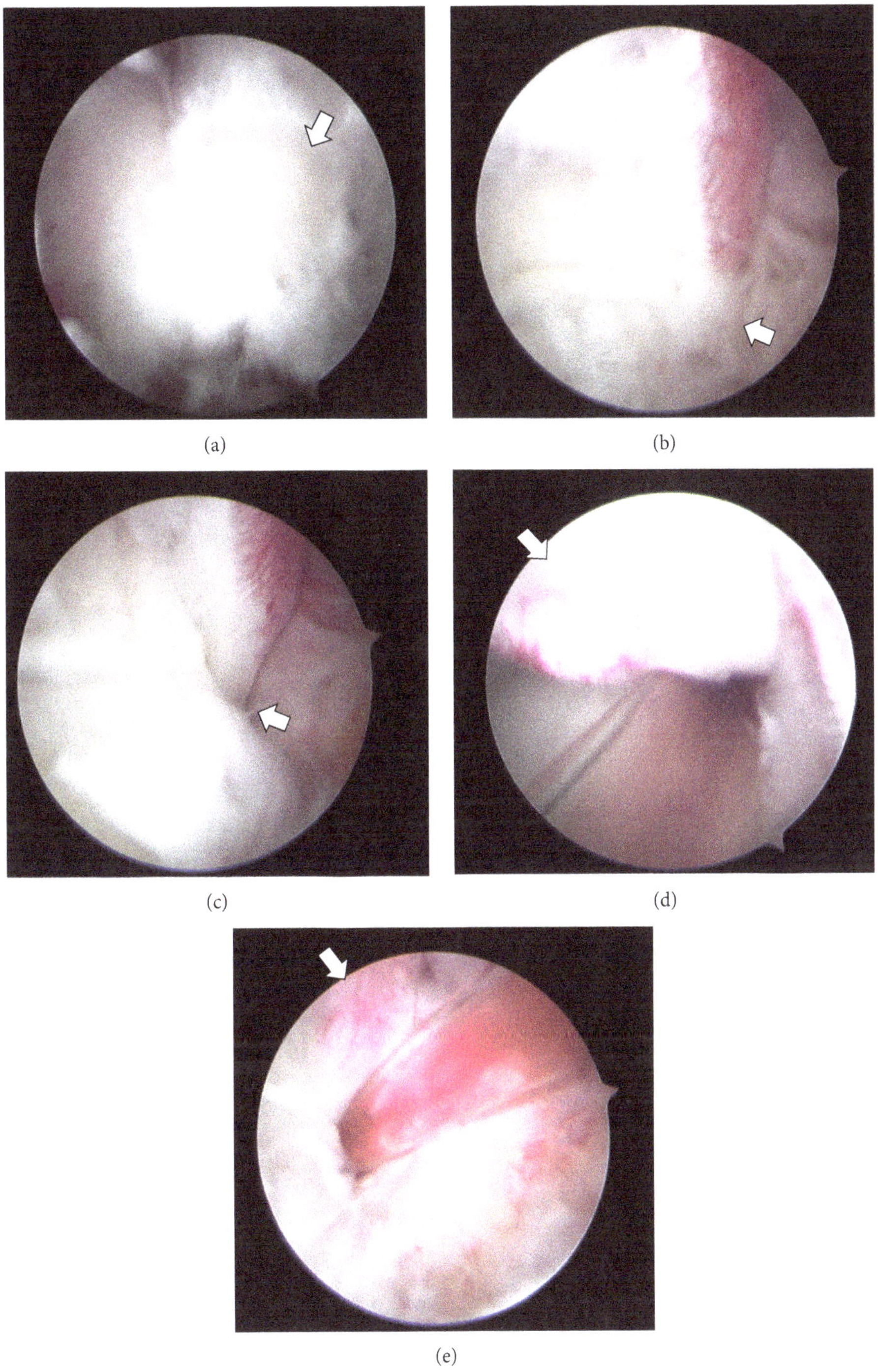


FIGURE 5: Arthroscopic views of the posterior aspect of the left ankle. (a) The posterior aspect of the os trigonum (arrow) can be visualized. (b) The fibrous portion of the tunnel compressed the flexor hallucis longus (FHL) tendon (arrow) after removal of the os trigonum. (c) Stenosis was not seen (arrow) after the release of the FHL tendon. Suction was performed along the FHL tendon (d) toward a level proximal to the ankle joint posteriorly and (e) anterior to the talar tubercles and the master knot of Henry.

when she sustained a severe left ankle sprain. Alternatively, she might have an anatomic feature whereby the FHL tendon enters the tunnel at an oblique angle, predisposing it to irritation. As documented by Sammarco and Cooper [6], FHL tendinitis is not uncommon, even in nonathletes, and should always be considered in the differential diagnosis of posteromedial ankle pain.

The os trigonum syndrome with stenosing FHL tenosynovitis is a common cause of posterior ankle impingement, as encountered in our patient. Conservative treatment is the recommended first line of treatment. Secondary treatment options are open or arthroscopic excision of the os trigonum with release of the FHL tendon. Open surgery for the os trigonum associated with tenosynovitis of the FHL has been

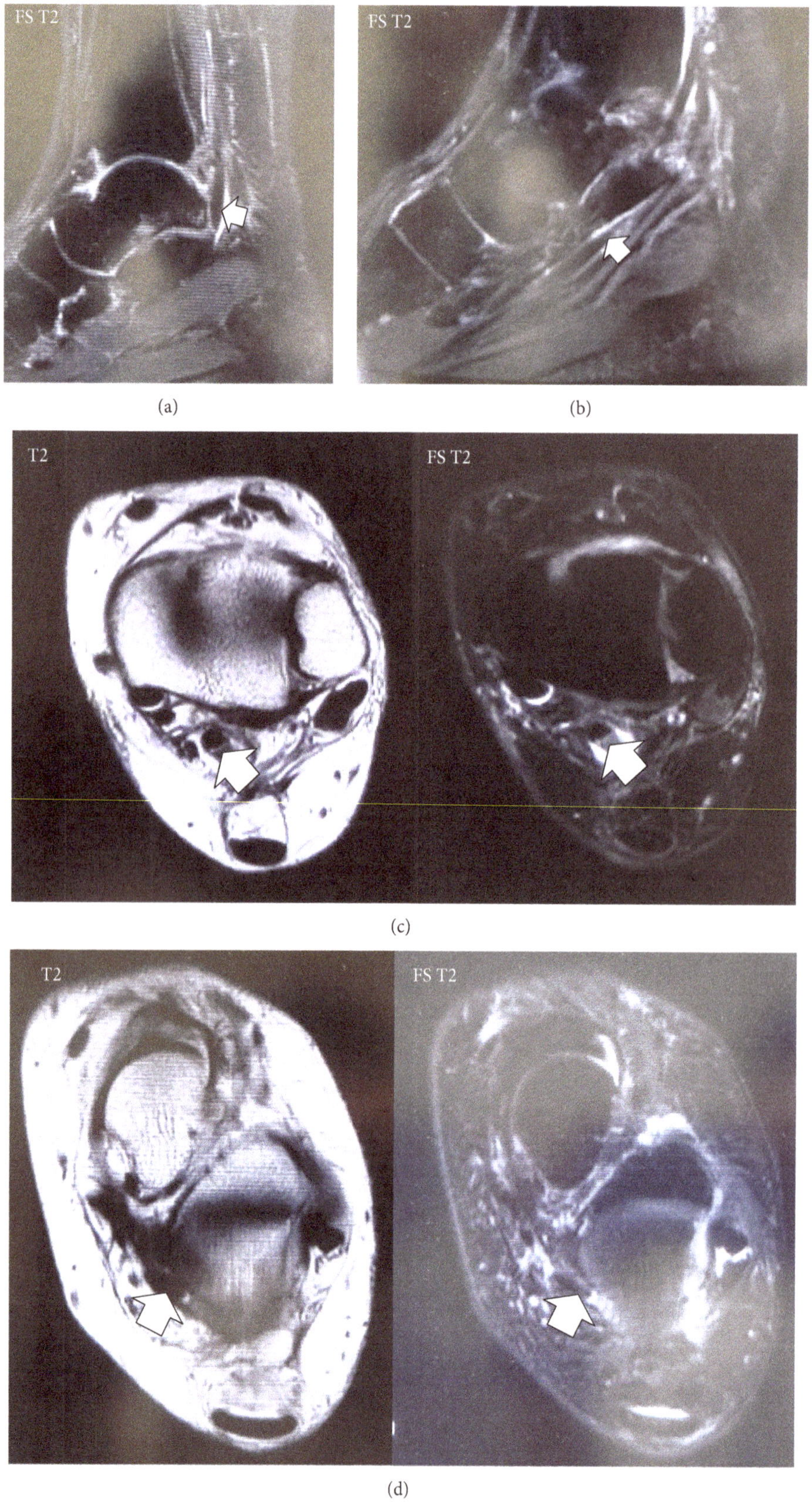


Figure 6: Fat saturation T2-weighted magnetic resonance images showing no effusion along the flexor hallucis longus (FHL) tendon at a level proximal to the ankle joint posteriorly in the (a) sagittal and (b) axial planes. T2-weighted and fat saturation T2-weighted images showing no accumulation of effusion along the FHL between the talar tubercles and the master knot of Henry in the (c) sagittal and (d) axial planes.

reported [15]. However, arthroscopic approaches have gained popularity in the past decade because they produce less scarring and are associated with less postoperative pain, minimal overall morbidity, and an earlier return to daily activity. A more rapid return to activity, improved visualization of pathology, less postoperative pain, and a decreased risk of complications have been noted as advantages of the endoscopic approach to the posterior hindfoot and ankle [16]. Moreover, some authors have reported the effectiveness of posterior ankle arthroscopy for FHL stenosing tenosynovitis with the os trigonum [17, 18]. Therefore, we selected posterior ankle arthroscopy in this case and found it to be an effective procedure for the treatment of massive effusion caused by stenosing tenosynovitis of the FHL with the os trigonum.

There are several articles of similar reports of massive effusion in the FHL tendon sheath. Qu et al. reported cases of diffuse FHL tenosynovitis with effusion at a level proximal to the ankle joint posteriorly and/or between the talar tubercles and the master knot of Henry, although it was treated by open extensive tenosynovectomy [19]. Lee also reported cases of effusion with the FHL tendon sheath at a level of the interphalangeal joint and/or the metatarsophalangeal joint, although it was treated by an open procedure [20]. However, we treated a massive effusion in the FHL tendon sheath with stenosing tenosynovitis involving an os trigonum via posterior ankle arthroscopy. This point might be different from reports by Qu et al. [19] and Lee et al. [20].

One limitation of this report is the short follow-up period. Although the effusion has not recurred as of the latest follow-up visit 1 year after surgery, further follow-up is necessary.

In conclusion, we encountered a rare case of massive effusion along the FHL tendon associated with stenosing tenosynovitis and os trigonum that was treated by removal of the os trigonum and release of the stenosing fibrous tunnel via a posterior arthroscopic procedure. Surgical treatment was successful in this case even with massive effusion along the FHL tendon sheath.

## Disclosure

The level of evidence is 4.

## References

[1] C. N. van Dijk, P. E. Scholten, and R. Krips, "A 2-portal endoscopic approach for diagnosis and treatment of posterior ankle pathology," *Arthroscopy: The Journal of Arthroscopic & Related Surgery*, vol. 16, no. 8, pp. 871–876, 2000.

[2] M. Tey, J. C. Monllau, J. M. Centenera, and X. Pelfort, "Benefits of arthroscopic tuberculoplasty in posterior ankle impingement syndrome," *Knee Surgery, Sports Traumatology, Arthroscopy*, vol. 15, no. 10, pp. 1235–1239, 2007.

[3] J. A. Russell, R. M. Shave, H. Yoshioka, D. W. Kruse, Y. Koutedakis, and M. A. Wyon, "Magnetic resonance imaging of the ankle in female ballet dancers en pointe," *Acta Radiologica*, vol. 51, no. 6, pp. 655–661, 2010.

[4] J. A. Russell, D. W. Kruse, Y. Koutedakis, I. M. McEwan, and M. Wyon, "Pathoanatomy of posterior ankle impingement in ballet dancers," *Clinical Anatomy*, vol. 23, no. 6, pp. 613–621, 2010.

[5] G. H. Theodore, G. J. Kolettis, and L. J. Micheli, "Tenosynovitis of the flexor hallucis longus in a long-distance runner," *Medicine and Science in Sports and Exercise*, vol. 28, no. 3, pp. 277–279, 1996.

[6] G. J. Sammarco and P. S. Cooper, "Flexor hallucis longus tendon injury in dancers and nondancers," *Foot & Ankle International*, vol. 19, no. 6, pp. 356–362, 1998.

[7] W. Hamilton and W. Chao, "Posterior ankle pain in athletes and dancers," *Foot and Ankle Clinics*, vol. 4, pp. 811–832, 1999.

[8] C. W. Spoor, J. L. van Leeuwen, C. G. Meskers, A. F. Titulaer, and A. Huson, "Estimation of instantaneous moment arms of lower-leg muscles," *Journal of Biomechanics*, vol. 23, no. 12, pp. 1247–1259, 1990.

[9] B. Hintermann, B. M. Nigg, and C. Sommer, "Foot movement and tendon excursion: an in vitro study," *Foot & Ankle International*, vol. 15, no. 7, pp. 386–395, 1994.

[10] P. Klein, S. Mattys, and M. Rooze, "Moment arm length variations of selected muscles acting on talocrural and subtalar joints during movement: an in vitro study," *Journal of Biomechanics*, vol. 29, no. 1, pp. 21–30, 1996.

[11] J. B. Carr, "Complications of calcaneus fractures entrapment of the flexor hallucis longus: report of two cases," *Journal of Orthopaedic Trauma*, vol. 4, no. 2, pp. 166–168, 1990.

[12] L. Ferris, N. A. Sharkey, T. S. Smith, and D. K. Matthews, "Influence of extrinsic plantar flexors on forefoot loading during heel rise," *Foot & Ankle International*, vol. 16, no. 8, pp. 464–473, 1995.

[13] P. H. Leitschuh, J. P. Zimmerman, J. M. Uhorchak, R. A. Arciero, and L. Bowser, "Hallux flexion deformity secondary to entrapment of the flexor hallucis longus tendon after fibular fracture," *Foot & Ankle International*, vol. 16, no. 4, pp. 232–235, 1995.

[14] W. G. Hamilton, "Stenosing tenosynovitis of the flexor hallucis longus tendon and posterior impingement upon the os trigonum in ballet dancers," *Foot & Ankle*, vol. 3, no. 2, pp. 74–80, 1982.

[15] M. Uzel, E. Cetinus, E. Bilgic, A. Karaoguz, and Y. Kanber, "Bilateral os trigonum syndrome associated with bilateral tenosynovitis of the flexor hallucis longus muscle," *Foot & Ankle International*, vol. 26, no. 10, pp. 894–898, 2005.

[16] C. Rungprai, J. N. Tennant, and P. Phisitkul, "Disorders of the flexor hallucis longus and os trigonum," *Clinics in Sports Medicine*, vol. 34, no. 4, pp. 741–759, 2015.

[17] N. M. Corte-Real, R. M. Moreira, and F. Guerra-Pinto, "Arthroscopic treatment of tenosynovitis of the flexor hallucis longus tendon," *Foot & Ankle International*, vol. 33, no. 12, pp. 1108–1112, 2012.

[18] H. Funasaki, H. Hayashi, K. Sakamoto, R. Tsuruga, and K. Marumo, "Arthroscopic release of flexor hallucis longus tendon sheath in female ballet dancers: dynamic pathology, surgical technique, and return to dancing performance," *Arthroscopy Techniques*, vol. 4, no. 6, pp. e769–e774, 2015.

[19] W. Qu, T. Liu, W. Chen, Z. Sun, S. Dong, and M. Chen, "Effect of extensive tenosynovectomy on diffuse flexor hallucis longus tenosynovitis combined with effusion," *Journal of Orthopaedic Surgery*, vol. 27, no. 3, 2019.

[20] J. W. Lee, M. W. Joo, J. K. Sung, J. H. Ahn, and Y. K. Kang, "Origin of satellite ganglion cysts with effusion in the flexor hallucis longus tendon sheath around the hallux," *Clinics in Orthopedic Surgery*, vol. 10, no. 1, pp. 94–98, 2018.

# 37

# Traumatic Fracture: Dislocation of Cervicothoracic Junction—Grand Round Presentation of C7-T1 Instabilities and Different Instrumentation Techniques

**Mohammad A. Alsofyani,[1,2] Soufiane Ghailane,[1] Sultan Alsalmi,[3,4] Sreenath Jakinapally,[1] Louis Boissière,[1] Ibrahim Obeid,[1] and Jean-Marc Vital[1]**

[1]*Department of Spinal Surgery Unit, Bordeaux University, Bordeaux University Hospital, C.H.U Tripode Pellegrin, Place Amélie Raba Léon, 33076 Bordeaux, France*
[2]*Orthopedic Department, College of Medicine and University Hospital, University of Hail, P.O. Box 2440, Hail City, Saudi Arabia*
[3]*Department of Neurosurgery, Amiens University Medical Center, Amiens University, Amiens, France*
[4]*Department of Neurosurgery, Imam Abdulrahman Bin Faisal University, Dammam City, Saudi Arabia*

Correspondence should be addressed to Mohammad A. Alsofyani; mohd.alsofyani@gmail.com

Academic Editor: Eyal Itshayek

*Introduction.* Acute traumatic cervicothoracic junction spinal lesions are rare disorders and poorly documented. We report a case of a traumatic cervicothoracic fracture-dislocation. We present our experience in the operative treatment of an unstable fracture-dislocation at the cervicothoracic junction. *Materials and Method.* A seventy year old man was transferred to our hospital. We found paresthesia in the corresponding dermatome of C7 and C8 bilaterally. Initial CT scan shows vertebral body fracture of T1 with retropulsion into the spinal canal and anteroposterior dislocation of cervicothoracic junction type C according to AOSpine subaxial injury. Traumatic disc material at C7-T1 was removed by anterior cervical discectomy and fusion of C6-T2. Fixation was done from C6 to T2 in the prone position. *Results.* At one-year postoperative follow-up, radiographs revealed bony fusion at the level of C7-T1, and the patient had no major functional disability. *Conclusion.* We opted for the ventral-dorsal approach in our case for maximum stabilization and to prevent mechanical complications.

## 1. Introduction

Traumatic injuries at the cervicothoracic junction (CTJ) are a relatively rare event and considered as a significant cause of paraparesis or paraplegia posttraumatic. As young people are most commonly injured, it is considered as a significant economic burden to the family and society. In CTJ injuries, surgical techniques and associated complications have been extensively described in the literature during the past decade, whereas the choice of anterior versus posterior or double-stage fixation has been given little attention [1–3]. The purpose of this study is to discuss different instrumentation techniques of this rare injury.

## 2. Case Presentation

A seventy-year-old male was transferred to our hospital after sustaining trauma falling down into a watercourse. The initial Glasgow Coma Scale score was 15. Upon examination, he was hemodynamically stable and breathing spontaneously; we found paresthesia corresponding with dermatomes C7 and C8 bilaterally. The rest of the neurological physical

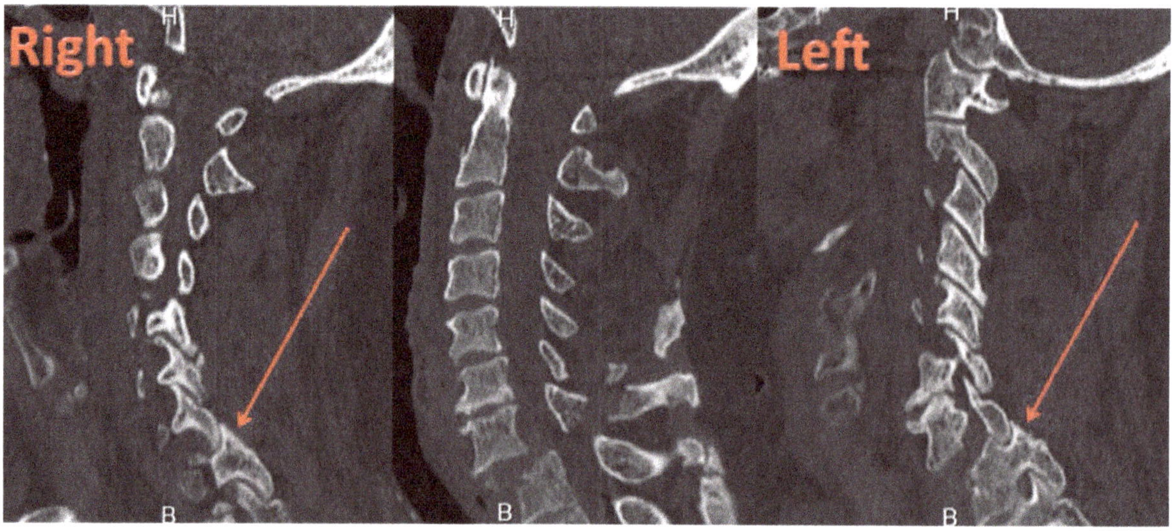


Figure 1: Preoperative CT scan of the patient shows vertebral body fracture of T1 and biarticular dislocation of the cervicothoracic junction.

examination was normal, and the patient was categorized grade E based on the American Spinal Injury Association classification.

Cervical spine radiography and two-dimensional reconstructed computed tomography (CT) scans (Figure 1) showed vertebral body fracture of T1 and anteroposterior dislocation of CTJ type C according to AOSpine subaxial injury.

Under general anesthesia, an image intensifier was used, and 16 kilograms of halo traction was applied with full muscle relaxation; the dislocation was irreducible. Iliac crest autogenous bone grafting was harvested. A left long presternocleidomastoid to the midline approach was then made for exposing the T2 vertebral body. Traumatic disc material at C7-T1 was removed by anterior cervical discectomy. Then, as the patient had biarticular dislocation, we placed the Caspar distractor on the medial line. The dislocation was reduced partially by increasing gently the distraction. When the facets were point to point on the oblique fluoroscopic view, we pushed gently on the upper vertebra, and the reduction was achieved on the oblique fluoroscopic. Anterior fusion from C6 to T2 was performed by iliac crest bone graft and anterior plate. This technique of reduction is successful in 34% of uniarticular dislocations and 27% of biarticular dislocations [4].

Secondly, for increasing the stability of CTJ, the patient was turned to the ventral position. Fixation was done without facetectomy associated with instrumentation from C6 to T2. Screws were placed in the lateral mass of C6 and pedicular screws from C7 to T2. Cervical spine radiography (Figure 2) and computed tomography (CT) scans (Figure 3) postoperative showed complete reduction of CTJ. In the immediate postoperative period, the patient complained of transient paraplegia; postoperative magnetic resonance imaging (MRI) (Figure 4) did not show mechanical compression or epidural hematoma. The transient paraplegia disappeared on the first postoperative day. The patient was discharged to the rehabilitation center with an immobilisation collar for 2 months.

At one-year follow-up, cervical spine radiography (Figure 5) revealed a well-reduced CTJ with bone graft healing; the patient had no major functional trouble.

## 3. Discussion

CTJ is a region in the vertebral column where biomechanically, it represents a region where there is an inflection from mobile cervical lordosis to rigid thoracic kyphosis. Radiographically, it is not easy to visualize especially in traumatic cases. Traumatic injuries to the CTJ usually include fracture-dislocation or isolated fracture [5–7]. Immediate treatment includes closed reduction, followed by surgical fixation [6, 8]. The different anatomical features of CTJ [3, 9], with the peculiar biomechanical characteristics [10], require the need of a suitable surgical technique for maximum stabilization.

Nichols et al. [11] reported a 9% incidence of CTJ injury, described as unilateral and bilateral facet dislocations or true fracture-subluxation of C7-T1. Evans [12] in 1983 published one of the largest reviews to date, where he investigated 14 cases determined from 587 cervical spinal cord injuries (SCIs) during a 26-year period, providing an incidence of 2.4% of cervical SCIs.

Dislocations of the CTJ are frequently missed especially in simple cervical trauma cases visiting the emergency department. Evans [12] confirms that almost two-thirds were not well diagnosed on admission. Similar arguments have already been focused and discussed in a series of three-hundred cervical spine traumas by Bohlman [13], published over forty years ago. Traumatic lesions at the CTJ are easily missed, due to poor visualization in this area; other imaging studies such as swimmer's view, CT reconstruction, or MRI should be carried out in suspicious cases [7].

Following trauma at CTJ, neurological problems are commonly seen. This may be due to the anatomical features of the upper thoracic spine through the small canal size, even though vascular insufficiency through the low blood supply

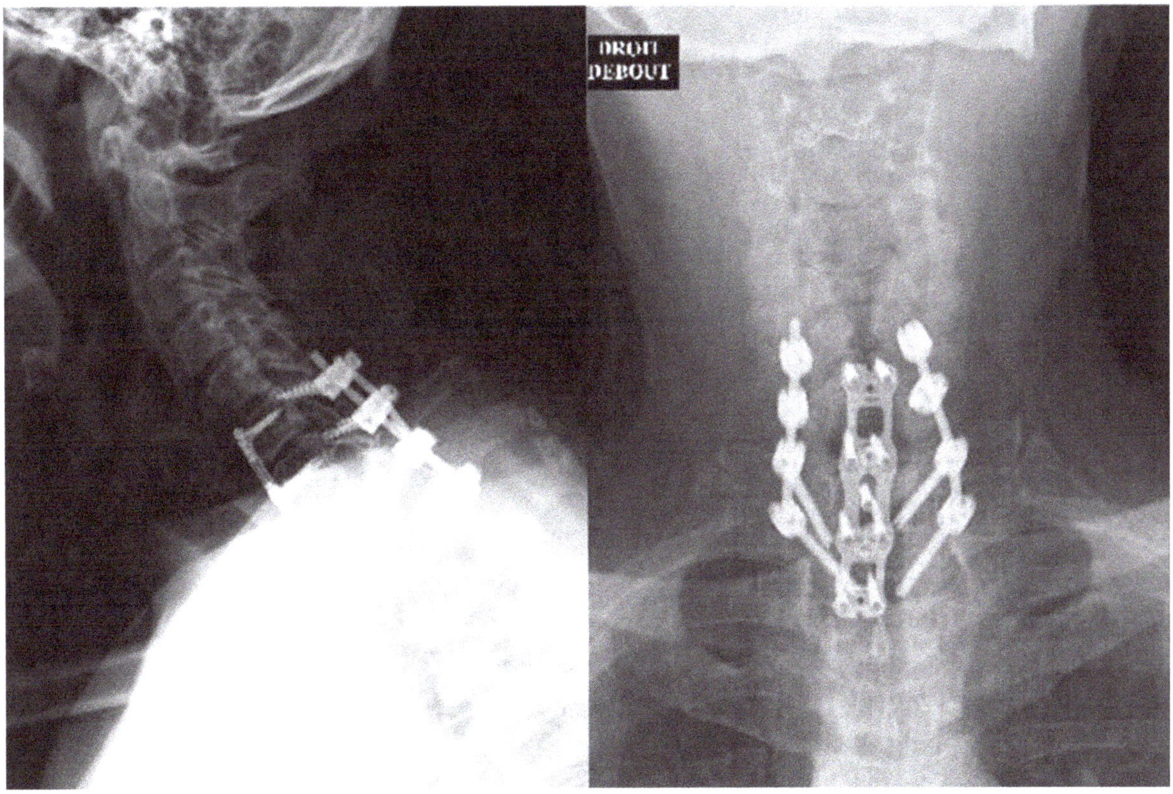


FIGURE 2: The patient underwent a C6-T2 fixation, followed by posterior C6-T2 arthrodesis.

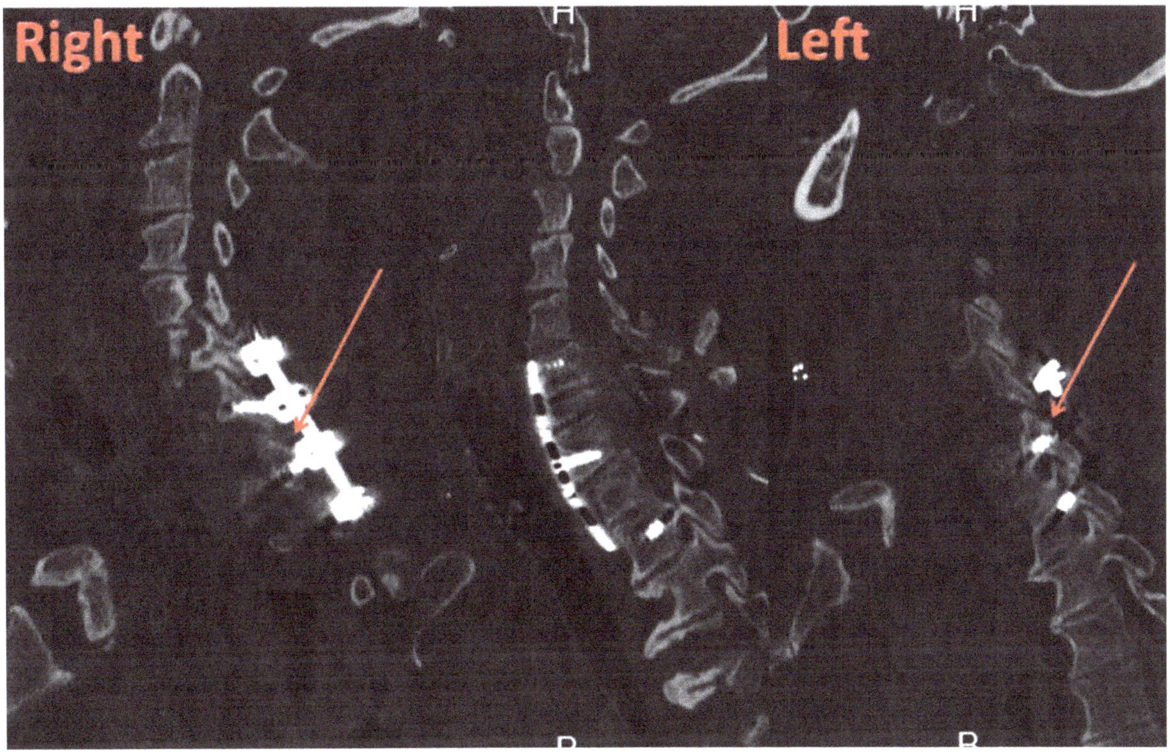


FIGURE 3: Postoperative CT scan shows complete reduction of cervicothoracic dislocation.

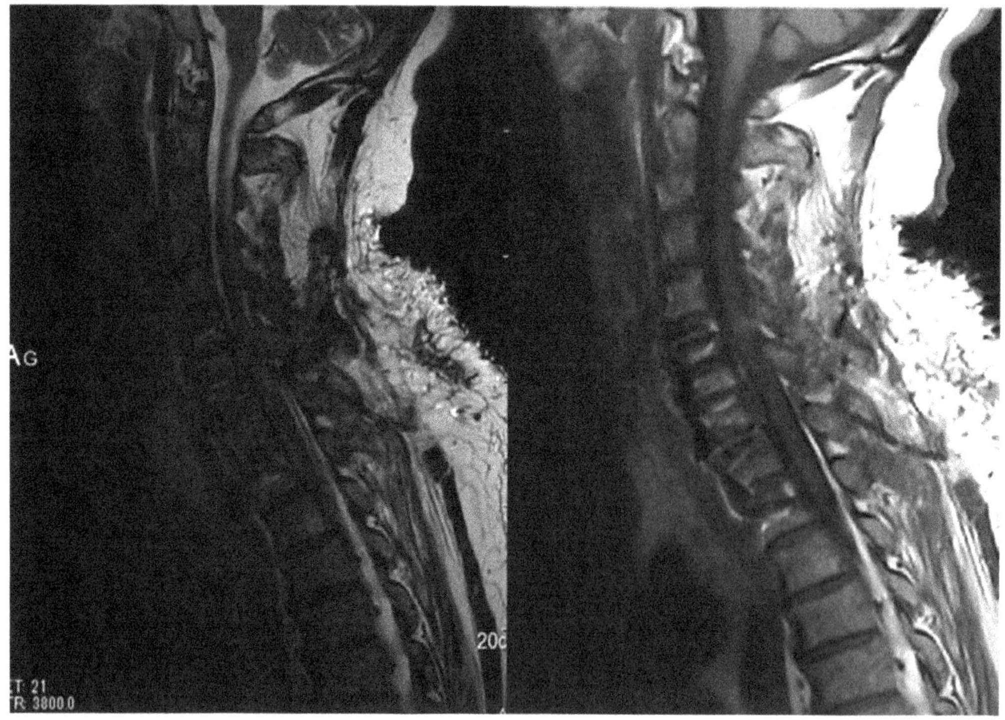


FIGURE 4: MRI postoperative does not show any abnormality of the spine canal.

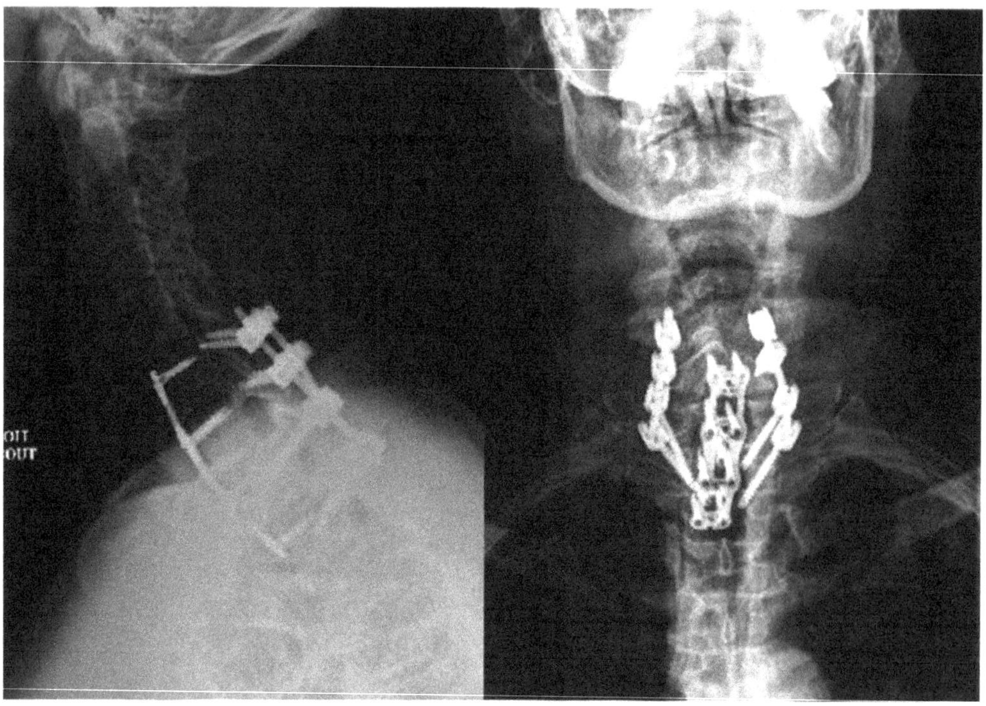

FIGURE 5: X-ray at one-year follow-up shows a well bony fusion.

of the lower cervical spine makes it more susceptible to ischemic injury.

A large and growing body of literature has investigated the successful results for anterior instrumentation for pathological fractures of the CTJ; the reported results of anterior instrumentation for traumatic fractures and dislocations are limited [14]. More recent attention has focused on biomechanical features regarding the adequacy of anterior instrumentation for stabilizing posterior element injuries of the cervical spine [15, 16]. Bueff et al. [17] reported in a cadaveric study that anterior fixation techniques had less stiffness than posterior fixation, especially in resisting flexion-distraction forces. Boockvar et al. [2] demonstrated that anterior instrumentation alone may not be enough biomechanically for CTJ and that combined anterior-posterior fixation and fusion may be considered to increase stabilization for fusion success.

Anterior approaches can be practically classified into a low anterolateral cervical approach, a transmanubrial-transsternal approach, and a thoracotomy [14]. The way of choosing the approach depends on the level of lesion and the surgeon's experience. The low cervical approach is widening of the classical cervical approach medial to sternocleidomastoid (SCM); this allows access to the first and the second thoracic vertebral body [14, 18]. The transmanubrial-transsternal approach is required for the lesion down to T3 [14]. It can be done with low cervical approach for accessing the lower cervical spine. Several modifications were done for decreasing the high risk of morbidity by this approach [14]. Pointillart et al. [19] modified the approach by extending the standard anterolateral cervical approach caudally. Preoperative planning of MRI sagittal slices is mandatory as described by Sharan et al. [20]. If the sternum restricts the access, a median manubriotomy gives adequate access to the spine. The advantages of this modified approach are to protect the clavicles, sternoclavicular joints, and sternal body. If the lesion is below the T4 level, a thoracotomy has to be performed.

Posterior approach to the CTJ has been performed largely because of the technical difficulty of the anterior approach. Practically posterior instrumentation of the CTJ should always be fused, because of the instability of the CTJ. In the cervical spine, lateral mass screws are often performed in the posterior fixations. The thickness of the lateral mass is decreased from C5 to C7 from 11 to 8.7 mm [21]. Inversely, the size of the pedicle increases progressively from the low cervical spine to the thoracic spine. The pedicle width increases from C5 to C7 from 5.2 mm to 6.5 mm [21]. The angle decreases from 4 to 6 in each level from C5 to T1 between the vertebral body and the axis of the pedicle, decreasing from 50 at the C5 to 34 at the T1 [21]. Instrumentation of pedicle screws must estimate these differences in angulation. Posterior instrumentation can bring back most of the stability in a two-column but not a three-column injury [22].

Collectively, in our case, we started with the anterior approach to reduce the dislocation from the front as it is less invasive comparing with posterior facetectomy and we have direct exposure of the body and disc. Then, we have instrumented the cervical spine posteriorly to decrease the risk of instability and mechanical complications as the patient had a three-column injury of CTJ. Our case report with the grand round presentation of the literature outlines the importance of anterior versus posterior or double-stage fixation at the CTJ. Our case presented with a three-column injury and has shown the importance of previous literature for understanding the stability at this unique region [15–17, 22].

## Consent

The authors certify that they have obtained all appropriate patient consent forms. In the form, the patient(s) has/have given his/her/their consent for his/her/their images and other clinical information to be reported in the journal. The patients understand that their names and initials will not be published and due efforts will be made to conceal their identity, but anonymity cannot be guaranteed.

## Authors' Contributions

The authors contributed equally to this work.

## Acknowledgments

We would also like to show our gratitude to the 5th International Conference on Spine and Spinal Disorders and the 15th International Conference and Exhibition on Alzheimers Disease, Dementia & Ageing which were held in Rome from April 22 to 23, 2019, for giving us a chance to present this case report.

## References

[1] V. Krishnamoorthy, *Surgical management of traumatic cervico thoracic junction fracture subluxation – a single centre experience*, International Journal of Current Research, 2015.

[2] J. A. Boockvar, M. F. Philips, A. E. Telfeian, D. M. O'Rourke, and P. J. Marcotte, "Results and risk factors for anterior cervicothoracic junction surgery," *Journal of Neurosurgery*, vol. 94, no. 1, pp. 12–17, 2001.

[3] V. Y. Wang and D. Chou, "The cervicothoracic junction," *Neurosurgery Clinics of North America*, vol. 18, no. 2, pp. 365–371, 2007.

[4] J. M. Vital, O. Gille, J. Sénégas, and V. Pointillart, "Reduction technique for uni- and biarticular dislocations of the lower cervical spine," *Spine*, vol. 23, no. 8, pp. 949–954, 1998, discussion 955.

[5] A. Amin and A. Saifuddin, "Fractures and dislocations of the cervicothoracic junction," *Journal of Spinal Disorders & Techniques*, vol. 18, no. 6, pp. 499–505, 2005.

[6] J. R. Chapman, P. A. Anderson, C. Pepin, S. Toomey, D. W. Newell, and M. S. Grady, "Posterior instrumentation of the unstable cervicothoracic spine," *Journal of Neurosurgery*, vol. 84, no. 4, pp. 552–558, 1996.

[7] G. Sapkas, S. Papadakis, P. Katonis, N. Roidis, and G. Kontakis, "Operative treatment of unstable injuries of the cervicothoracic junction," *European Spine Journal*, vol. 8, no. 4, pp. 279–283, 1999.

[8] P. Korovessis, P. Katonis, A. Aligizakis et al., "Posterior compact Cotrel-Dubousset instrumentation for occipitocervical, cervical and cervicothoracic fusion," *European Spine Journal*, vol. 10, no. 5, pp. 385–394, 2001.

[9] T. Vanden Hoek and D. Propp, "Cervicothoracic junction injury," *The American Journal of Emergency Medicine*, vol. 8, no. 1, pp. 30–33, 1990.

[10] V. K. Goel, C. R. Clark, D. McGowan, and S. Goyal, "An in-vitro study of the kinematics of the normal, injured and stabilized cervical spine," *Journal of Biomechanics*, vol. 17, no. 5, pp. 363–376, 1984.

[11] C. G. Nichols, D. H. Young, and W. R. Schiller, "Evaluation of cervicothoracic junction injury," *Annals of Emergency Medicine*, vol. 16, no. 6, pp. 640–642, 1987.

[12] D. K. Evans, "Dislocations at the cervicothoracic junction," *Journal of Bone and Joint Surgery. British Volume*, vol. 65, no. 2, pp. 124–127, 1983.

[13] H. H. Bohlman, "Acute fractures and dislocations of the cervical spine. An analysis of three hundred hospitalized patients and review of the literature," *The Journal of Bone and Joint Surgery. American Volume*, vol. 61, no. 8, pp. 1119–1142, 1979.

[14] R. A. Kaya, O. N. Türkmenoğlu, Ö. N. Koç et al., "A perspective for the selection of surgical approaches in patients with upper thoracic and cervicothoracic junction instabilities," *Surgical Neurology*, vol. 65, no. 5, pp. 454–463, 2006.

[15] Y. Do Koh, T. H. Lim, J. Won You, J. Eck, and H. S. An, "A biomechanical comparison of modern anterior and posterior plate fixation of the cervical spine," *Spine*, vol. 26, no. 1, pp. 15–21, 2001.

[16] P. C. McAfee, H. H. Bohlman, T. B. Ducker, S. M. Zeidman, and J. A. Goldstein, "One-stage anterior cervical decompression and posterior stabilization. A study of one hundred patients with a minimum of two years of follow-up," *The Journal of Bone & Joint Surgery*, vol. 77, no. 12, pp. 1791–1800, 1995.

[17] H. U. Bueff, J. C. Lotz, O. K. Colliou et al., "Instrumentation of the cervicothoracic junction after destabilization," *Spine*, vol. 20, no. 16, pp. 1789–1792, 1995.

[18] D. K. Resnick, "Anterior cervicothoracic junction corpectomy and plate fixation without sternotomy," *Neurosurgical Focus*, vol. 12, no. 1, article E7, 2002.

[19] V. Pointillart, N. Aurouer, N. Gangnet, and J.-M. Vital, "Anterior approach to the cervicothoracic junction without sternotomy: a report of 37 cases," *Spine*, vol. 32, no. 25, pp. 2875–2879, 2007.

[20] A. D. Sharan, G. J. Przybylski, and L. Tartaglino, "Approaching the upper thoracic vertebrae without sternotomy or thoracotomy: a radiographic analysis with clinical application," *Spine*, vol. 25, no. 8, pp. 910–916, 2000.

[21] A. B. Bayoumi, I. E. Efe, S. Berk, E. M. Kasper, Z. O. Toktas, and D. Konya, "Posterior rigid instrumentation of C7: surgical considerations and biomechanics at the cervicothoracic junction. A review of the literature," *World Neurosurgery*, vol. 111, pp. 216–226, 2018.

[22] J. L. Kreshak, D. H. Kim, D. P. Lindsey, A. C. Kam, M. M. Panjabi, and S. A. Yerby, "Posterior stabilization at the cervicothoracic junction: a biomechanical study," *Spine*, vol. 27, no. 24, pp. 2763–2770, 2002.

# 38

# Treatment of Infected Pseudoarthrosis in a Subtrochanteric Fracture in a Patient with Osteopetrosis

**Llano Lionel, Jorge D. Barla, Campelo Diego, Taype Danilo, Carlos F. Sancineto, and Guido Carabelli**

*Instituto de Ortopedia y Traumatología "Carlos E. Ottolenghi", Hospital Italiano de Buenos Aires, Argentina*

Correspondence should be addressed to Llano Lionel; lionel.llano@hospitalitaliano.org.ar

Academic Editor: Eyal Itshayek

Osteopetrosis is a disease of osteoclasts that results in failure of bone remodeling. Despite the sclerotic radiographic appearance of the thickened cortices and its material hardness, osteopetrotic bone is weak and prone to fracture by minor trauma. We report a case of a subtrochanteric fracture in an osteopetrotic patient, with further pseudoarthrosis and infection. Several surgical procedures were required, with further complications. The outcome of each procedure and the final result are also described.

## 1. Introduction

Osteopetrosis was first described by Albers-Schoenberg when he marked the increased radiographic density of the bones in 1904 [1]. Despite the sclerotic radiographic appearance of the thickened cortices and its material hardness, osteopetrotic bone is weak and prone to fracture by minor trauma. Areas of concentrated stress such as the femoral neck and subtrochanteric areas are especially susceptible [2, 3]. The internal fixation is difficult to perform due to bone fragility; therefore, orthopedists may prefer to use conservative treatment with skeletal traction or plaster application [4]. There is paucity of literature comparing the effectiveness of the conservative versus operative treatment of fractures of long bones in patients with osteopetrosis. Furthermore, the main complications reported in the operative treatment of fractures in patients with osteopetrosis are pseudoarthrosis and osteomyelitis [1, 4]. In the present report, we will describe the surgical management of a patient with an infected pseudoarthrosis associated with a subtrochanteric fracture.

## 2. Case Report

A 64-year-old patient with the diagnosis of osteopetrosis came to external consult with right hip pain and limping. He presented with subtrochanteric fracture in the year 2013. Radiographic images evidenced a failure of osteosynthesis and pseudoarthrosis of the fracture (Figure 1). A biopsy is performed, and the culture result is an Enterococcus Cloacae, sensitive to vancomycin. Surgery is decided and the previous material is removed. We use a long plate in the lateral aspect of the femur (LCP) and an intramedullary nail Expert (Depuy Synthes). Both implants are covered with polymethyl methacrylate cement (PMMA) with local vancomycin (Figure 2).

After 10 months of follow-up, the patient presents with relapse of the pain and limping again. Radiographs evidence a new failure of the material previously used and no consolidation of the previous fracture. A new biopsy is performed with negative results (Figure 3).

A second revision surgery is done, previous implants are retired, and a femoral neck fracture is evidenced

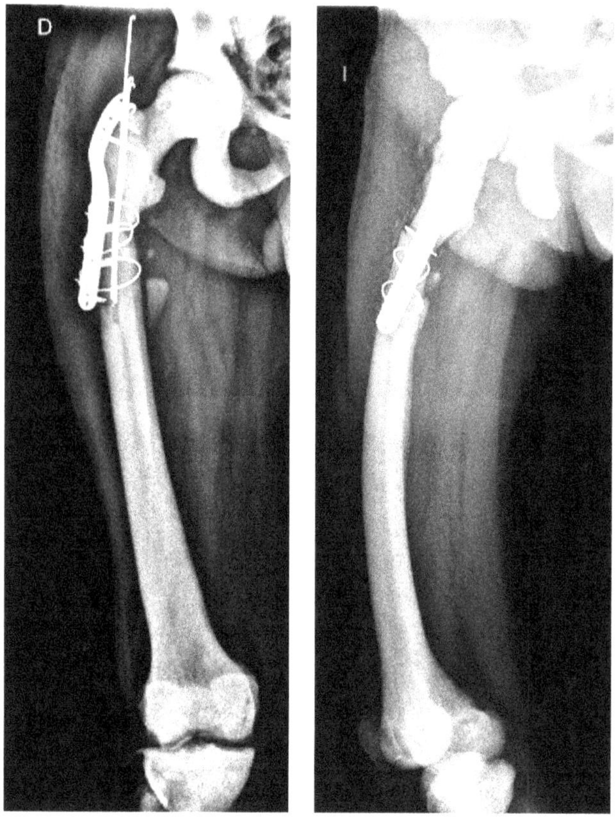


(a) (b)

Figure 1: Anteroposterior (a) and lateral (b) radiographs of the femur showing the failure of osteosynthesis of the subtrochanteric fracture.

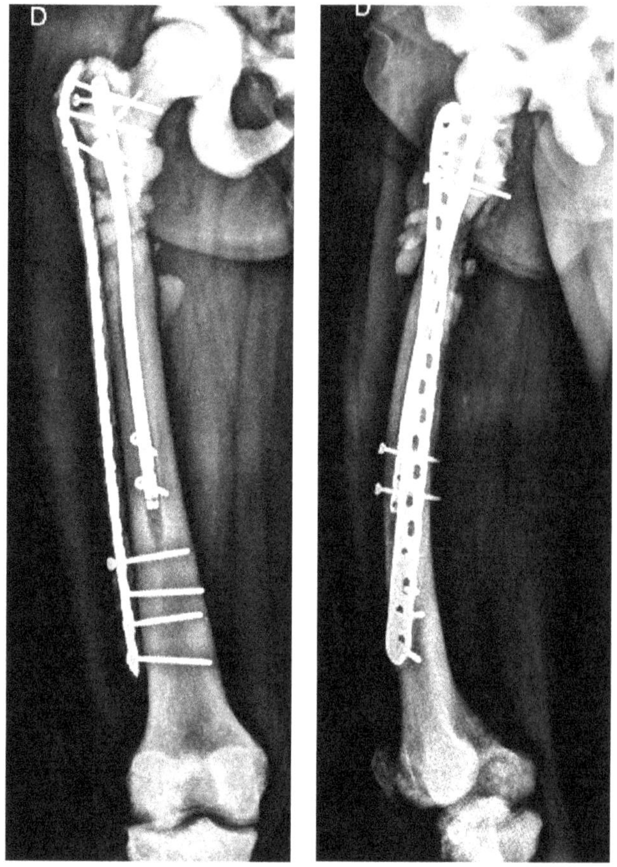


(a) (b)

Figure 2: Postoperative anteroposterior (a) and lateral (b) radiographs of the first revision surgery described.

during fluoroscopy. We decided to use a long intramedullary nail (LFN, Depuy Synthes) covered with PMAA and vancomycin (considering previous cultures) and bone allograft for the pseudoarthrosis. Also a reconstruction plate of 3.5 mm is used for the femoral neck fracture, applying compression on the focus (Figure 4).

After 6 months of follow-up, in a new radiographic control, we observed a pull out of the nail previously used. Biopsy cultures remain negative, with no reactivation of the previous infection (Figure 5).

A final procedure is performed; we proceeded with new nailing and 2 blocking screws to the femoral neck. Also a T plate is used to gain lateral stability. The femoral neck fracture is consolidated, and no new surgeries were needed (Figure 6).

After 2 years of follow-up, the patient has no new complications; he is painless and with no limping. New radiologic studies evidence signs of fracture consolidation of the subtrochanteric fracture (Figure 7). No signs of infection are also evidenced.

## 3. Discussion

Osteopetrosis is a disease of osteoclasts that results in failure of bone remodeling. Histologically, mature osteopetrotic fracture callus contains no Haversian organization and has a paucity of osteoclasts [5]. Fractures occur frequently in patients with osteopetrosis, and there are several difficulties associated with operative treatment, including the extreme hardness of the bone, which impedes drilling and cutting, hardware failure, periprosthetic fractures, coxa vara deformity, delayed union, pseudoarthrosis, refracture, and periprosthetic infection [2, 6]. The use of blocked plate is the most reported strategy for the management of diaphyseal fractures in patients with osteopetrosis; the said indication is associated with a lower technical difficulty, despite the high nonunion rate presented by these cases [6, 7]. Endomedular nailing in diaphyseal fractures in patients with osteopetrosis presents great technical difficulties but greater mechanical stability in relation to the use of plaque [8]; we consider that the combined use of implants increases fracture focus stability after the first failure of implants. There are fewer reports describing treatment of femoral neck fractures in adults. Armstrong et al. treated seven patients nonoperatively with nonweightbearing, and all had developed coxa vara that subsequently was treated with a valgus osteotomy. In three patients, the fractures were treated with either pins or a compression screw and all united. One patient was treated nonoperatively with nonweightbearing, but a developed nonunion was treated with pins at 6 months, after which the fracture

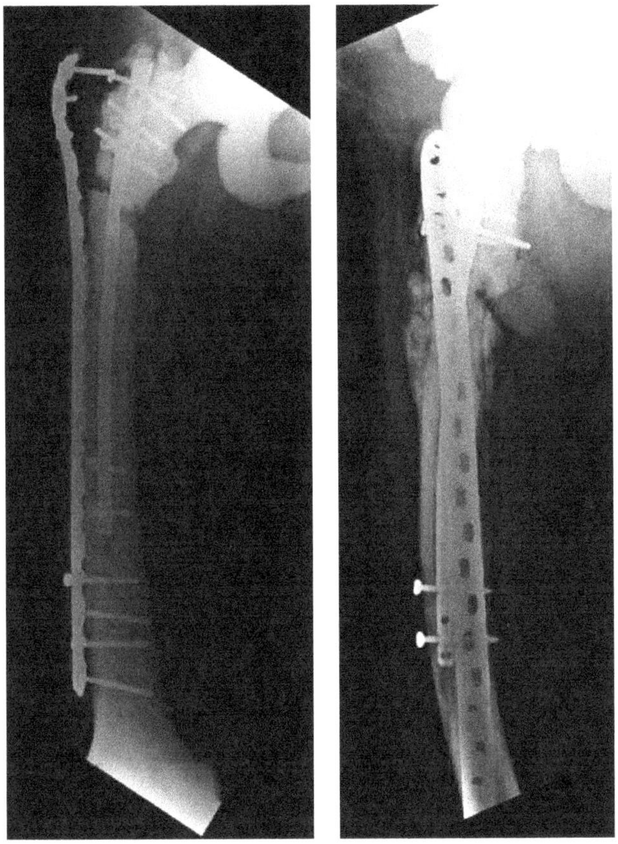

(a) (b)

Figure 3: Anteroposterior (a) and lateral (b) radiographs of the femur showing the failure of the first revision configuration.

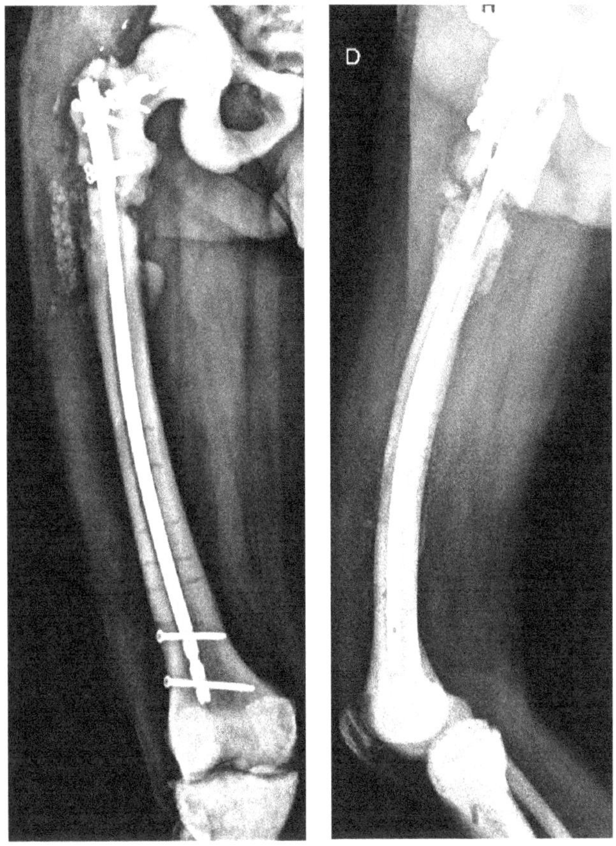


(a) (b)

Figure 4: Postoperative anteroposterior (a) and lateral (b) radiographs of the third revision surgery described.

united [2]. Rolauffs et al. reported a 39-year-old man with a femoral neck fracture treated with multiple parallel screws [9]. Three of the four screws broke, the fracture settled into varus, and osteomyelitis of the femur subsequently developed. In our patient, we decided to use a 3.5 mm blocked plate to grant absolute stability to the fracture site, associated with an endomedular nail for the pseudoarthrosis site. There were no signs of nonunion or osteosynthesis failure associated with the femoral neck fracture. The complex management of osteoporotic bone infection is directly associated with its poor bone quality. There is no literary consensus regarding the management of such infections [10]. It was decided to use an endomedular nail coated with PMMA with antibiotic (vancomycin) for the local treatment of the infection associated with intravenous antibiotic treatment prolonged for 6 weeks (vancomycin). In spite of the osteosynthesis failure, there was no recurrence of the infection after such treatment. Park et al. reported good results using blocked plates for the treatment of long bone pseudoarthrosis, using it as an augmentation technique associated with an endomedular nail [11]. However, there are no current reports that refer to the use of this technique for the treatment of infected pseudoarthrosis in the context of a patient with osteopetrosis.

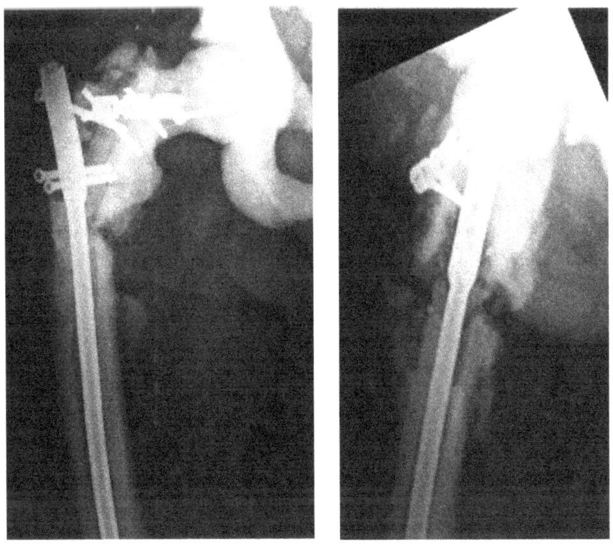

(a) (b)

Figure 5: Anteroposterior (a) and lateral (b) radiographs showing the pull out of the intramedullary nail of the femur.

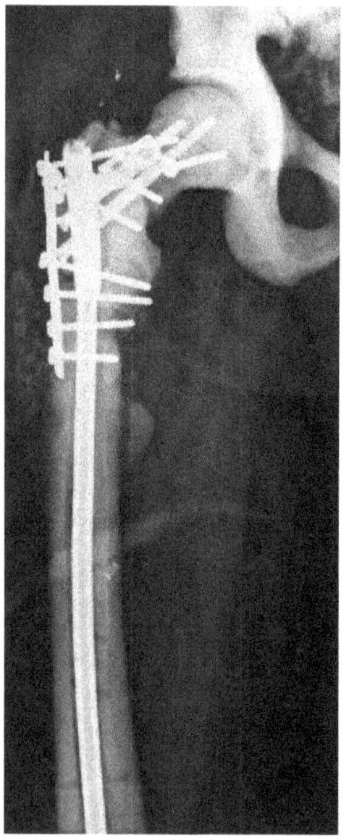

FIGURE 6: Postoperative anteroposterior radiograph of the femur after the last revision surgery.

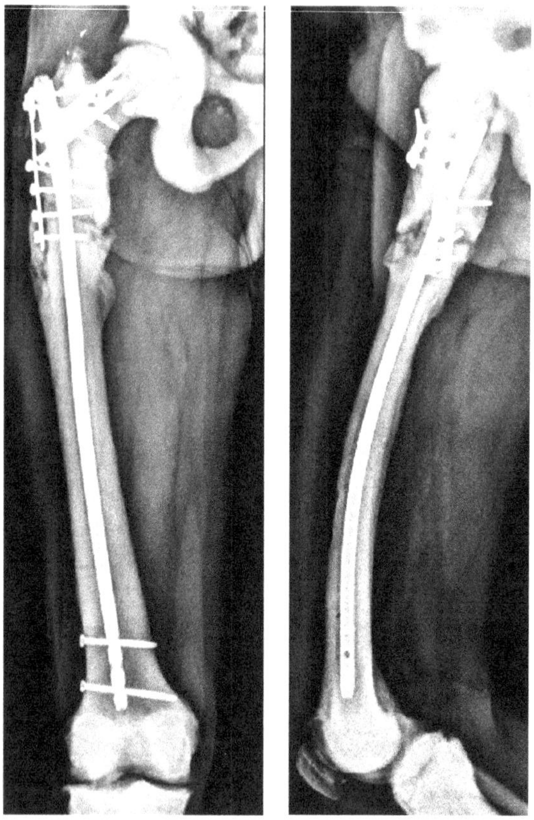

(a) (b)

FIGURE 7: Two-year follow-up. Anteroposterior (a) and lateral (b) radiographs of the femur.

## 4. Conclusion

Despite the difficult management of the patient and the multiple surgeries required, we consider that the use of PMAA-coated endomedular nail and antibiotics, associated with a blocked plate as an augmentation, is a technique to be considered for the management of infected pseudoarthrosis of long bones in patients with osteopetrosis.

## References

[1] H. Albers-Schonberg, "Roentgenbilder einer seltenen Knochen-nerkrankung," *Münchener Medizinische Wochenschrift (1950)*, vol. 51, p. 365, 1904.

[2] D. G. Armstrong, J. T. Newfield, and R. Gillespie, "Orthopedic management of osteopetrosis: results of a survey and review of the literature," *Journal of Pediatric Orthopedics*, vol. 19, no. 1, pp. 122–132, 1999.

[3] A. Chhabra, L. Erik Westerlund, A. J Kline, and R. McLaughlin, "Management of proximal femoral shaft fractures in osteopetrosis: a case series using internal fixation," *Orthopedics*, vol. 28, no. 6, pp. 587–592, 2005.

[4] T. Huang, Q. Liang, H. Qian, X. Li, and C. Zou, "Surgical treatment of an osteopetrotic patient with postoperative fractures: lessons from siblings with osteopetrosis," *The Tohoku Journal of Experimental Medicine*, vol. 230, no. 2, pp. 93–96, 2013.

[5] L. de Palma, A. Tulli, G. Maccauro, S. P. Sabetta, and M. del Torto, "Fracture callus in osteopetrosis," *Clinical Orthopaedics and Related Research*, vol. 308, no. 308, pp. 85–89, 1994.

[6] L. W. Breck, R. C. Cornell, and J. E. Emmett, "Intramedullary fixation of fractures of the femur in a case of osteopetrosis," *The Journal of Bone and Joint Surgery American Volume*, vol. 39, no. 6, pp. 1389–1394, 1957.

[7] R. K. Sen, N. R. Gopinathan, R. Kumar, and U. C. Saini, "Simple reproducible technique in treatment for osteopetrotic fractures," *Musculoskeletal Surgery*, vol. 97, no. 2, pp. 117–121, 2013.

[8] M. Kumbaraci, L. Karapinar, M. Incesu, and A. Kaya, "Treatment of bilateral simultaneous subtrochanteric femur fractures with proximal femoral nail antirotation (PFNA) in a patient with osteopetrosis: case report and review of the literature," *Journal of Orthopaedic Science*, vol. 18, no. 3, pp. 486–489, 2013.

[9] B. Rolauffs, T. M. Bernhardt, C. von Eiff, M. L. Hart, and D. Bettin, "Osteopetrosis, femoral fracture, and chronic osteomyelitis caused by Staphylococcus aureus small colony variants (SCV) treated by Girdlestone resection: 6-year follow-up," *Archives of Orthopaedic and Trauma Surgery*, vol. 122, no. 9-10, pp. 547–550, 2002.

[10] C. Sobacchi, A. Schulz, F. P. Coxon, A. Villa, and M. H. Helfrich, "Osteopetrosis: genetics, treatment and new insights into osteoclast function," *Nature Reviews Endocrinology*, vol. 9, no. 9, pp. 522–536, 2013.

[11] K. C. Park, C. W. Oh, J. W. Kim et al., "Minimally invasive plate augmentation in the treatment of long-bone nonunions," *Archives of Orthopaedic and Trauma Surgery*, vol. 137, no. 11, pp. 1523–1528, 2017.

# Symptomatic Medial Bone Excrescence in the Distal Phalanx of the Hallux after the First Metatarsophalangeal Joint Arthrodesis: A Case Report and Radiographic Reviews

**Yuji Maenohara, Ryutaro Takeda, Song Ho Chang, Yasunori Omata, Sakae Tanaka, and Takumi Matsumoto**

*Department of Orthopaedic Surgery, Faculty of Medicine, The University of Tokyo, 7-3-1 Hongo, Bunkyo-ku, Tokyo 113-8655, Japan*

Correspondence should be addressed to Takumi Matsumoto; matumot-tky@umin.ac.jp

Academic Editor: Robert U. Ashford

Medial bone excrescence at the base of the distal phalanx of the hallux is a common manifestation which is rarely painful. In this case report, we described the first case of the excrescence becoming symptomatic one year after a metatarsophalangeal (MTP) joint arthrodesis of the great toe in a 74-year-old female. The medial bony excrescence which was obscure preoperatively became obvious postoperatively in the anteroposterior foot radiographs. The patient was successfully treated by an excision of the excrescence. In order to clarify the pathology of the excrescence, we reviewed the radiographs with respect to the excrescence before and after hallux surgeries including 97 metatarsal osteotomies and 33 MTP joint arthrodesis. The width of the excrescence measured in the anteroposterior foot radiographs displayed substantial increment one month after the hallux surgeries (osteotomy group: $0.9 \pm 0.7$ vs. $1.5 \pm 0.7$ mm, $p < 0.01$; arthrodesis group: $1.3 \pm 0.8$ vs. $1.8 \pm 1.0$ mm, $p < 0.01$). However, there was no significant difference in the width of the excrescence between one month after surgery and at the most recent follow-up of around 20 months in average after the surgery (osteotomy group: $1.5 \pm 0.7$ vs. $1.4 \pm 0.7$ mm, $p = 0.62$; arthrodesis group: $1.8 \pm 1.0$ vs. $1.8 \pm 0.7$ mm, $p = 0.37$). The present case and our radiographic review suggested that the postoperative medial bony excrescence was not the result of change of position of the preexisting excrescence. The correction of pronation deformity through hallux surgeries could emphasize the medial bony excrescence and cause symptomatic irritation upon shoe contact.

## 1. Introduction

The medial bone excrescence at the base of the distal phalanx of the hallux does not often garner attention as it is rarely symptomatic. Histologically, it is considered to be reactive bone formation and is present in most people with a prevalence rate of up to 88.5% [1]. However, there is a case report in which excrescence became symptomatic after corrective osteotomy for hallux valgus deformity was performed [2]. We present a case in which the excrescence became symptomatic after hallux metatarsophalangeal (MTP) joint arthrodesis was conducted. While speculating on the probable reasons for the development of the new symptoms due to the excrescence after hallux procedures, we noticed that the excrescence that was earlier obscure in the preoperative foot radiograph became conspicuous after surgery in some patients (Figure 1). Because the hallux valgus is a multiplanar deformity including the pronation deformity of the first ray [3], the surgical correction of the deformity might alter the position of the excrescence. However, there has been no literature to explain whether the medial bony excrescence is caused by postoperative growth or rotational change of position of the preexisting excrescence. Therefore, we reviewed the series of foot radiographs before and after hallux surgeries to resolve this question.

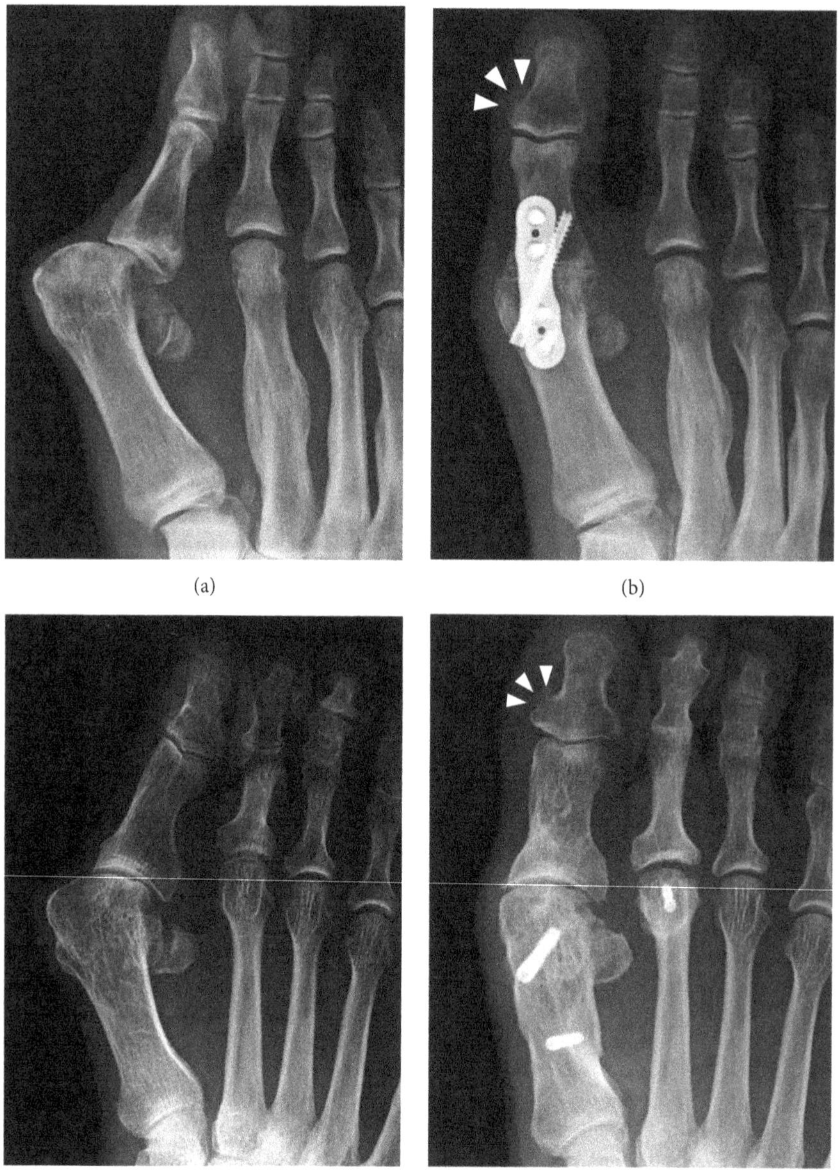


Figure 1: Representative anteroposterior foot radiographs of the cases showing increased width of medial bone excrescence at the distal phalanx of the hallux after the metatarsophalangeal arthrodesis (a, b) or metatarsal osteotomy (c, d) performed to rectify hallux valgus deformity. Arrowheads indicate the protruded bone excrescence after the procedures.

## 2. Case Report

The patient was a 74-year-old female with a 32-year history of seropositive rheumatoid arthritis (RA). The patient underwent the first MTP joint arthrodesis for hallux valgus deformity and MTP joint destruction due to RA. The MTP joint arthrodesis was performed through dorsal longitudinal incision using flat cut joint preparation technique [4]. The arthrodesis site was fixed with a headless compression screw and a dorsal locking plate. Hallux valgus angle and intermetatarsal angle between 1st and 2nd improved from 48 to 16 degrees and from 21 to 16 degrees after the surgery, respectively (Figure 2). Although the postoperative course was uneventful, the patient began to complain of localized pain at the medial aspect of the distal phalanx of the hallux during walking with shoes, one year after the procedure. Weight-bearing anteroposterior foot radiographs revealed increased width of medial excrescence at the base of the distal phalanx of the hallux as compared to the preoperative radiographs. Since there was tenderness on palpation and callosity just above the excrescence, the symptom was considered to be caused by this excrescence. Surgical excision of the excrescence was performed with the removal of the metal implant for the MTP joint arthrodesis (Figure 2). Thereafter, the pain disappeared, and there was no recurrence of the symptom at the recent follow-up that was conducted two years after the excision.

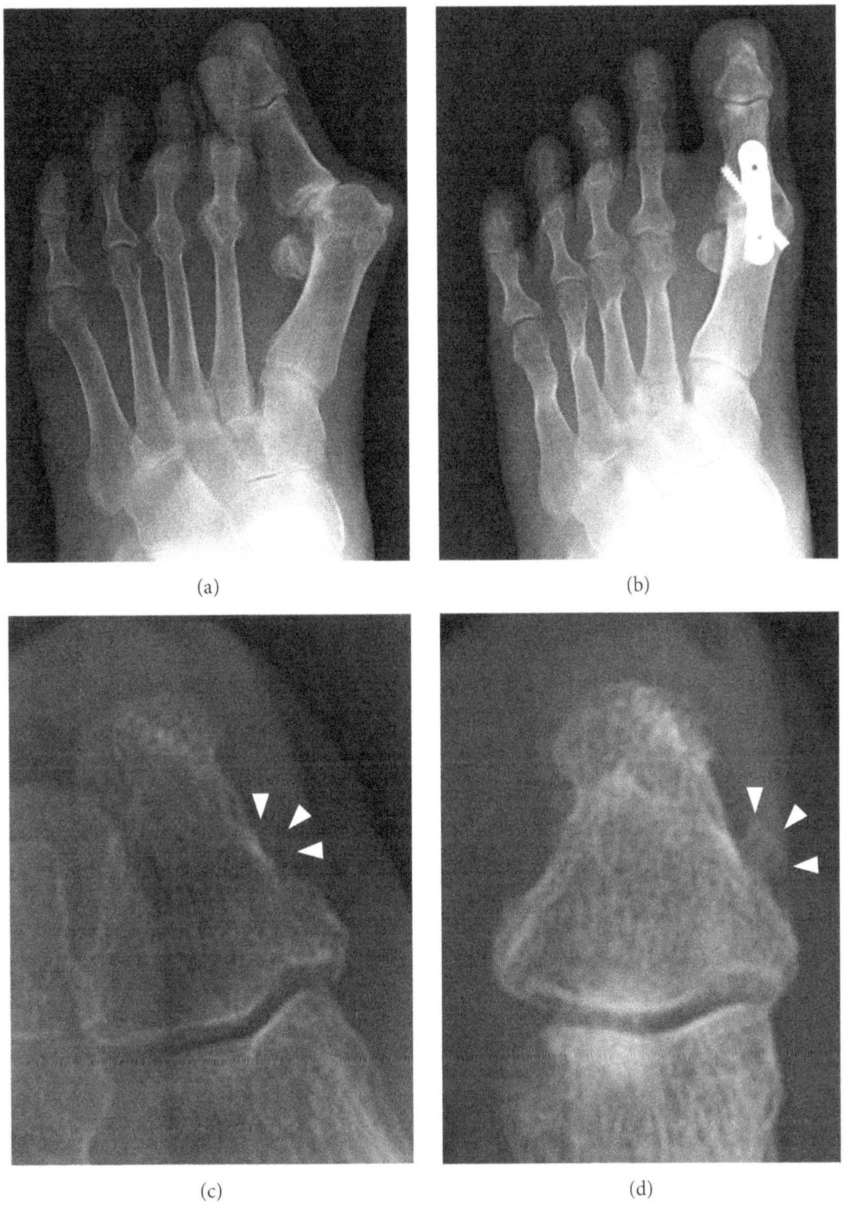

(a) (b) (c) (d)

FIGURE 2: Continued.

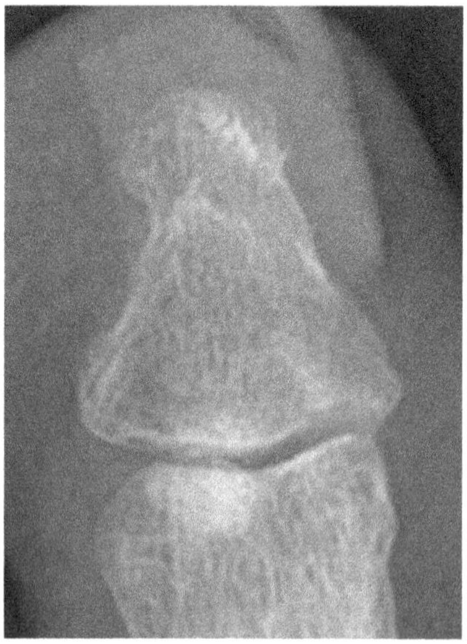

(e)

FIGURE 2: A case of symptomatic medial bone excrescence of the distal phalanx of the hallux after the metatarsophalangeal joint arthrodesis. Anteroposterior foot radiographs before surgery (a) and one year after surgery (b). Magnified images showing obscure excrescence before surgery (c), defined excrescence after arthrodesis (d), and disappeared excrescence after excision (e). Arrowheads indicate the bone excrescence.

## 3. Discussion

A bony excrescence at the medial aspect of the base of the distal phalanx of the hallux is a frequent radiographic finding; however, on rare occasions, it becomes symptomatic. In a review of 157 foot radiographs by Lee et al., including 117 adult and pediatric patients who visited the hospital with foot problems, a specific bone excrescence was observed in 88.5% of the feet [1]. In this study, an outgrowth of 0.4 mm or less was judged as negative excrescence and that of 0.5 mm or more as positive. Another radiographic study by Montiel et al. analyzed unilateral feet of 254 patients who visited the clinic with foot problems and reported a prevalence of 51.9% excrescence, with no description about the judgment criterion [5]. In the present study including a specified cohort of patients who underwent surgery for their hallux disorders, excrescence was observed in 72% of the patients preoperatively and in 93% cases, one month after the surgery as per the judgement criterion by Lee et al. [1].

The clinical implication of the presence of medial excrescence of the base of the distal phalanx of the hallux has been proposed in a case report by Villas et al. that indicated preexisting bony excrescence becomes symptomatic after bunion surgery [2]. This case report by Villas et al. described a 54-year-old woman who developed a painful compression lesion localized to the excrescence after a scarf and Akin osteotomy, which was aggravated by shoe contact and direct pressure. This was successfully treated by surgical excision of the excrescence [2]. Villas et al. attributed this postoperative complication to overcorrection of the hallux deformity with a change in the hallux valgus angle from 33° to 8° and the intermetatarsal angle from 12° to 2°. However, we did not recognize overcorrection of the first ray in the present case.

The bony excrescence at the medial aspect of the base of the distal phalanx of the hallux has been identified as a reactive bone across various literature, suggesting chronic or repetitive stress as a causative factor [1, 5]. In proof of this theory, the absence of excrescence in the juvenile population has been reported [1, 5]. Lee et al. reported the absence of excrescence in the radiographs from patients younger than 18 years. This study also noted a significant correlation between the width of the excrescence and the age of the patient ($r = 0.57$, $p < 0.0001$) in the cohort consisting of 117 patients (6-81 years, mean 37.5) [1]. Montiel et al. reported in their radiographical study which included the patients aged between 2 and 81 years that the prevalence of the excrescence was 1.3% in the patients under 16 years and 65% in those over 60 years [5].

As for the postoperative symptomatic medial bone excrescence, there has been no discussion about its pathology. Thus, we investigated the width of the excrescence in the foot radiographs and compared the results before and after hallux surgeries. Radiographic measurements were performed using the preoperative, one month postsurgery, and most recent anteroposterior weight-bearing foot radiographs for the patients who underwent hallux surgeries including metatarsal osteotomy (osteotomy group, 97 cases in 82 patients) and MTP joint arthrodesis (arthrodesis group, 33 cases in 29 patients) between January 2015 and December 2019 in our facility. The mean follow-up periods were $22.3 \pm 13.4$ months in the osteotomy group and $20.3 \pm 11.2$ months in the arthrodesis group. The maximum width of the excrescence in the mediolateral direction was measured as per the method described by Lee et al. (Figure 3) [1]. The patients' backgrounds and radiographic measurements are shown in Table 1. The comparison between the preoperative

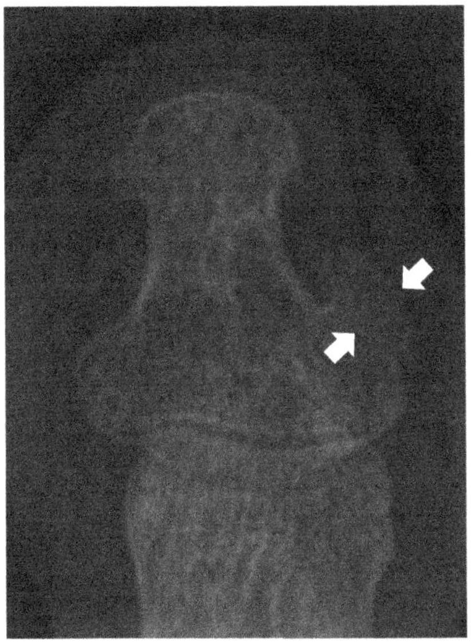

FIGURE 3: Measurement of the maximal width of the medial bone excrescence of the distal phalanx of the hallux (arrows).

TABLE 1: Patients' backgrounds and radiographic measurements in the osteotomy and arthrodesis groups.

| | Osteotomy ($n = 97$) | Arthrodesis ($n = 33$) |
|---|---|---|
| Sex F : M (% female) | 89 : 8 (92%) | 29 : 4 (88%) |
| Follow-up periods (months) | $22.3 \pm 13.4$ | $20.3 \pm 11.2$ |
| RA as underlying pathology (% patients) | 30 (31%) | 22 (67%) |
| Radiographic parameters | | |
| Hallux valgus angle (degrees) | | |
| Preoperative | $40.5 \pm 10.8$ | $39.5 \pm 22.5$ |
| Recent follow-up | $11.5 \pm 8.7^*$ | $9.7 \pm 7.0^*$ |
| Intermetatarsal angle (degrees) | | |
| Preoperative | $17.9 \pm 4.3$ | $15.0 \pm 6.4$ |
| Recent follow-up | $8.0 \pm 4.3^*$ | $11.2 \pm 3.8^*$ |
| Width of excrescence (mm) | | |
| Preoperative | $0.9 \pm 0.7$ | $1.3 \pm 0.8$ |
| Postop 1 month | $1.5 \pm 0.7^*$ | $1.8 \pm 1.0^*$ |
| Recent follow-up | $1.4 \pm 0.7^*$ | $1.8 \pm 0.7^*$ |

RA: rheumatoid arthritis. All continuous variables were presented as mean ± standard deviation. A paired $t$ -test was used to compare the radiographic measurements between preoperative and postoperative conditions. $^*p < 0.05$ vs. preoperative condition.

condition and one month after surgery demonstrated the significant increase of the width of excrescence after surgery in both the groups (osteotomy group: $0.9 \pm 0.7$ vs. $1.5 \pm 0.7$ mm, $p < 0.01$; arthrodesis group: $1.3 \pm 0.8$ vs. $1.8 \pm 1.0$ mm, $p < 0.01$). There was no significant difference in the width of excrescence between one month after surgery and at the most recent follow-up in both the groups (osteotomy group: $1.5 \pm 0.7$ vs. $1.4 \pm 0.7$ mm, $p = 0.62$; arthrodesis group: $1.8 \pm 1.0$ vs. $1.8 \pm 0.7$ mm, $p = 0.37$). These radiographic reviews suggested that the postoperative medial bony excrescence was not the result of postoperative growth but just a rotational change of position of the preexisting excrescence following the surgeries. Surgeons must be aware that the excrescence arising from the medial border and plantar aspect of the distal phalanx can be underestimated in the foot with hallux valgus.

To the best of our knowledge, this report is the first to identify a case in which the preexisting asymptomatic excrescence became symptomatic after the MTP joint arthrodesis. There were several possible causes of the preexisting asymptomatic excrescence becoming symptomatic after the procedure: (1) the change in position of the excrescence after the procedure, (2) overload around the IP joint with weight-bearing secondary to the immobile MTP joint, and (3) excessive pressure at the skin over the excrescence by shoe contact, which could be aggravated by the immobile MTP joint.

## 4. Conclusions

The correction of pronation deformity by hallux surgeries could enhance the medial bony excrescence at the medial aspect of the base of the distal phalanx of the hallux. This can cause symptomatic irritation between the excrescence and shoes. Since such occurrences are rare, we consider that there is no need to remove the excrescence in every case in the first surgical intervention.

## References


[1] M. Lee, J. Hodler, P. Haghighi, and D. Resnick, "Bone excrescence at the medial base of the distal phalanx of the first toe: normal variant, reactive change, or neoplasia?," *Skeletal Radiology*, vol. 21, no. 3, pp. 161–165, 1992.

[2] C. Villas, J. Del Rio, A. Valenti, and M. Alfonso, "Symptomatic medial exostosis of the great toe distal phalanx: a complication due to over-correction following akin osteotomy for hallux valgus repair," *The Journal of Foot and Ankle Surgery*, vol. 48, no. 1, pp. 47–51, 2009.

[3] E. Wagner and P. Wagner, "Metatarsal pronation in hallux valgus deformity: a review," *JAAOS: Global Research and Reviews*, vol. 4, no. 6, 2020.

[4] T. Matsumoto, R. Takeda, T. Kasai et al., "Clinical outcomes after first metatarsophalangeal joint arthrodesis by flat cut joint preparation with individual adjustment for sagittal alignment," *The Journal of Foot and Ankle Surgery*, 2021.

[5] V. Montiel, M. Alfonso, C. Villas, and A. Valenti, "Medial and lateral exostoses of the distal phalanx of the hallux: A potentially painful *bunion-like* structure. Part 1: Incidence and clinical application," *Foot and Ankle Surgery*, vol. 25, no. 2, pp. 158–164, 2019.

# 40

# Resolution of Chronic Shoulder Pain after Repair of a Posttraumatic Diaphragmatic Hernia: A 22-Year Delay in Diagnosis and Treatment

**Brody W. King,[1] John G. Skedros,[2,3] Robert E. Glasgow,[4] and D. Glen Morrell[5]**

[1]*University of Utah School of Medicine, Salt Lake City, Utah, USA*
[2]*Utah Orthopaedic Specialists, Salt Lake City, Utah, USA*
[3]*Intermountain Medical Center, Salt Lake City, Utah, USA*
[4]*University of Utah Department of Surgery, Salt Lake City, Utah, USA*
[5]*Tanner Clinic, Layton, Utah, USA*

Correspondence should be addressed to John G. Skedros; jskedrosmd@uosmd.com

Academic Editor: Kiyohisa Ogawa

Diagnosing traumatic diaphragmatic rupture (TDR) due to penetrating rib fractures is challenging because the lesions are often too small to be detected and may present years after injury. Patients with delays in diagnosis of TDR rarely present with orthopaedic-related complaints of pain. We report the case of a 52-year-old female who presented with chronic left shoulder pain following a motor vehicle accident (MVA). In addition to left-side lower rib fractures, she also sustained a left-sided splenic laceration, pneumothorax, and two-part upper humerus fracture. Fracture treatment was percutaneous pinning; the other injuries were treated nonoperatively. Her shoulder pain could not be attributed to shoulder or neck pathology. Twenty years after the MVA, she began experiencing episodes of left-sided abdominal pain and nausea. A CT scan obtained two years later revealed a diaphragm hernia, which was repaired laparoscopically. Unique aspects of this case include (1) presentation to an orthopaedic surgeon with a chief complaint of chronic shoulder pain; (2) at 22 years, this is the fourth longest case of a delay in diagnosis of TDR; and (3) the unique symptom of ipsilateral referred shoulder pain, which immediately improved after hernia repair.

## 1. Introduction

Traumatic diaphragmatic rupture (TDR) is a common, likely underreported, consequence of blunt force trauma or penetrating injuries to the abdomen and chest and is often associated with multiple traumatic injuries [1]. Up to 90% of cases are caused by motor vehicle accidents (MVAs) [2], as was the cause of the case that we report here. Up to 66% of TDRs are not diagnosed during initial workup [3], which is most likely explained by absent, nonspecific, and/or intermittent symptoms that are often delayed in onset [4]. Most TDRs are diagnosed either incidentally or with nonspecific gastrointestinal/pulmonary symptoms. CT imaging can reveal a "collar sign" or a "funky fat sign", indicating herniation of abdominal viscera or omental fat, respectively [5].

Patients with intermittent, nonspecific symptoms may go undiagnosed for weeks, months, or even many years. Our review of the literature revealed that the majority of delayed diaphragmatic hernia diagnoses occurred within one year of initial injury; however, 17 cases were reported between two and eight years after initial injury [6–14], seven cases between 10 and 20 years [3, 7, 15–19], and three cases over 20 years [20–22]. There have been reports of incidental diagnosis in asymptomatic patients [23]; however, this is uncommon. Most patients present with symptoms of respiratory distress including dyspnea and shortness of breath, abdominal pain, and/or nausea/vomiting [6–22]. We report the

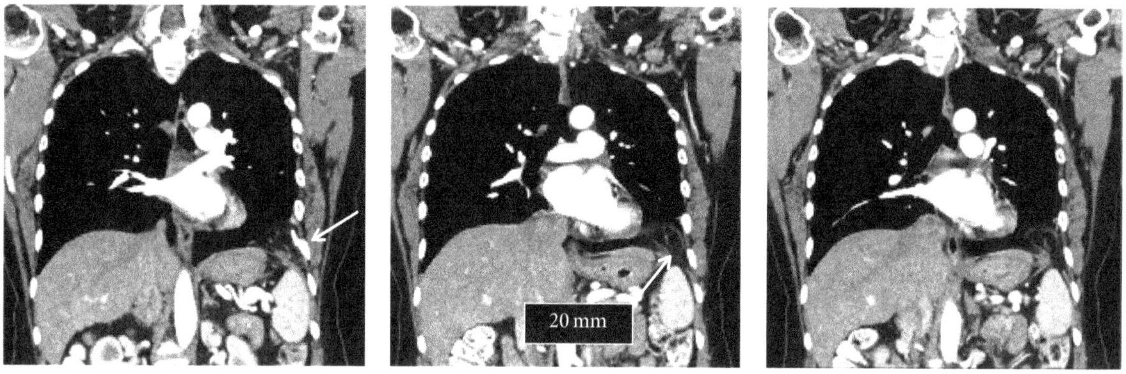


(a) (b) (c)

Figure 1: Coronal CT scan images showing diaphragmatic omental herniation (right side of each image). The arrow in (a) shows a healed rib fracture. The arrow in (b) indicates the hernia, which can be seen in each image.

fourth longest diagnosis delay at 22 years, with a unique presenting symptom of chronic left-sided shoulder pain, which was why our patient initially sought consultation with an orthopaedic surgeon.

## 2. Case Presentation

The patient is an otherwise healthy 52-year-old female (height 170 cm, weight 66 kg, BMI 22.8) with a long history of left shoulder pain following motor vehicle accident (MVA) 22 years prior. The MVA occurred on June 26, 1996, when she was hit on the driver's side of her car, which she was driving. She sustained multiple left-sided skeletal and visceral injuries including a splenic laceration, pneumothorax, two-part upper humerus fracture, and fractures of the sixth through eleventh ribs. Her initial treatment after the MVA included placement of a chest tube, admission to the intensive care unit for three days, left humerus fracture repair via percutaneous pinning, and nonoperative management of her splenic laceration. The patient was in the hospital for 10 days.

During the next few months, all apparent injuries healed; however, the left shoulder pain persisted and began radiating into the left mandible. The dull pain was never less than a 2/10 and intermittently increased to an 8/10 during cold weather and occasionally after large meals (0 = no pain, 10 = worst pain, determined with the visual analogue scale). Physical therapy and subacromial and glenohumeral corticosteroid injections were given in the first year following injury but were discontinued because there was no improvement in shoulder pain.

Ten years after the MVA, the patient consulted with one of us (orthopaedic surgeon, J.G.S.). CT scans and other radiology images and reports obtained during the initial evaluation following the MVA were unavailable at that time. This consultation was followed by serial orthopaedic physical examinations spanning several months. Possible diagnoses of a rotator cuff tear or glenohumeral injuries (e.g., labrum tear) and other sequelae (e.g., posttraumatic arthritis) were considered as possible causes of shoulder pain; however, the pain could not be recreated with provocative manual tests. Magnetic resonance scanning showed no significant pathology of the neck or shoulder. Cardiac etiologies were also ruled out. Surgery with arthroscopic evaluation was performed and the buried pins were removed from the left upper humerus, but relief of shoulder pain was not achieved.

Nearly 20 years after the MVA (10 years following orthopaedic consultation), the patient developed unpredictable episodes of sharp left-sided "gassy" abdominal pain and nausea. These episodes occurred 2-3 times per week, lasting 3-24 hours, and would resolve after vomiting or dry heaving. The patient denied associated fevers, chills, or diarrhea. The frequency and duration of these nausea spells also increased over the following two years. A work-up for gallbladder and hepatobiliary problems was negative (but no abdominal CT scan was ordered). Plain radiographs taken at an urgent care clinic in January 2018 showed findings suggestive of a left-side diaphragmatic hernia. A general surgeon (D.G.M.) was consulted, and a CT scan was done that confirmed the diagnosis of a left-sided, posttraumatic diaphragmatic hernia with a defect measuring 2-2.5 cm in the anterior-lateral left diaphragm juxtaposed to healed rib fractures. There were abdominal contents including omentum in the left pleural space (Figures 1 and 2).

The patient was then referred to another general surgeon specialist (R.E.G.) for laparoscopic repair. During laparoscopy, the hernia containing incarcerated omentum was visualized in the left anterior-lateral diaphragm. The omentum was reduced into the abdominal cavity. There was a focal adhesion to the lung that was divided through the defect. The diaphragmatic defect was closed primarily using polyester suture with Teflon pledgets incorporated in the stitches, and no mesh was required. A red rubber catheter was advanced into the defect prior to closure. After conclusion of the surgery and deinsufflation of the $CO_2$-inflated abdomen, the pleural space was aspirated to reduce the chance of pneumothorax, and the catheter was removed. A chest X-ray in the recovery room confirmed lung reexpansion and no pneumothorax. The patient was discharged on postoperative day #1 with an uneventful recovery. Immediately following diaphragmatic repair, the patient reported complete resolution of all symptoms including shoulder pain,

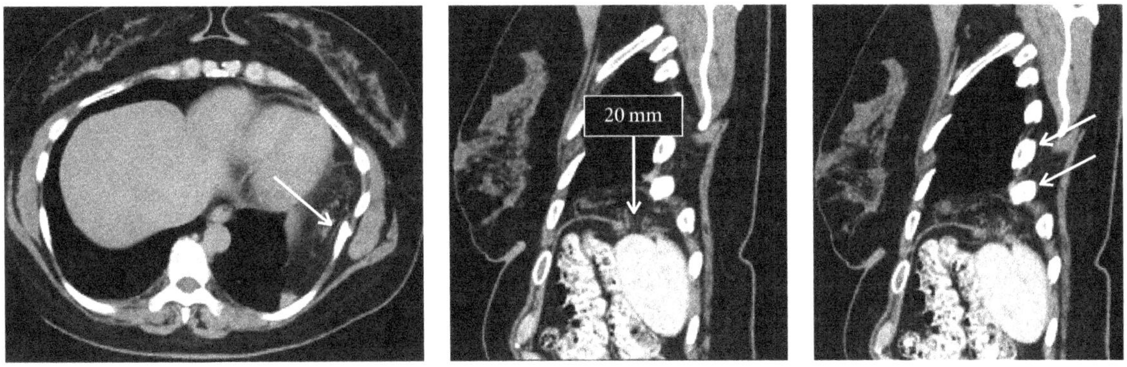


(a) (b) (c)

FIGURE 2: Axial (a) and sagittal (b and c) CT scan images showing diaphragmatic omental herniation. (a) also shows a healed rib fracture (arrow), which is adjacent to the herniated omentum. Two healed rib fractures are also indicated by arrows in (c).

mandibular pain, abdominal pain, and nausea. At 20 months after laparoscopy at her final follow-up appointment, she reported no recurrence of any symptoms.

## 3. Discussion

Acute diagnosis of TDR largely depends on the nature of the concomitant primary injuries, the size of the diaphragmatic defect, and the presenting symptoms [4]. Large TDRs (>10 cm) are associated with blunt force trauma, higher morbidity, and higher mortality, while small TDRs are more often associated with penetration by a displaced fractured rib, stabbing injury, or gunshot [2, 24]. When compared to small TDRs, large TDRs are also more likely to show herniation of abdominal contents into the thoracic cavity with imaging, leading to a more rapid repair [25]. Our patient's TDR was likely caused by penetration from a displaced rib fracture that was missed because it was too small to show signs of herniation. She also had splenic bleeding and a pneumothorax in the vicinity that likely impeded detection of the TDR. While multidetector CT imaging is more sensitive and specific than other imaging modalities for detecting diaphragmatic rupture [26], exploratory laparoscopy affords greater sensitivity and specificity [27, 28] and should be considered for multitrauma patients whose symptoms are not explained by CT results. Had our patient's splenic rupture been treated surgically, the TDR may have been visualized and repaired before any symptoms of shoulder pain began.

Our patient's atypical symptoms of left shoulder and mandibular pain likely also contributed to the delay in diagnosis. Irritation of the diaphragm can cause referred pain along the phrenic nerve, mostly along the C4 dermatome [29], which is a phenomenon known as Kehr's sign [30]. However, this has not been reported as a consequence of TDR. The most common presenting symptoms of diaphragmatic hernia include respiratory distress, dyspnea, shortness of breath, abdominal pain, nausea, and vomiting [6–22]. These symptoms arise when abdominal viscera or omental fat become incarcerated or herniate into the thoracic cavity through the unhealed diaphragmatic defect.

The diaphragm is not known to spontaneously heal, and defects can enlarge over time because the abdominal-thoracic pressure gradient of 9-12 mmHg draws abdominal contents through the defect into the pleural cavity [2, 31]. Our patient's TDR likely grew over time, eventually getting large enough for her abdominal contents to begin herniating into the thoracic cavity. This hernia resulted in episodes of epigastric and abdominal colicky pain, nausea, and vomiting, which progressively became more frequent and severe. At the time of diagnosis, only omental fat was found herniating through the diaphragmatic defect, which is referred to as the "funky fat" sign in CT scan images [5].

Surgical repair is indicated in nearly all cases of TDR. The surgical approach depends on the time of presentation following injury and the size of the defect. Acute presentations are often managed via laparotomy to assess other visceral damage, while delayed presentations with herniating viscera may be managed via thoracotomy to address intrathoracic adhesions [32]. Stable patients can be managed with laparoscopy, thoracoscopy, or video-assisted thoracoscopic surgery (VATS). Smaller diaphragmatic ruptures can be primarily repaired (as done in our patient), while larger defects may require incorporation of a mesh [32, 33]. Our patient's left shoulder and mandibular pain immediately and completely resolved following repair of the diaphragm, supporting our conclusion that these symptoms were caused by diaphragmatic irritation rather than intrinsic shoulder pathology.

## 4. Conclusion

This report describes the case of a female with a delay in diagnosis of a TDR with eventual herniation from a rib fracture sustained during an MVA 22 years prior. This case is unique because (1) she presented to an orthopaedic surgeon with a chief complaint of chronic shoulder pain, (2) it is the fourth longest delay in diagnosis of TDR that we could locate in our literature review, and (3) the unique symptoms of ipsilateral referred shoulder and mandibular pain were attributed to a diaphragmatic defect. Due to the high morbidity and mortality associated with diaphragmatic hernias, early diagnosis and subsequent repair of TDR are critical. Physicians should recognize that patients with rib fractures and adjacent visceral injuries are at a higher risk for TDRs that might not be revealed on CT scans or present typically. One of these atypical presentations includes chronic shoulder pain that does not improve with standard medical/surgical interventions. This report supports expanding the differential diagnosis to include TDRs in patients with persistent shoulder pain following rib fractures.

## Consent

Written informed consent was obtained from the patient.

## References


[1] T. Arak, K. Solheim, and J. Pillgram-Larsen, "Diaphragmatic injuries," *Injury*, vol. 28, no. 2, pp. 113–117, 1997.

[2] A. Desir and B. Ghaye, "CT of blunt diaphragmatic rupture," *RadioGraphics*, vol. 32, no. 2, pp. 477–498, 2012.

[3] C. Sala, M. Bonaldi, P. Mariani, F. Tagliabue, and L. Novellino, "Right post-traumatic diaphragmatic hernia with liver and intestinal dislocation," *Journal of Surgical Case Reports*, vol. 2017, no. 3, 2017.

[4] O. F. Grimes, "Traumatic injuries of the diaphragm: Diaphragmatic hernia," *The American Journal of Surgery*, vol. 128, no. 2, pp. 175–181, 1974.

[5] I. Ocak and D. C. Strollo, "Fractured ribs and the CT funky fat sign of diaphragmatic rupture," *Case Reports in Radiology*, vol. 2016, Article ID 6723632, 4 pages, 2016.

[6] F. Al-Mashat, A. Sibiany, A. Kensarah, and K. Eibany, "Delayed presentation of traumatic diaphragmatic rupture," *The Indian Journal of Chest Diseases & Allied Sciences*, vol. 44, pp. 121–124, 2002.

[7] J. Lu, B. Wang, X. Che et al., "Delayed traumatic diaphragmatic hernia," *Medicine*, vol. 95, no. 32, p. e4362, 2016.

[8] B. M. Gali, A. A. Bakari, D. W. Wadinga, and U. S. Nganjiwa, "Missed diagnosis of a delayed diaphragmatic hernia as intestinal obstruction: a case report," *Nigerian Journal of Medicine*, vol. 23, no. 1, pp. 83–85, 2014.

[9] S. Lal, Y. Kailasia, S. Chouhan, A. Gaharwar, and G. Shrivastava, "Delayed presentation of post traumatic diaphragmatic hernia," *Journal of Surgical Case Reports*, vol. 2011, no. 7, p. 6, 2011.

[10] A. Reina, E. Vidana, P. Soriano et al., "Traumatic intrapericardial diaphragmatic hernia: case report and literature review," *Injury*, vol. 32, no. 2, pp. 153–156, 2001.

[11] M. J. Ramdass, S. Kamal, A. Paice, and B. Andrews, "Traumatic diaphragmatic herniation presenting as a delayed tension faecopneumothorax," *Emergency Medicine Journal*, vol. 23, no. 10, p. e54, 2006.

[12] M. Kafih and R. Boufettal, "A late post-traumatic diaphragmatic hernia revealed by a tension fecopneumothorax (a case report)," *Revue de Pneumologie Clinique*, vol. 65, no. 1, pp. 23–26, 2009.

[13] T. R. de Nadai, J. C. Lopes, C. C. Inaco Cirino, M. Godinho, A. J. Rodrigues, and S. Scarpelini, "Diaphragmatic hernia repair more than four years after severe trauma: four case reports," *International Journal of Surgery Case Reports*, vol. 14, pp. 72–76, 2015.

[14] G. Aprea, A. Canfora, A. Ferronetti et al., "7 years-delayed presentation of a traumatic diaphragmatic rupture: laparoscopic repair," *BMC Surgery*, vol. 13, Suppl 1, p. A2, 2013.

[15] D. B. Christie III, J. Chapman, J. L. Wynne, and D. W. Ashley, "Delayed right-sided diaphragmatic rupture and chronic herniation of unusual abdominal contents," *Journal of the American College of Surgeons*, vol. 204, no. 1, p. 176, 2007.

[16] S. Kumar, S. Kumar, S. Bhaduri, S. More, and P. Dikshit, "An undiagnosed left sided traumatic diaphragmatic hernia presenting as small intestinal strangulation: a case report," *International Journal of Surgery Case Reports*, vol. 4, no. 5, pp. 446–448, 2013.

[17] A. L. Andreev, A. V. Protsenko, and A. V. Globin, "Laparoscopic repair of a posttraumatic left-sided diaphragmatic hernia complicated by strangulation and colon obstruction," *Journal of the Society of Laparoendoscopic Surgeons*, vol. 14, no. 3, pp. 410–413, 2010.

[18] M. Baldwin, A. Dagens, and B. Sgromo, "Laparoscopic management of a delayed traumatic diaphragmatic rupture complicated by bowel strangulation," *Journal of Surgical Case Reports*, vol. 2014, no. 7, 2014.

[19] G. L. Shreck and T. W. Toalson, "Delayed presentation of traumatic rupture of the diaphragm," *The Journal of the Oklahoma State Medical Association*, vol. 96, no. 4, pp. 181–183, 2003.

[20] D. Hariharan, R. Singhal, S. Kinra, and A. Chilton, "Post traumatic intra thoracic spleen presenting with upper GI bleed!-a case report," *BMC Gastroenterology*, vol. 6, no. 1, 2006.

[21] J. L. Faul, "Diaphragmatic rupture presenting forty years after injury," *Injury*, vol. 29, no. 6, pp. 479-480, 1998.

[22] S. Singh, M. M. H. Kalan, C. E. Moreyra, and R. F. Buckman Jr., "Diaphragmatic rupture presenting 50 years after the traumatic event," *The Journal of Trauma*, vol. 49, no. 1, pp. 156–159, 2000.

[23] J. Ruiz-Tovar, P. Calero García, V. Morales Castiñeiras, and E. Martínez Molina, "Post trauma diaphragmatic hernia," *Revista de Gastroenterología del Perú*, vol. 28, no. 3, pp. 244–247, 2008.

[24] K. L. Shackleton, E. T. Stewart, and A. J. Taylor, "Traumatic diaphragmatic injuries: spectrum of radiographic findings," *Radiographics*, vol. 18, no. 1, pp. 49–59, 1998.

[25] S. Iochum, T. Ludig, F. Walter, H. Sebbag, G. Grosdidier, and A. G. Blum, "Imaging of diaphragmatic injury: a diagnostic challenge?," *Radiographics*, vol. 22, suppl_1, pp. S103–S116, 2002.

[26] R. Kaur, A. Prabhakar, S. Kochhar, and U. Dalal, "Blunt traumatic diaphragmatic hernia: pictorial review of CT signs," *Indian Journal of Radiology and Imaging*, vol. 25, no. 3, pp. 226–232, 2015.

[27] Y. B. El-Bendary, J. Al-Adawi, and H. Al-Qadhi, "The use of laparoscopy in the management of trauma patients: brief review," *Sultan Qaboos University Medical Journal*, vol. 16, no. 1, pp. e9–e14, 2016.

[28] P. Nguyen, B. Davis, and D. D. Tran, "Laparoscopic repair of diaphragmatic rupture: a case report with radiological and surgical correlation," *Case Reports in Surgery*, vol. 2017, Article ID 4159108, 4 pages, 2017.

[29] J. A. Waxenbaum and B. Bordoni, "Anatomy, head and neck, cervical nerves," in *StatPearls*, StatPearls Publishing, Treasure Island (FL), 2019, https://www.ncbi.nlm.nih.gov/books/NBK538136/.

[30] S. Soyuncu, F. Bektas, and Y. Cete, "Traditional Kehr's sign: left shoulder pain related to splenic abscess," *Turkish Journal of Trauma and Emergency Surgery*, vol. 18, no. 1, pp. 87-88, 2012.

[31] U. H. Bhatti and S. Dawani, "Large bowel obstruction complicating a posttraumatic diaphragmatic hernia," *Singapore Medical Journal*, vol. 56, no. 04, pp. e56–e58, 2015.

[32] Q. A. Ain Atif and T. Khaliq, "Traumatic right diaphragmatic hernia; a delayed presentation," *Journal of Ayub Medical College Abbottabad*, vol. 28, no. 3, pp. 625-626, 2016.

[33] C. C. Jadlowiec and L. U. Sakorafas, "Delayed presentation of traumatic right-sided diaphragmatic hernia after abdominoplasty," *Case Reports in Surgery*, vol. 2014, Article ID 949531, 4 pages, 2014.

# 41

# Tulip-Screw Head Disjunction from Posterior C2 Fracture Fixation Instrumentation

**Halle E. K. Burley,[1,2] Darius S. Ansari,[1,3] Alexander von Glinski,[1,4,5,6] Ryan Goodmanson,[1,4] Benjamin Schell,[1,4] Jens R. Chapman,[1,4] and Rod J. Oskouian[1,4]**

[1]*Seattle Science Foundation, Seattle, Washington, USA*
[2]*Western University of Health Sciences, College of Osteopathic Medicine of the Pacific-Northwest, 200 Mullins Dr., Lebanon OR 97355, USA*
[3]*University of Illinois College of Medicine, 1835 W Polk St., Chicago, IL 60612, USA*
[4]*Swedish Neuroscience Institute, Swedish Medical Center, Seattle, Washington, USA*
[5]*Department of Trauma Surgery, BG University Hospital Bergmannsheil, Ruhr University Bochum, Bochum, Germany*
[6]*Hansjörg Wyss Hip and Pelvic Center, Swedish Hospital, Seattle, Washington, USA*

Correspondence should be addressed to Halle E. K. Burley; halle.burley@westernu.edu

Academic Editor: Elke R. Ahlmann

This report presents an unusual case of instrumentation failure after posterior fixation of a C2 fracture and reviews currently available treatment alternatives. The patient, a 53-year-old female, initially presented to the emergency department at an outside facility with acute alcohol intoxication and acute neck pain following a fall from a ladder. CT demonstrated bilateral C2 pars fractures and unstable posteroinferior displacement of the posterior elements. She underwent an emergent C2 open-reduction internal fixation (ORIF) at the outside facility with 3.5 mm polyaxial synapse pedicle screws (DePuy Synthes, Switzerland). There were no known complications and the patient was discharged. Two years after the index operation, cervical CT scan at a different facility revealed that although the fracture was fully healed, bilateral tulip caps had detached from the pedicle screw heads at C2. All implants were removed without postoperative complications. Industry review of alternate lag screws approved for the cervical spine demonstrated that there is not currently an ideal implant for fixation of C2 fractures without fusion. Cannulated trauma screws, which are low profile and would have avoided the instrumentation failure seen here, are not currently FDA approved for the cervical spine.

## 1. Introduction

Traumatic spondylolisthesis of the axis, also known as a Hangman's fracture, is a common injury following motor vehicle accidents [1–3]. Effendi and colleagues classified these injuries into three groups based on mechanism. Type I fractures occur with axial loading and hyperextension. Type II fractures are hyperextension injuries with rebound hyperflexion. Type III fractures are primarily flexion injuries with rebound extension [4]. Levine and Edwards modified the system by adding a type IIA, which represents flexion-distraction injuries. These combined forces produce a characteristic bilateral fracture of the pars interarticularis, sparing the odontoid, with or without associated anterolisthesis of the vertebral body [2, 5]. Affected patients may or may not present with neurological symptoms, and if the fracture is nondisplaced and stable, it can be treated nonoperatively with external immobilization [3, 5, 6]. Type I and II fractures generally fall into this category and can be treated conservatively with a collar. In cases of excessive angulation of C2 on C3, disruption of the C2-3 disc space, extensive displacement (<4-6 mm), or failure of external orthoses, surgical fixation and/or fusion is indicated [5, 6]. The typical operation for an isolated C2 fracture involves posterior reduction and fixation with pars screws [7, 8]. Further ventral C2-3 discectomy and fusion is performed for fractures that demonstrate

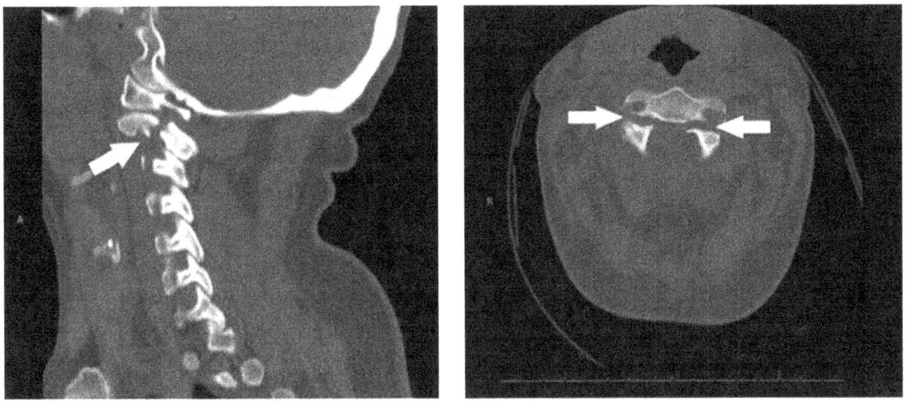

(a) (b)

Figure 1: Fracture of C2 pedicles shown with white arrows. Sagittal view (a) and axial view (b).

sufficient instability to warrant more extensive fixation or in cases of neurological deficit. In cases where an anterior approach is contraindicated, the construct will be subject to excess stress, or bone quality is poor and posterior fusion to C1 or even the occiput may be indicated. The anterior approach is preferred because it preserves rotation at the atlantoaxial joint [1]. Presented here is an unusual case of bilateral tulip detachment from the screw heads two years status post C2 open-reduction internal fixation (ORIF) with polyaxial pedicle screws for a type I traumatic C2 fracture without known additional trauma.

## 2. Case Material

A 53-year-old female presented to the emergency department of an outside facility with acute alcohol intoxication and acute neck pain following a fall from a ladder. Computed tomography (CT) imaging of her cervical spine demonstrated bilateral C2 pars fractures. There was no listhesis of the body of C2, but the posterior elements were displaced posteroinferiorly and determined to be unstable by the outside hospital's radiologist (Figure 1). Physical examination demonstrated intact cranial nerves II-XII, intact sensation, and full motor strength in all extremities. Given the displacement of the fracture and her physically active lifestyle, it was determined by her care team at the outside facility that surgical treatment was warranted. She underwent an emergent C2 open-reduction internal fixation (ORIF) at the outside facility. According to the operative report, the procedure was performed from a posterior approach via standard midline incision at C1-4 with the patient prone. Polyaxial 3.5 mm pedicle screws (SYNAPSE System, DePuy Synthes, Switzerland) were implanted bilaterally. There were no known complications and the patient was discharged home after the operation. It is unclear whether she followed up with her surgeon after the index operation, but she did participate in a course of physical therapy.

Eight months after the index operation at the outside facility, she presented to our clinic for reevaluation, complaining of posterior neck pain that had not improved since surgery. She was experiencing frequent headaches, new onset vertigo, and limited range of motion unresponsive to conservative management. A CT scan of the cervical spine revealed a healed C2 fracture with intact instrumentation. The patient was referred to further physical therapy with massage and scheduled for a repeat CT scan in 1 year.

She instead returned at 9 months with concerns of a firm, mobile bump at the posterior aspect of her neck accompanied by shooting pain radiating to the head. X-rays performed at this visit demonstrated stable C2 lateral mass screws with no other interval changes, and she continued conservative management at this time.

At her scheduled 2-year follow up, she continued to complain of a posterior neck mass and pain. A CT scan revealed that bilateral tulip caps had detached from the pedicle screw heads at C2. The patient's original fracture had healed, without any evidence of pseudarthrosis. Due to her discomfort, surgical removal of the instrumentation was recommended. One month prior to the planned instrumentation removal, flexion and extension radiographs of the cervical spine were obtained in order to visualize the overall bony anatomy and to assess the stability of the cervical spine (Figure 2). These images reaffirmed the findings of the previous CT, demonstrating detached bilateral screw heads with a stable, healed C2 fracture. No grossly mobile segments or listhesis was appreciated on these films.

The patient underwent an elective instrumentation removal. She was positioned prone and the C2 level was exposed through a midline incision. The tulip heads were visibly disengaged from their respective screws and extensive metallosis was observed in the surrounding tissue. Upon inspection of the implant, there was erosion of the coupling portion of the tulip head (Figure 3). Once the tulips were removed, the pedicle screws were removed at C2 bilaterally and the incision was closed. Postoperative CT scan (Figure 4) demonstrated removal of instrumentation with complete healing of the original C2 fracture. The postoperative course was uncomplicated and she was discharged in stable condition.

## 3. Discussion

This case demonstrates a unique instance of instrumentation failure after successful osteosynthesis of a traumatic avulsion

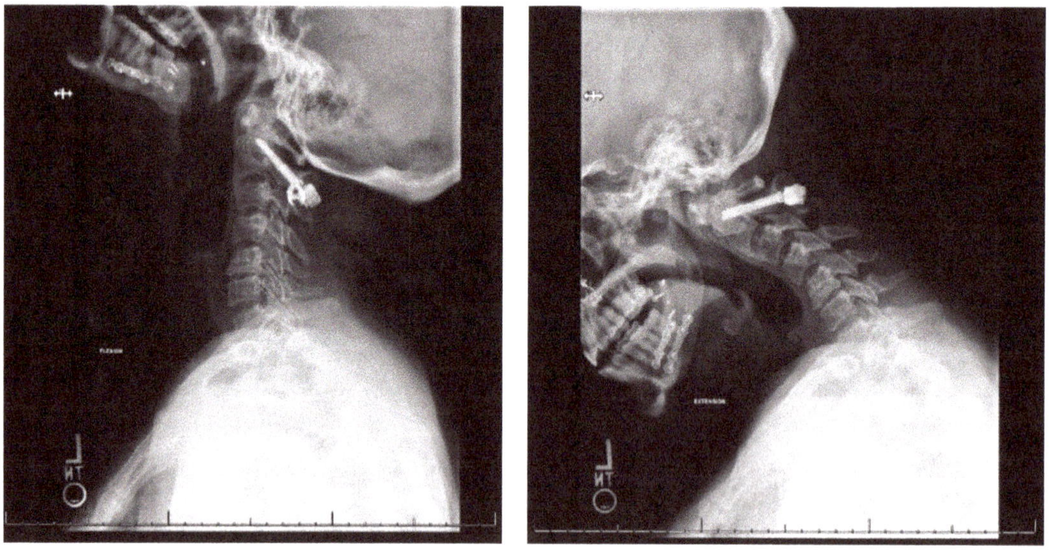

(a) (b)

FIGURE 2: Radiographs of the cervical spine in extension (a) and flexion (b) display complete detachment of the tulip from the screw.

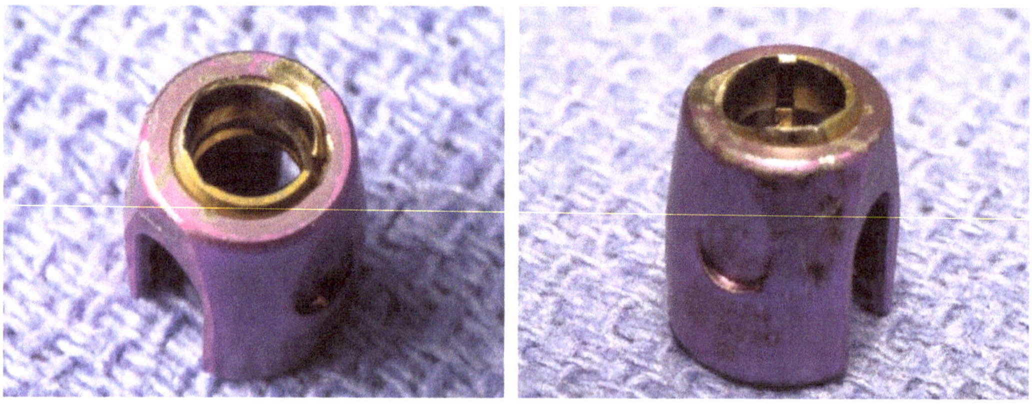

FIGURE 3: Erosion of the coupling portion of the tulip head from motion at the tulip-screw junction.

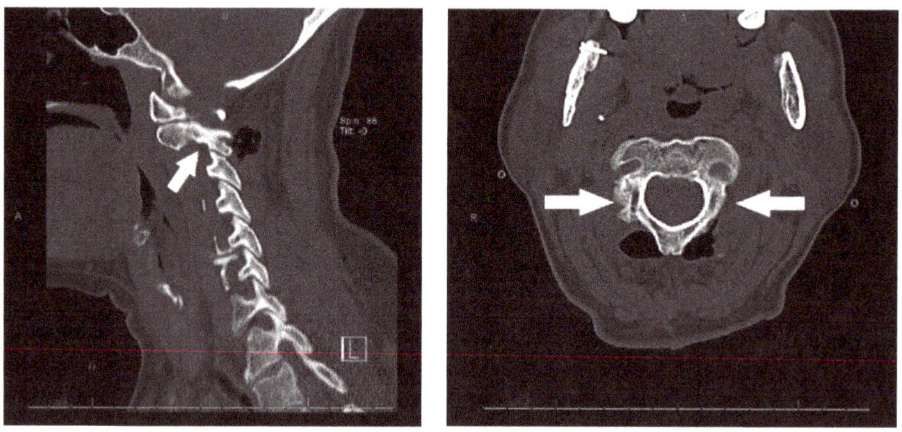

(a) (b)

FIGURE 4: Healing of original C2 pedicle fractures shown with white arrows. Sagittal view (a) and axial view (b).

fracture of the neural arch of C2 in a physically active, otherwise healthy 52-year-old female. Instrumentation failures most commonly occur at points of maximum biomechanical stress. These can occur at the fracture lines or at the junction between multiple components, like the junction between the tulip head and pedicle screw head [9, 10]. In the absence of

Table 1: Currently available posterior cervical screws.

| Company | Device/system | Modular | Removeable tulip | Partially threaded component | Other features |
|---|---|---|---|---|---|
| Stryker | OASYS | Yes | No | Yes | n/a |
| | YUKON | No | No | No | n/a |
| Medtronic | Infinity | Yes | No | No | n/a |
| Zimmer Biomet | Virage | No | No | Yes | Varying thread forms |
| | Lineum | No | No | Yes | Translational tulip |
| Globus | QUARTEX | No | No | Yes | n/a |
| | ELLIPSE | No | No | Yes | Nonthreaded locking cap |
| DePuy Synthes | SYNAPSE | No | No | Yes | n/a |
| | MOUNTAINEER | No | No | Yes | Laminoplasty-capable |

known trauma during the postoperative period, we hypothesize that the repetitive stress of the suboccipital muscle mass against the polyaxial screw when the patient extended her neck eroded the junction between the screw and polyaxial head due to repetitive cycling of the polyaxial head on the pedicle screw over time, causing it to dislodge. Alternately, the patient's extensive course of physical therapy and massage may have caused the tulip heads to dislodge. The prominence of the implants likely irritated the paraspinal muscles, causing the patient greater than usual postoperative muscle tension and discomfort. This would prompt her to undergo more intensive physical therapy and massage, thereby stressing the tulip-screw junction more than it was designed to withstand as an independent unit.

Prominent spinal instrumentation, while not necessarily problematic for the success of a fusion, can cause a considerable amount of discomfort for the patient postoperatively. For instance, in patients with prominent instrumentation following scoliotic deformity correction, skin irritation at the site of prominence is a potential cause of dissatisfaction and even reoperation [11]. Such complaints are less commonly reported in the cervical region [12]. More commonly, this is reported with instrumentation of the thoracolumbar and pelvic regions. The lower rate of complaints postcervical fusion is likely due to local soft tissue coverage and/or the infrequency of direct pressure to the cervical region in the course of daily activities [13]. In this clinical vignette, the prominence of the instrumentation likely caused irritation that prompted continued office visits, imaging, and therapy for the patient which could have led to the instrumentation failure.

The pedicle screws selected by the outside facility for this procedure, while unorthodox as a stand-alone unit, did serve their purpose of reducing the fracture. According to industry-provided information, the section of nonthreaded shaft adjacent to the screw head was originally designed to protect surrounding soft tissues. Although they were not intended to be used as lag screws, this feature incidentally resulted in effective reduction of the fracture fragments and produced a solid, bony fusion. However, despite the generally favorable outcome of the fixation technique, in retrospect, the use of a lag or positional screw without a tulip may have prevented the complications that this patient faced before ultimately undergoing an additional procedure.

The challenge, of course, is in the availability of such implants. Bilateral C2 arch fractures that are unstable enough to require surgical fixation but do not occur concomitantly with fractures to surrounding vertebrae are relatively rare, making the development of specialized implants for their repair not financially feasible [14]. The ideal screw for this type of repair would be a lag screw, not a polyaxial pedicle screw. Many orthopedic implant companies offer cervical spinal screws with fracture-reducing capabilities, but all come with a nonremoveable tulip head (Table 1). At this point in time, there is not an ideal, approved device on the market for posterior approach C2 arch fracture fixations not involving a fusion. This is likely why a screw with a superfluous, and later symptomatic, tulip head was used in this case. In typical cases of fracture fixation where a lag screw is used to create compression at the fracture site and bony union, 3.5-4.0 mm cortical- or cancellous-type trauma screws can be used with success [15, 16]. In theory and in practice, these could also be used to reduce and stabilize cervical fractures, but currently, they are not FDA approved for cervical spine use.

This case demonstrates that implants can still fail despite solid bone healing. Best practices would be to solve problems by using implants as they have been designed and intended. However, sometimes proper implants may not be available or exist to solve the problem in a way that is best for the patient. This case highlights the value of conservative use of instrumentation in surgery and the need for specialized implants for the fixation of isolated traumatic C2 fractures.

## References


[1] W. R. Francis, J. W. Fielding, R. J. Hawkins, J. Pepin, and R. Hensinger, "Traumatic spondylolisthesis of the axis," *The Journal of Bone and Joint Surgery British volume*, vol. 63, pp. 313–318, 1981.

[2] M. Montalbano, C. Fisahn, M. Loukas, R. J. Oskouian, J. R. Chapman, and R. S. Tubbs, "Pediatric hangman's fracture: a

comprehensive review," *Pediatric Neurosurgery*, vol. 52, no. 3, pp. 145–150, 2017.

[3] R. C. Schneider, K. E. Livingston, A. J. Cave, and G. Hamilton, ""Hangman's fracture" of the cervical spine," *Journal of Neurosurgery*, vol. 22, no. 2, pp. 141–154, 1965.

[4] B. Effendi, D. Roy, B. Cornish, R. G. Dussault, and C. A. Laurin, "Fractures of the ring of the axis: a classification based on the analysis of 131 cases," *The Journal of Bone and Joint Surgery British volume*, vol. 63, pp. 319–327, 1981.

[5] R. Al-Mahfoudh, C. Beagrie, E. Woolley et al., "Management of typical and atypical hangman's fractures," *Global Spine Journal*, vol. 6, no. 3, pp. 248–256, 2016.

[6] A. M. Levine and C. C. Edwards, "The management of traumatic spondylolisthesis of the axis," *The Journal of Bone and Joint Surgery American Volume*, vol. 67, no. 2, pp. 217–226, 1985.

[7] R. Bristol, J. S. Henn, and C. A. Dickman, "Pars screw fixation of a hangman's fracture: technical case report," *Operative Neurosurgery*, vol. 56, article ONS-E204, Supplement 1, 2005.

[8] H. Murphy, G. D. Schroeder, W. J. Shi et al., "Management of Hangman's Fractures," *Journal of Orthopaedic Trauma*, vol. 31, pp. S90–S95, 2017.

[9] M. M. M. Eldin and A. M. A. Ali, "Lumbar transpedicular implant failure: a clinical and surgical challenge and its radiological assessment," *Asian Spine Journal*, vol. 8, no. 3, pp. 281–297, 2014.

[10] Z. S. Jager, S. Inceoglu, D. Palmer, Y. T. Akpolat, and W. K. Cheng, "Preventing instrumentation failure in three-column spinal osteotomy: biomechanical analysis of rod configuration," *Spine Deformity*, vol. 4, no. 1, pp. 3–9, 2016.

[11] K. Bagchi, A. Mohaideen, J. D. Thomson, and C. L. Foly, "Hardware complications in scoliosis surgery," *Pediatric Radiology*, vol. 32, no. 7, pp. 465–475, 2002.

[12] S. W. Kim, C. I. Ju, C. G. Kim, S. M. Lee, and H. Shin, "Efficacy of spinal implant removal after thoracolumbar junction fusion," *Journal of Korean Neurosurgical Society*, vol. 43, no. 3, pp. 139–142, 2008.

[13] M. Hume, D. A. Capen, R. W. Nelson, S. Nagelberg, and J. C. Thomas, "Outcome after Wiltse pedicle screw removal," *Journal of Spinal Disorders*, vol. 9, no. 2, pp. 121–124, 1996.

[14] E. J. Muller, M. Wick, and G. Muhr, "Traumatic spondylolisthesis of the axis: treatment rationale based on the stability of the different fracture types," *European Spine Journal*, vol. 9, no. 2, pp. 123–128, 2000.

[15] B. Au, J. Groundland, T. K. Stoops, B. G. Santoni, and H. C. Sagi, "Comparison of 3 methods for maintaining inter-fragmentary compression after fracture reduction and fixation," *Journal of Orthopaedic Trauma*, vol. 31, no. 4, pp. 210–213, 2017.

[16] L. Oberkircher, C. Bliemel, F. Flossdorf, T. Schwarting, S. Ruchholtz, and A. Krüger, "Biomechanical evaluation of 2 insertion points for ventral screw fixation of C-2 dens fractures," *Journal of Neurosurgery Spine*, vol. 18, no. 6, pp. 553–557, 2013.

# Nontraumatic Spondylolisthesis of the Axis with Cervical Kyphosis

**Shuhei Mizobuchi, Nobuaki Tadokoro, Shogo Takaya, Katsuhito Kiyasu, Ryuichi Takemasa, and Masahiko Ikeuchi**

*Department of Orthopaedic Surgery, Kochi Medical School, Kochi University, Kohasu, Oko-cho, Nankoku 783-8505, Japan*

Correspondence should be addressed to Shuhei Mizobuchi; buchika3@gmail.com

Academic Editor: Akio Sakamoto

This study aimed at presenting a rare nontraumatic spondylolisthesis of the axis and considering its possible cause. Traumatic spondylolisthesis of the axis, called hangman's fracture, frequently occurs as a high-energy trauma. However, nontraumatic spondylolisthesis of the axis is quite rare, and relevant literature on this condition is scarce. We reported a case of a 49-year-old man who had spondylolisthesis of the axis without experiencing a traumatic episode. Plain radiograph and CT image showed 7.0 mm anterolisthesis of the axis. Both C2 and C3 facet joints positioned asymmetrically, and the unilateral side oriented coronally, which was less resistant to rotational motion. These facet joint abnormalities could cause segmental instability and spondylolisthesis of the axis. Due to the resultant myelopathy, the slip with cord compression was surgically corrected by posterior decompression with instrumented fusion.

## 1. Introduction

Hangman's fracture is known as traumatic spondylolisthesis of the axis. It occurs due to a bilateral fracture of the C2 pars interarticularis. This fracture is typically a result of high-energy trauma and hyperextension [1, 2]. It accounts for 20 to 22% of all axis fractures [3]. Reports on hangman's fracture frequently appear in publications. However, there are very few reports describing spondylolisthesis of the axis without a traumatic event. In this report, we present a rare case of a 49-year-old man with nontraumatic spondylolisthesis of the axis.

## 2. Case Presentation

A 49-year-old man was referred to our clinic, complaining of bilateral numbness in the hands, a disorder affecting hand dexterity and gait disturbance. He had no history of any traumatic accidents or such, including in his childhood. He was an agricultural engineer and had neither comorbidities nor the history of notable sport activities. The neurological examination revealed bilateral-hand muscle weakness and hypesthesia. Plain radiograph showed a marked case of spondylolisthesis of the axis. The axis had slipped 7 mm anteriorly. There was no slippage reduction in the flexion and extension positions according to the radiographs (Figure 1). We observed cervical kyphosis with -20 degrees on the C2-7 angles. CT images revealed no fractures at the pars interarticularis indicating hangman's fracture (Figure 2). The C2-3 facet joints were spatially asymmetrical and coronally oriented on the left side. Furthermore, the C2 vertebra had rotated clockwise compared to the lower level (Figure 3). By contrast, C3-4 facet joints were symmetrical, and both facing C3-4 facet joints formed a bowl-shaped plane, which was resistant to rotational movement. MRI images demonstrated spinal cord compression at the C2-3 level with spinal cord edema, the following multilevel cervical spinal cord decompression, and facet joint edema at C2-3 (Figure 4).

We performed C2-5 posterior decompression with C2 partial laminectomy and C3-5 laminectomy and C6-7

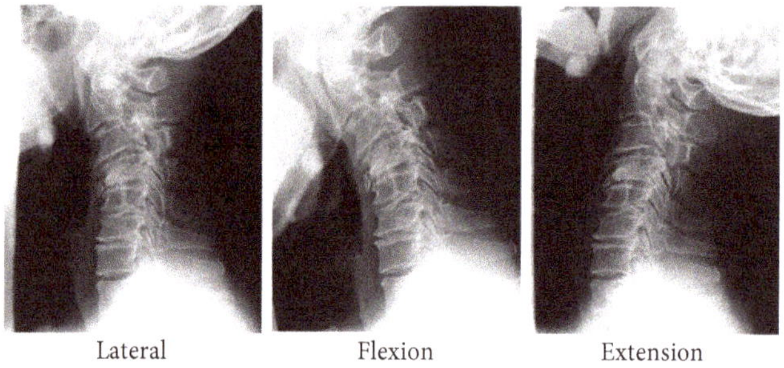


FIGURE 1: Preoperative X-ray. Axis slipped anteriorly by 7 mm. No change in slippage was observed in the flexion and extension positions.

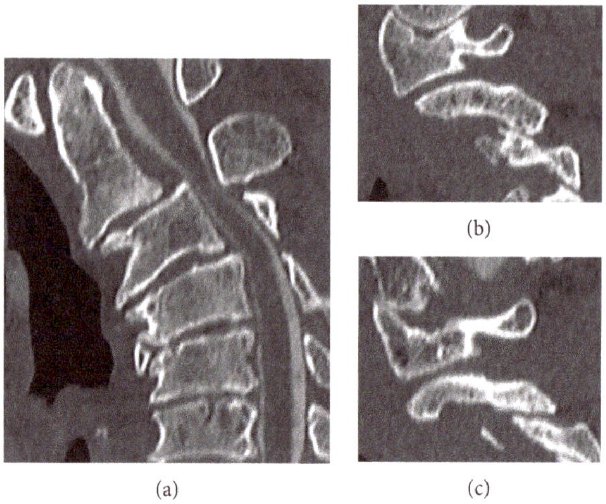


FIGURE 2: Preoperative CT myelography images. (a) Sagittal view. (b) Right view and (c) Left view of the C2-3 facet joint. CT images show that the bilateral pars interarticularis were not fractured.

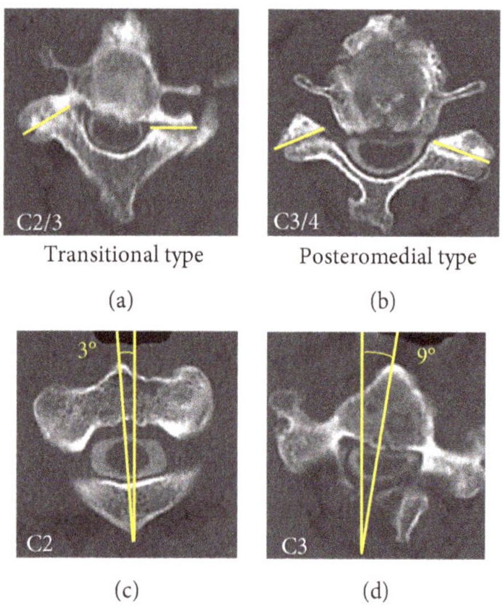


FIGURE 3: (a) The facet joint of C2/3 was transitional. (b) The facet joint of C3/4 was posteromedial, (c, d) C2 vertebra rotated to the right and to the lower vertebra.

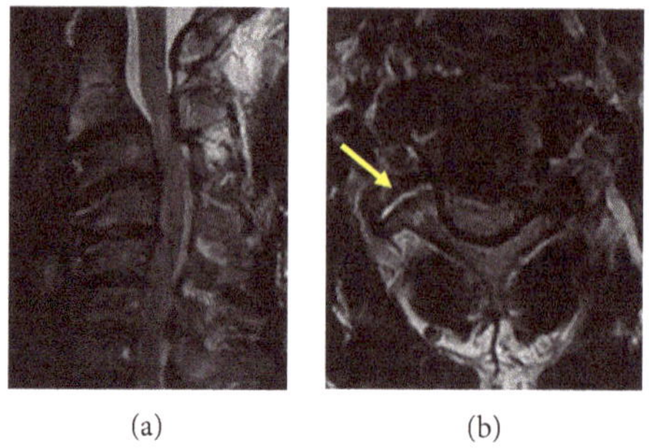


FIGURE 4: Preoperative MRI images. (a) Preoperative MRI images showed spinal cord compression at C2-3 level with spinal edema. (b) Axial MRI images of C2-3 right facet joint indicate an articular edema.

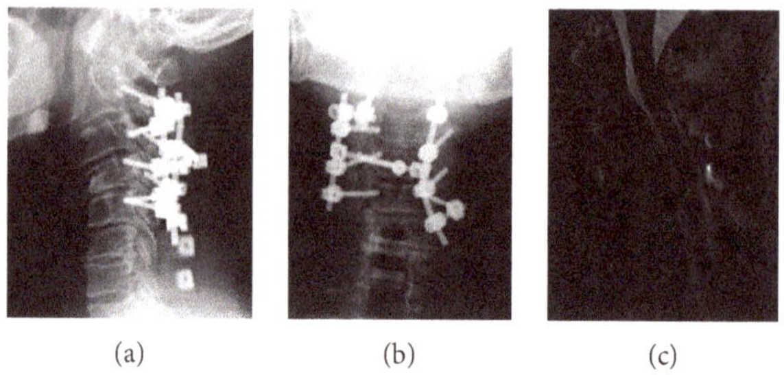


FIGURE 5: (a, b) Postoperative X-ray. X-ray shows C2-5 posterior fusion. Anterior spondylolisthesis of the axis was corrected. (c) Postoperative MRI image. MRI image shows that decompression had been performed and that the central cord deficit had been improved.

laminoplasty for progressive myelopathy. Then, we inserted the pedicle screws as possible for strong fixation except for left C3 and C4 that were inserted lateral mass screws for instrumented fusion. The anterior slip and rotational deformity of axis were fully corrected (Figure 5). Cervical kyphosis was corrected from -20 degrees to -15 degrees. Bilateral numbness in the hands and the disorder affecting hand dexterity were completely resolved. The JOA score improved from its preoperative score of 11.5 to its postoperative score of 17. Two years following surgery, the corrected alignment had been maintained without any instability. We observed no symptoms of any recurrence.

## 3. Discussion

Traumatic spondylolisthesis of the axis is a failure in the pars interarticularis of the neural arch and a separation from the C2 vertebral body [4]. On the other hand, the main cause of degenerative cervical spondylolisthesis is arthrosis of the facet joints, disc degeneration, and cervical sagittal malalignment [5]. Cervical spondylolisthesis is not a rare condition in the elderly. The most frequently involved levels were C3/4 (46%) and C4/5 (49.4%). In contrast, the cervical spondylolisthesis occurring at C2/3 was reported to less frequent (6.8%) [6]. We presented a 49-year-old patient with nontraumatic spondylolisthesis of the axis and cervical kyphosis. The presented case had the morphological asymmetry of C2-3 facet joints in addition to degenerative changes including facet joint arthrosis, disc degeneration, and kyphotic deformity. Takano et al. suggested that thinning of the facets and narrowing of the joint space may be the primary causes of degenerative cervical spondylolisthesis rather than disc involvement [7]. Furthermore, Pal and colleagues analyzed the orientation of the superior articular surfaces from C3 to T3 using axial CT slices and categorized orientation of the facet joints into posteromedial, posterolateral, and transitional types [8]. All C2-3 facet joints were reported to show posteromedially facing superior articular facets [8–10]. In this case, the C2-3 facet joint showed transitional type and posteromedial type on the left and right sides, respectively. Rong suggested posteromedially oriented facet joints could restrict the axial rotation by the contralateral facet, acting as a barricade. The posteromedially oriented facet joints at C2-3 level thus were of significant importance for the stabilization of the C2 vertebra during rotational movement, facilitating the C1-2 rotation [10]. The transitionally oriented facets restrict rotation and lateral bending only on one side, by both superior articular facets facing in the same direction. This suggests that morphological abnormalities at the C2-3 facet joint in our current case may have affected rotational stability. In addition, the C2-3 facet joint had articular edema and vertebral rotation compared to the lower level. These findings also indicate a segmental instability at the C2-3 level.

In conclusion, we have presented a rare case of nontraumatic spondylolisthesis of the axis, which is relevant to facet joint pathology. The abnormal orientation and asymmetry of the C2-3 facet joints points to segmental instability, which lead to spondylolisthesis of the axis in the absence of a traumatic event.

## References


[1] H. Murphy, G. D. Schroeder, W. J. Shi et al., "Management of Hangman's Fractures," *Journal of Orthopaedic Trauma*, vol. 31, no. 4, pp. S90–S95, 2017.

[2] J. A. Gehweiler Jr., W. M. Clark, R. E. Schaaf, B. Powers, and M. D. Miller, "Cervical spine trauma: the common combined conditions," *Radiology*, vol. 130, no. 1, pp. 77–86, 1979.

[3] R. Al-Mahfoudh, C. Beagrie, E. Woolley et al., "Management of typical and atypical hangman's fractures," *Global Spine Journal*, vol. 6, no. 3, pp. 248–256, 2016.

[4] P. Schleicher, M. Scholz, A. Pingel, and F. Kandziora, "Traumatic spondylolisthesis of the axis vertebra in adults," *Global Spine Journal*, vol. 5, no. 4, pp. 346–358, 2015.

[5] H. S. Jun, J. H. Kim, J. H. Ahn et al., "T1 slope and degenerative cervical spondylolisthesis," *Spine*, vol. 40, no. 4, pp. E220–E226, 2015.

[6] S.-D. Jiang, L.-S. Jiang, and L.-Y. Dai, "Degenerative cervical spondylolisthesis: a systematic review," *International Orthopaedics*, vol. 35, no. 6, pp. 869–875, 2011.

[7] M. Takano, S. Nishimura, H. Nagahari, and M. Kamata, "Posterior correction surgery of progressive degenerative cervical spondylolisthesis- a case report," *Journal of Spine*, vol. 5, no. 3, 2016.

[8] G. P. Pal, R. V. Routal, and S. K. Saggu, "The orientation of the articular facets of the zygapophyseal joints at the cervical and upper thoracic region," *Journal of Anatomy*, vol. 198, no. 4, pp. 431–441, 2001.

[9] R. Aoyama, T. Shiraishi, M. Kato et al., "Characteristic findings on imaging of cervical spondylolisthesis: analysis of computed tomography and X-ray photography in 101 spondylolisthesis patients," *Spine Surgery and Related Research*, vol. 2, no. 1, pp. 30–36, 2018.

[10] X. Rong, Z. Liu, B. Wang, H. Chen, and H. Liu, "The facet orientation of the subaxial cervical spine and the implications for cervical movements and clinical conditions," *Spine*, vol. 42, no. 6, pp. E320–E325, 2017.

# Spinal Subdural Abscess following Transforaminal Lumbar Interbody Fusion

**Isamu Miura,[1,2] Motoo Kubota,[1] Oji Momosaki,[1,2] Kento Takebayashi,[2] Takakazu Kawamata,[2] and Masahito Yuzurihara[1]**

[1]*Department of Spinal Surgery, Kameda Medical Center, 929 Higashi-cho, Kamogawa-shi, Chiba 296-8602, Japan*
[2]*Department of Neurosurgery, Tokyo Women's Medical University, 8-1 Kawada-cho, Shinjuku-ku, Tokyo 162-8666, Japan*

Correspondence should be addressed to Isamu Miura; isamu2345@yahoo.co.jp

Academic Editor: Bayram Unver

Spinal subdural abscesses are rare lesions. We report the case of surgical site infection complicated with meningitis and rapidly progressive spinal subdural abscess caused by *P. aeruginosa* following transforaminal lumbar interbody fusion (TLIF). A 72-year-old woman was admitted to our hospital complaining of drop foot syndrome and sciatica caused by stenosis of the L5/6 intervertebral foramen accompanied by L5 lumbar vertebral fracture. Accordingly, TLIF of L5-L6 and balloon kyphoplasty of L5 were performed. On the 3rd postoperative day (POD), she was diagnosed with surgical site infection complicated with bacterial meningitis. Subcutaneous fluid, blood, and cerebrospinal fluid cultures indicated *P. aeruginosa*. On the $7^{th}$ POD, a repeat MRI showed a large dorsal fluid collection consistent with a subdural infection and massive cauda equina compression. We performed debridement and instrument removal and found a dural laceration that was not observed during the first operation. An intraoperative insensible dural laceration may cause bacteria intrusion into the subdural space.

## 1. Introduction

Subdural abscesses are suppurative infections of the space between the dura and arachnoid. Spinal subdural abscesses are rare lesions [1]. Bacterial abscesses involving the spinal canal are associated with high morbidity and mortality [2]. The most common pathogen in spinal subdural abscesses is *Staphylococcus aureus*, and *Pseudomonas aeruginosa* is rarely detected in such lesions [3]. Herein, we report the case of surgical site infection complicated with meningitis and rapidly progressive spinal subdural abscess caused by *P. aeruginosa* following transforaminal lumbar interbody fusion (TLIF). Our findings showed that an intraoperative insensible dural laceration can cause bacteria intrusion into the subdural space.

## 2. Case Report

A 72-year-old woman with no significant medical history including diabetes started suffering from back pain and leg pain in the lower parts of her left leg at 16 weeks and 8 weeks prior to admission, respectively. She visited our hospital and was suspected to have an L5 vertebral fracture. She experienced left drop foot syndrome 1 week prior to admission and was admitted to our hospital for treatment. She had lumbago and left sciatica. Manual muscle testing of the tibialis anterior and extensor hallucis longus decreased to 1/5 each. The lumbar computed tomography showed a decreased height of L5 and L6 vertebral bodies (Figure 1(a)). Lumbar magnetic resonance images (MRI) of the L5 vertebral body showed slightly low intensity on T1-weighted images and slightly high intensity on the STIR images (Figures 1(b) and 1(c)). The left L5 nerve root was compressed within the L5/6 intervertebral foramen on the T2-weighted images (Figure 1(d)). Myelography was performed via the L2-L3 interlaminar space eight days before TLIF. The patient was considered to present left L5 radiculopathy caused by stenosis of the L5/6 intervertebral foramen accompanied by L5 lumbar vertebral fracture. Accordingly, TLIF of L5-L6 and balloon kyphoplasty of

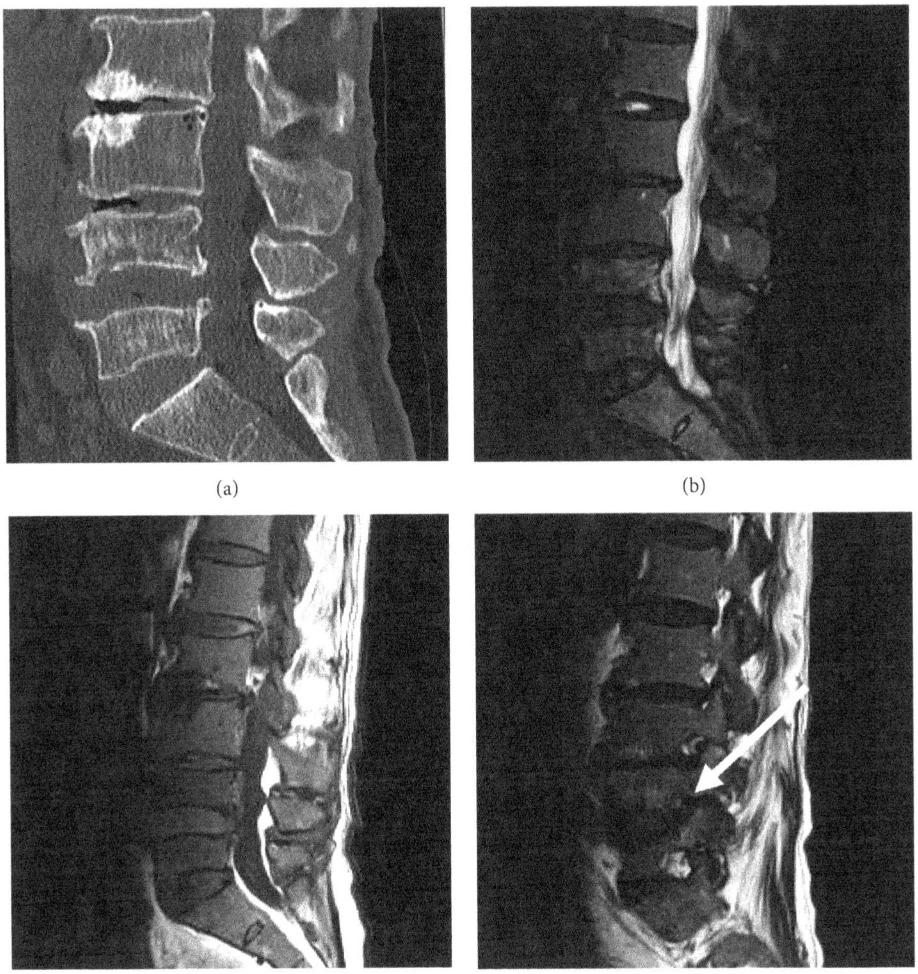

FIGURE 1: CT axial image demonstrating the decreased height of the L5 and L6 vertebral bodies (a). Sagittal magnetic resonance images showing iso- to low-intensity change in L5 vertebral body on a FLAIR (b), and low-intensity change on a T1-weighted image (c). T2 sagittal image showing compression of the left L5 nerve root at the L5/6 intervertebral foramen (d).

L5 were performed. Postoperatively, the patient had no neurological deterioration.

On the 3rd postoperative day (POD), she had a high fever of 39 degrees Celsius. She had neck stiffness and back pain with tenderness on pressure. Her white blood cell count and C-reactive protein level were over 60,000/mm$^3$ and 23 mg/dL, respectively. Her cell count in cerebrospinal fluid (CSF) was over 5600/$\mu$L (with 87% neutrophils). Lumbar MRI showed subcutaneous fluid without any findings of a subdual abscess or leakage of CSF. A gram stain of subcutaneous fluid showed gram-negative rods. Later, subcutaneous fluid cultures, CSF cultures, and blood cultures indicated *P. aeruginosa*. She was diagnosed with surgical site infection (SSI) complicated with bacterial meningitis. Cefepime and vancomycin were administrated. On the 7$^{th}$ POD, a repeat MRI showed a large dorsal fluid collection consistent with a subdural infection and massive cauda equina compression (Figures 2(a) and 2(b)). Fluid on the anterior part of the L5 vertebral body and subcutaneous fluid had increased compared to the previous MRI finding. Debridement and instrument removal were performed under general anesthesia. All rods and pedicle screws were removed, but the titanium cages were left. A dural laceration on the edge of the residual L6 lamina was found (Figure 2(c)). The arachnoid was conserved, and there was no leakage of CSF. This laceration was not recognized during the first operation. The intravenous antibiotic therapy was continued and switched to an oral antibiotic six weeks after debridement. MRI showed no findings of subdural infection (Figure 3). Although we planned additional fixation surgery, fortunately, 8 months later, the patient had no neurological deterioration following conservative treatment using a lumbar corset and administration of romosozumab to prevent new compression fractures and promote bone fusion. We need further follow-up because of the possibility of a slip or subsidence. If the slip progresses, we will consider surgical intervention using percutaneous pedicle screws with a different trajectory.

## 3. Discussion

*P. aeruginosa* is an important pathogen of SSI [4]. Hey et al. reported that the prevalence rate of *P. aeruginosa* in SSI was

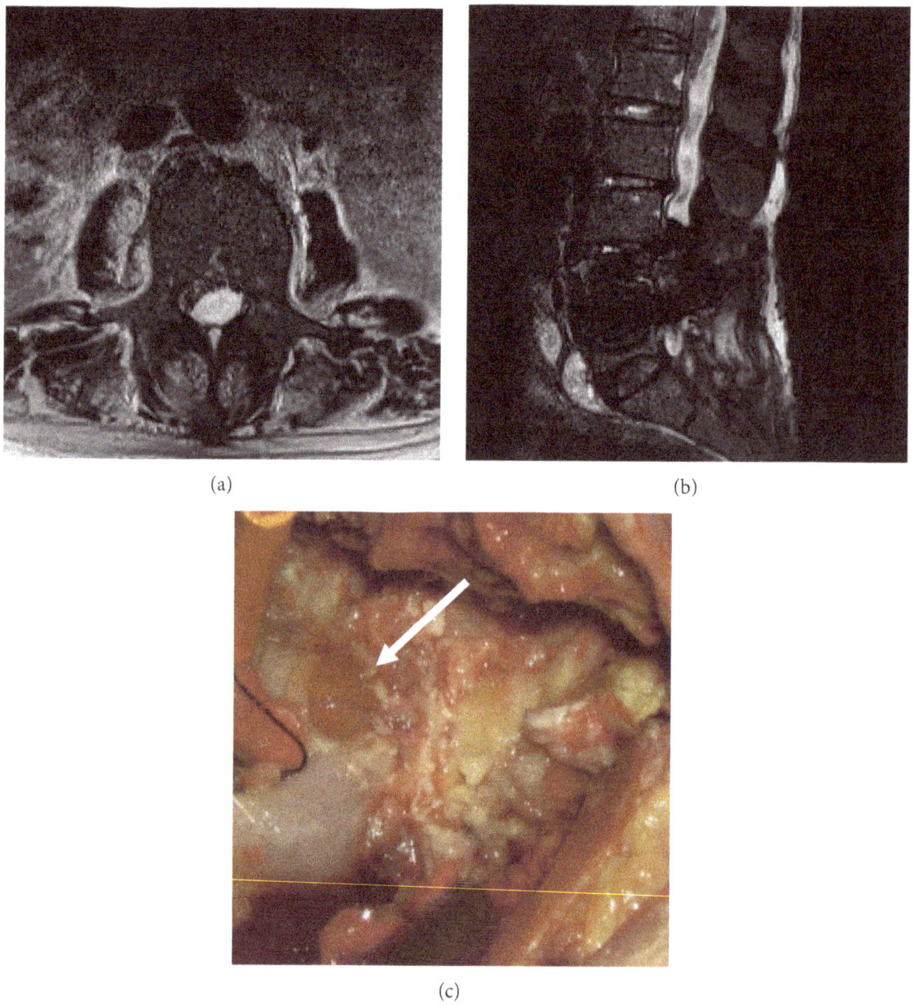

FIGURE 2: T2 axial image showing intradural high intensity mass compressing the cauda equina (a). T2 sagittal imaging showing high intensity areas of the anterior L5 vertebral, intradural space, and subcutaneous space (b). Operative view (c). Arrow showing arachnoid and laceration of dura at the edge of the residual L6 lamina.

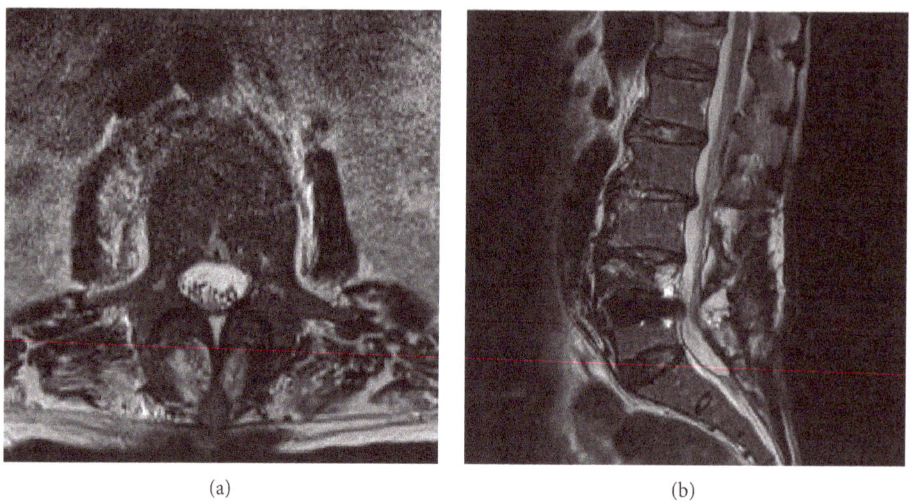

FIGURE 3: Postoperative MRI imaging after debridement. T2 axial image (a) and sagittal image (b) showing disappearance of mass compressing the cauda equina.

35%. On the other hand, most pathogens involved methicillin-susceptible *S. aureus* and methicillin-resistant *S. aureus* in spinal subdural abscess [1, 2, 5]. Velissaris et al. reviewed 65 cases of spinal subdural abscess and found only one case of spinal lumber abscess due to *P. aeruginosa* [2]. Therefore, our case is thought to be rare.

In our case, a dural laceration that was not observed during the first operation was found during wound debridement and instrument removal. Wu et al. reported a case of spinal subdural empyema after a dural tear during thoracic laminectomy [6]. They considered that the anatomical barrier of the dura was disrupted during the initial surgery via a dural tear, facilitating subdural extension of the infection. In our case, bacterial meningitis preceded the appearance of subdural abscess on the MRI. Wu et al. reported the case of spinal subdural abscess following meningitis caused by *S. aureus* [6]. In our patient, myelography was performed via the L2-L3 interlaminar space eight days before TLIF. The patient had no fever and no headache after myelography, and the puncture level was different from the operation level. Although the possibility of infection by the puncture for myelography cannot be completely excluded, it is thought that, in this instance, dural laceration during TLIF allowed bacteria to intrude into the subdural space. A spinal CSF fistula may develop into bacterial meningitis although we could not find CSF leakage. This indicates that there may be an unnoticed dural tear or laceration in cases of postoperative spinal subdural abscesses.

Subdural abscess is a serious condition, and Bartels et al. reported a mortality rate of 25% [7]. Fortunately, we could treat the patient in our case. Early diagnosis and emergent treatment are vital to prevent the formation and progression of neurologic deficits and death [2].

This case involves left L5 foraminal stenosis after an L5 compression fracture. The most widely used surgical approach for osteoporotic spinal fractures is fusion surgery including vertebroplasty and kyphoplasty [8]. For foraminal stenosis, decompression surgery is commonly used via facetectomy and elevation of the disc height by interbody fusion [9]. Sasaki et al. reported a case of vertebroplasty and posterior interbody fusion (PLIF) for radiculopathy caused by osteoporotic vertebral fractures [10]. They reported that the surgical outcome of PLIF is better than that of other surgical methods without fixation because spinal stabilization is preserved. We performed TLIF. However, the surgical site infection rate in instrumentation surgery is higher. Recently, a report has described foraminal decompression via a lateral approach using spinal endoscopy [11]. In this case, minimally invasive endoscopic surgery may be better.

*P. aeruginosa* can cause a rapidly progressive spinal subdural abscess when a dural laceration occurs during spinal surgery because bacteria can directly intrude into the subdural space.

## Consent

Informed consent was obtained from the patient for the publication of this case report and any accompanying images.

## Acknowledgments

We would like to thank Editage and EIGO EXPERTS for editing and reviewing this manuscript for English language.

## References

[1] A. D. Ramos, J. D. Rolston, G. E. Gauger, and P. S. Larson, "Spinal subdural abscess following laminectomy for symptomatic stenosis: a report of 2 cases and review of the literature," *American Journal of Case Reports*, vol. 17, no. 17, pp. 476–483, 2016.

[2] D. Velissaris, D. Aretha, F. Fligou, and K. S. Filos, "Spinal subdural Staphylococcus aureus abscess: case report and review of the literature," *World Journal of Emergency Surgery*, vol. 4, no. 1, p. 31, 2009.

[3] J. V. Coumans and B. P. Walcott, "Rapidly progressive lumbar subdural empyema following acromial bursal injection," *Journal of Clinical Neuroscience*, vol. 18, no. 11, pp. 1562-1563, 2011.

[4] H. W. Hey, D. W. Thiam, Z. S. Koh et al., "Is intraoperative local vancomycin powder the answer to surgical site infections in spine surgery?," *Spine*, vol. 42, no. 4, pp. 267–274, 2017.

[5] M. J. Kraeutler, J. D. Bozzay, M. P. Walker, and K. John, "Spinal subdural abscess following epidural steroid injection," *Journal of Neurosurgery Spine*, vol. 22, no. 1, pp. 90–93, 2015.

[6] A. S. Wu, R. W. Griebel, K. Meguro, and D. R. Fourney, "Spinal subdural empyema after a dural tear. Case report," *Neurosurgical Focus*, vol. 17, no. 6, article E10, 2004.

[7] R. H. Bartels, T. R. de Jong, and J. A. Grotenhuis, "Spinal subdural abscess. Case report," *Journal of Neurosurgery*, vol. 76, no. 2, pp. 307 311, 1992.

[8] M. Shen and Y. Kim, "Osteoporotic vertebral compression fractures: a review of current surgical management techniques," *American Journal of Orthopedics*, vol. 36, no. 5, pp. 241–248, 2007.

[9] S. Fujibayashi, M. Neo, M. Takemoto, M. Ota, and T. Nakamura, "Paraspinal-approach transforaminal lumbar interbody fusion for the treatment of lumbar foraminal stenosis," *Journal of Neurosurgery Spine*, vol. 13, no. 4, pp. 500–508, 2010.

[10] M. Sasaki, M. Aoki, K. Nishioka, and T. Yoshimine, "Radiculopathy caused by osteoporotic vertebral fractures in the lumbar spine," *Neurologia Medico-Chirurgica*, vol. 51, no. 7, pp. 484–489, 2011.

[11] Y. Ishimoto, H. Yamada, E. Curtis et al., "Spinal endoscopy for delayed-onset lumbar radiculopathy resulting from foraminal stenosis after osteoporotic vertebral fracture: a case report of a new surgical strategy," *Case Reports in Orthopedics*, vol. 2018, Article ID 1593021, 4 pages, 2018.

# 44

# Extensor Tendon Dislocation at the Metacarpophalangeal Joint of Both Ring Fingers Caused by a Specific Hand Posture in a Shiatsu Therapist

**Mariko Kamiya, Gen Sasaki, Kensuke Ikuta, Hideaki Miyamoto, Michio Kimura, and Hirotaka Kawano**

*Department of Orthopaedic Surgery, Teikyo University School of Medicine, 2-11-1 Kaga, Itabashi-ku, Tokyo 173-8606, Japan*

Correspondence should be addressed to Hideaki Miyamoto; miyamotoh@med.teikyo-u.ac.jp

Academic Editor: John Nyland

A 43-year-old female shiatsu therapist complained of sudden snapping of the metacarpophalangeal joints (MCPjs) of both ring fingers during a specific hand posture. The extensor tendon of the ring finger was dislocated ulnarly when the MCPj of the ring finger was flexed and deviated ulnarly and the MCPj of the middle finger was extended. Surgical exploration revealed an attenuated radial sagittal band. We plicated the juncturae tendinum of the extensor digitorum communis between the middle and ring fingers and released the ulnar sagittal band partially to centralise the extensor tendon excursion. Twenty-six months postoperatively, the patient regained full active and passive range of motion of all fingers without extensor tendon dislocation or snapping in either hand during work.

## 1. Introduction

Extensor tendon dislocation at the metacarpophalangeal joint (MCPj) of the hand has four etiologies: congenital origin, degenerative, traumatic, or spontaneous sagittal band rupture [1–3]. Degenerative dislocation of the middle finger extensor tendon, which is the most frequent etiology, usually occurs in patients with rheumatoid arthritis [3]. We report a rare case of spontaneous dislocation of the extensor tendons of both ring fingers caused by a specific hand posture in a shiatsu therapist.

## 2. Case Presentation

A 43-year-old female shiatsu therapist with 20 years of experience complained of sudden snapping of the MCPj of the left ring finger (her nondominant hand) and pain in the dorsum of the MCPj. The patient did not have any conditions that would predispose her to sagittal band laxity including prior trauma to the hand. Two weeks later, the snapping and pain occurred in the right ring finger. On physical examination, the extensor tendons at the dorsum of the MCPjs of both ring fingers dislocated with a specific hand posture (Figure 1). On actively extending the MCPjs of the ring fingers, the extensor tendons reduced with snapping. However, the ring finger extensor tendon did not dislocate if both the middle and ring finger MCPjs were flexed together. Radiography revealed no MCPj deformity. The patient did not comply with nonoperative treatment such as MCPj extension bracing because she could not continue work with bracing.

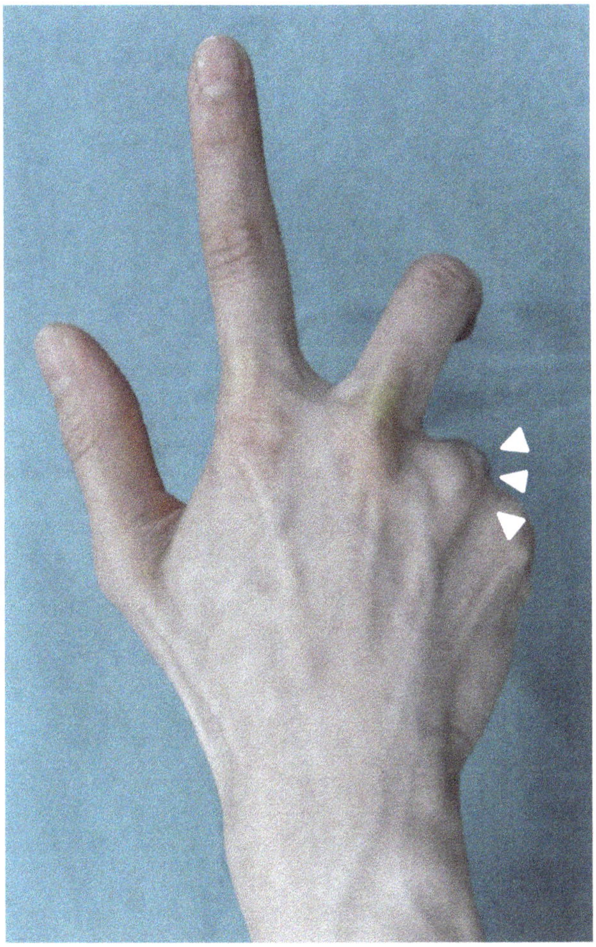

FIGURE 1: (a) Shiatsu-specific hand posture. (b) When the metacarpophalangeal joint (MCPj) of the ring finger is flexed and deviated ulnarly with concurrent extension of the MCPj of the middle finger, the extensor tendon of the ring finger dislocates ulnarly (white arrowheads).

Four weeks after the first visit, we performed reconstruction of the extensor tendons of the both ring fingers with wrist blocks. Surgical exploration through a longitudinal curved skin incision at the dorsum of the MCPj of the ring finger revealed a markedly attenuated radial sagittal band and ulnarly dislocated extensor tendons bilaterally (Figure 2). We plicated the juncturae tendinum of the extensor digitorum communis between the middle and ring fingers and released the ulnar sagittal band partially to centralise the extensor tendon excursion without dislocation, through the full range of motion of the MCPj intraoperatively. We also tested the range of motion of the active finger.

Postoperatively, we applied a bulky hand dressing with a forearm-based volar plaster splint to the MCPj in the extended position in order to prevent inadvertent passive flexion of the MCPj. Active flexion and extension exercises were performed from 1 to 6 weeks postoperatively. Six weeks postoperatively, we removed the splint and allowed all MCPj movements. Six months postoperatively, the patient resumed work as a shiatsu therapist without extensor tendon dislocation and snapping at the MCPjs. All finger movements were performed with no limitations in either hand. Twenty-six months postoperatively, the patient remained pain-free during work without extensor tendon dislocation or snapping in either hand.

## 3. Discussion

Dislocation of the extensor tendon usually presents with symptoms of pain and snapping at the MCPj during MCPj flexion. In our case, however, the extensor tendon was dislocated only when the MCPj of the middle finger was extended and the MCPj of the ring finger was flexed with ulnar deviation. In acute injuries, conservative treatment may provide satisfactory results [4]. When nonsurgical treatment fails to correct the subluxation, surgical treatment may be required. Reconstructive techniques include methods using an extensor digitorum communis tendon slip, juncturae tendinum, lumbrical tendon, and palmaris longus with a suture anchor [5]. Because chronic or spontaneous cases are associated with degenerative insufficiency of the injured sagittal band, various reconstructive techniques have been described using a variety of graft sources and attachment sites [6, 7]. Reconstructive techniques using grafts are associated with a number of potential problems such as donor site morbidity and dysfunction at the MCP joint because of ineffective graft pathways or attachment sites. In chronic cases, a concern might be raised that the ruptured sagittal band will be atrophied and difficult to use. On the other hand, some authors report satisfactory results with only reefing and imbrication of the extensor hood in these chronic cases [8, 9]. Although prior reconstructive techniques have reported satisfactory results, this technique is simpler than those reconstructive techniques and may offer the additional advantage of not substantially altering adjacent anatomy.

The sagittal band is the primary stabilizer of the extensor tendon at MCPj, keeping the tendon in position during flexion and extension. Failure of the sagittal band to centralise the tendon, which may be the result of trauma, laxity, or congenital absence, causes dislocation of the extensor tendon [10]. Usually, the dislocation occurs on the ulnar side of the middle finger because the radial component of the sagittal band is more prone to injury than the ulnar component. In addition, the metacarpal head of the middle finger is more prominent, and the attachment of its extensor tendon to the transverse fibers, compared to those of the three other fingers, is loosen [11, 12].

Contrary to most reports, our case indicated that excessive traction stress by repetitive use of a specific posture may contribute to rupture of the radial component of the sagittal band of the ring finger (Figure 3). This rare case of spontaneous tendon dislocation at the MCPj of the ring finger highlights that shiatsu-specific hand posture is a possible cause of sagittal band tear, in which the MCPj of the middle finger is extended and the MCPj of the ring finger is flexed.

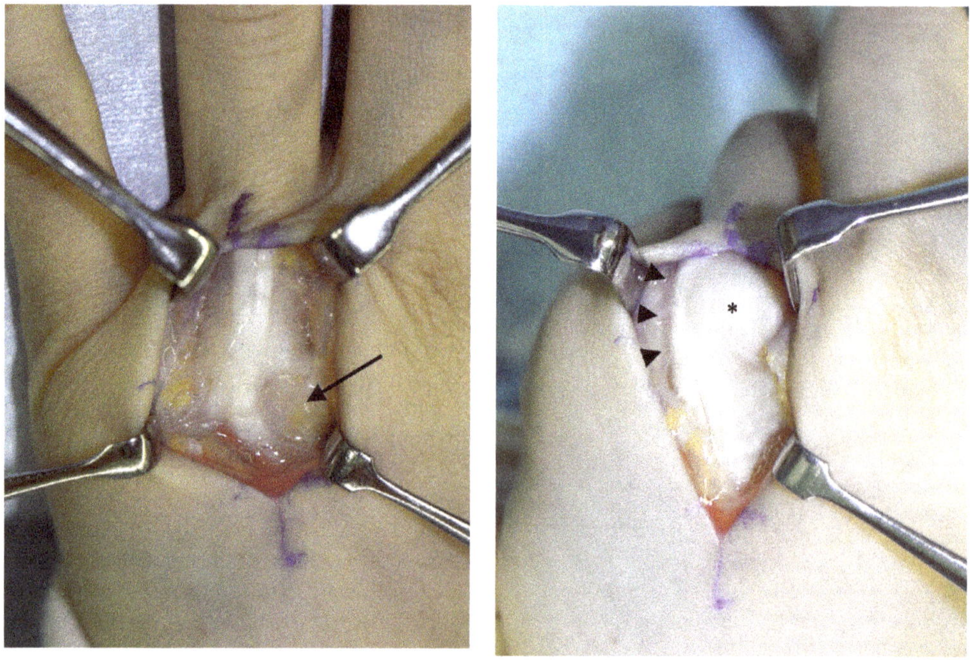

(a) (b)

Figure 2: Surgical image for the extensor tendon of the ring finger of the left hand. (a) Attenuated radial sagittal band (black arrow). (b) The metacarpal head of the ring finger pops through the attenuated sagittal band (asterisk) with the extensor tendon dislocated ulnarly (black arrowheads) in the shiatsu-specific hand posture.

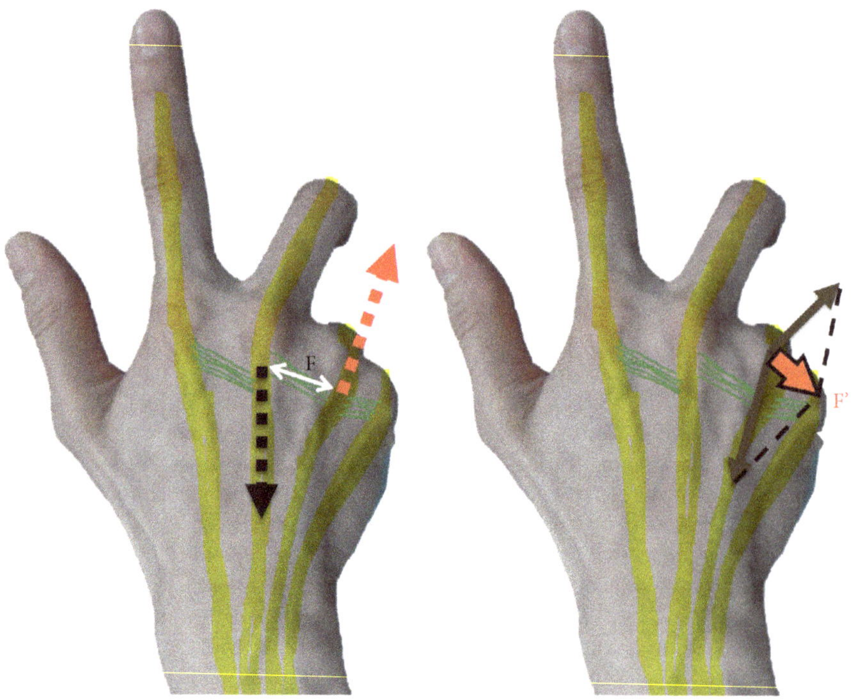


(a) (b)

Figure 3: Schematic images of an ulnarward translation force to the extensor tendon of the ring finger. (a) Force to the sagittal band between the middle and ring fingers. In the middle finger, when the metacarpophalangeal joint (MCPj) was extended, the extensor tendon was retracted proximally (black arrow). However, in the ring finger, when the MCPj was flexed, the extensor tendon was retracted distally (red arrow). The traction force to the sagittal band and the juncturae tendinum between the middle and ring fingers (F) may become larger and result in sagittal band and juncturae tendinum attenuation. (b) Force-vector combination to the extensor tendon at the MCPj of the ring finger resulting from MCPj flexion and ulnar deviation may develop an ulnarward translation force ($F'$).

## Consent

Written informed consent was obtained from the patient for the publication of this paper and any accompanying images.

## References

[1] N. Kang and P. Smith, "Congenital absence of the juncturae tendini contributing to dislocation of the extensor tendons," *The Journal of Hand Surgery*, vol. 26, no. 3, pp. 501–505, 2001.

[2] M. Ishizuki, "Traumatic and spontaneous dislocation of extensor tendon of the long finger," *The Journal of Hand Surgery*, vol. 15, no. 6, pp. 967–972, 1990.

[3] G. Inoue and Y. Tamura, "Dislocation of the extensor tendons over the metacarpophalangeal joints," *The Journal of Hand Surgery*, vol. 21, no. 3, pp. 464–469, 1996.

[4] L. W. Catalano III, S. Gupta, R. Ragland III, S. Z. Glickel, C. Johnson, and O. A. Barron, "Closed treatment of nonrheumatoid extensor tendon dislocations at the metacarpophalangeal joint," *The Journal of Hand Surgery*, vol. 31, no. 2, pp. 242–245, 2006.

[5] J. H. Lee, J. H. Baek, and J. S. Lee, "A reconstructive stabilization technique for nontraumatic or chronic traumatic extensor tendon subluxation," *The Journal of Hand Surgery*, vol. 42, no. 1, pp. e61–e65, 2017.

[6] R. E. Bunata, "Sagittal band reconstruction," *Journal of Hand Surgery*, vol. 24, no. 1, p. 198, 1999.

[7] H. K. Watson, J. Weinzweig, and P. M. Guidera, "Sagittal band reconstruction," *The Journal of Hand Surgery*, vol. 22, no. 3, pp. 452–456, 1997.

[8] M. A. Posner and M. S. McMahon, "Congenital radial subluxation of the extensor tendons over the metacarpophalangeal joints: a case report," *The Journal of Hand Surgery*, vol. 19, no. 4, pp. 659–662, 1994.

[9] M. J. Saldana and R. A. McGuire, "Chronic painful subluxation of the metacarpal halangeal joint extensor tendons," *The Journal of Hand Surgery*, vol. 11, no. 3, pp. 420–423, 1986.

[10] C. M. Young and G. M. Rayan, "The sagittal band: anatomic and biomechanical study," *The Journal of Hand Surgery*, vol. 25, no. 6, pp. 1107–1113, 2000.

[11] D. B. Kettelkamp, A. E. Flatt, and R. Moulds, "Traumatic dislocation of the long-finger extensor tendon," *The Journal of Bone and Joint Surgery. American Volume*, vol. 53, no. 2, pp. 229–240, 1971.

[12] G. M. Rayan, D. Murray, K. W. Chung, and M. Rohrer, "The extensor retinacular system at the metacarpophalangeal joint. Anatomical and histological study," *Journal of Hand Surgery*, vol. 22, no. 5, pp. 585–590, 2016.

# 45

# Nonunion of a Stress Fracture at the Base of the Second Metatarsal in a Soccer Player Treated by Osteosynthesis with the Bridging Plate Fixation Technique

**Futoshi Morio, Shota Morimoto, Shintaro Onishi, Toshiya Tachibana, and Tomoya Iseki**

*Department of Orthopedic Surgery, Hyogo College of Medicine, 663-8501, 1-1 Mukogawa-cho, Nishinomiya City, Hyogo, Japan*

Correspondence should be addressed to Tomoya Iseki; tomoya.i.0119@gmail.com

Academic Editor: Werner Kolb

*Background.* A stress fracture of the second metatarsal base in soccer players is extremely rare. In this case study, we report a nonunion of a stress fracture at the base of the second metatarsal in a female soccer player who had persistent pain despite continued conservative treatment, who then was treated with the bridging plate fixation technique. *Case Report.* A 19-year-old female college soccer player complained of pain on the dorsum of her right midfoot during a game without history of trauma and was conservatively treated for 6 months. Radiographic examination showed an oblique fracture with small bone fragment at the proximal base of the second metatarsal and computed tomography demonstrated sclerotic change around the fracture site. We diagnosed her with nonunion of a stress fracture at the base of the second metatarsal and performed operative treatments using autogenous cancellous iliac bone grafting and plate fixation bridging a second metatarsal and medial cuneiform with a locking plate. At 4 months after the initial surgery, she was able to return to playing soccer at preinjury level without complications or pain. *Conclusion.* We report a rare case of nonunion of a stress fracture at the base of the second metatarsal in a female soccer player without underlying diseases. Surgical treatment was applied, because the conservative treatment was ineffective for 6 months and led to nonunion. The plate fixation technique bridging the second metatarsal and medial cuneiform was a useful option to attain the bone fusion for small fracture fragment for a treatment of nonunion of a stress fracture at the base of the second metatarsal.

## 1. Introduction

Stress fractures occur in around 20% of elite level athletes [1–5], most commonly in the lower limb [6]. Metatarsal stress fractures account for 38% of all stress fractures of the lower limb, and especially, the second and third metatarsal are the most common [7], accounting for 80-90% of all metatarsal fractures [4]. In terms of stress fracture sites, the second metatarsal, the shaft and neck are the most common locations [8]. In regard to the type of sports, stress fractures of the second metatarsal most commonly occur in classical ballet dancers [9].

As for treatment for stress fractures at the base of the second metatarsal base, conservative treatment such as immobilization, restricted weight bearing, and physical therapy is generally recommended as initial treatment [10], and good results have been reported [11–14]. In cases of persistent pain and delayed or nonunion despite these treatments, an operative treatment such as plate fixation with bone grafting is considered as a treatment option [9, 15, 16]. However, it is still unclear which surgical treatment is the optimal choice.

We report a rare case of nonunion of a stress fracture at the base of the second metatarsal in a female soccer player who had persistent pain despite continued conservative treatment, who then was treated with the bridging plate fixation technique. She was able to return to playing soccer at preinjury level at 4 months after surgery, and no recurring symptoms nor refracture were present at the 2 years follow-up. Written informed consent was obtained from the patient for publishing this report. For author contribution, SM, FM, and SO performed surgery. They were involved in data acquisition and followed patients in clinics. TI and TT helped to draft the manuscript and participated in the design of the study. All authors read and approved the final manuscript.

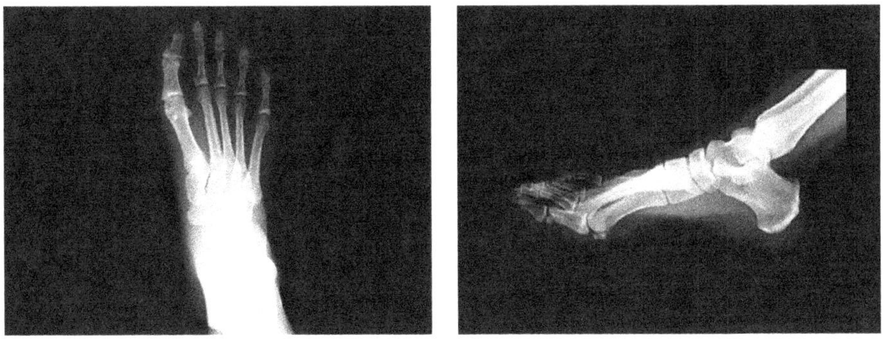

(a) (b)

FIGURE 1: Preoperative foot radiograph at an initial visit to our institution. An oblique fracture line at the base of the second metatarsal was identified on (a) anteroposterior and (b) lateral views.

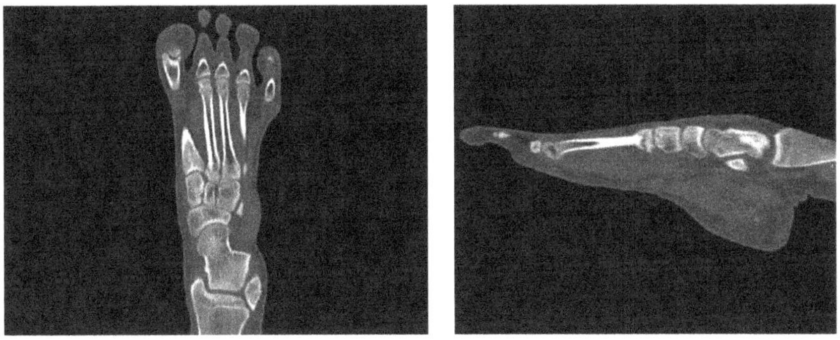

(a) (b)

FIGURE 2: Preoperative CT demonstrated a fracture line at the base of the second metatarsal and sclerotic change around the fracture site on (a) coronal and (b) sagittal views.

## 2. The Case

A 19-year-old female college soccer player complained of pain on the dorsum of her right midfoot during a game without history of trauma. Her height, weight, and body mass index were 158 cm, 58 kg, and 23.2 kg/m$^2$, respectively. She did not have any medical history or menstrual abnormalities. Furthermore, she trained 5 times a week for 3 hours each and played as a defender in games once a week. After her midfoot pain developed, she visited a local clinic and was diagnosed with stress fracture at the base of the second metatarsal. Although she was treated with conservative treatment including rest, restricted weight bearing, and physical therapy for 6 months, her midfoot pain remained, and radiological findings demonstrated no evidence of bone union at the fracture site, which led her to visiting our institution. At the first visit to our institution, she could not play soccer due to her midfoot pain, and physical examination revealed tenderness at the base of the second metatarsal. The American Orthopedic Foot and Ankle Society Midfoot Scale (AOFAS) score (100 points) was 70 points at that time. Radiographic examination showed an oblique fracture line at the base of the second metatarsal (Figure 1). Magnetic resonance imaging (MRI) showed a linear hypointense fracture line on T1-weighted and T2-weighted images and a bone marrow edema around the fracture site on STIR. Computed tomography (CT) demonstrated sclerotic change around the fracture site (Figure 2). In addition, laboratory examination revealed no abnormal findings such as iron deficiency anemia and vitamin D deficiency. According to clinical history, physical examination, and radiological findings, we diagnosed her with nonunion of a stress fracture at the base of the second metatarsal. Owing to the fact that the conservative treatment was ineffective for 6 months, we recommended operative treatment.

## 3. Surgical Technique

The operation was performed under general anesthesia in the supine position. An air tourniquet and a fluoroscopy were used for the operation. An approximately 4 cm straight incision was placed at the dorsal side of the tarsometatarsal joint. After confirming the nonunion lesion at the second metatarsal, the bone lesion was removed. An autogenous cancellous bone was harvested from the ipsilateral iliac bone using a minimally invasive technique with the Autograft OATS System (Arthrex, NJ, USA), then inserted into the union site, and subsequently fixed using the bridging plate fixation technique with a locking plate (T-fusion Plate, DePuySynthes, NJ, USA), which was placed between the distal fragment of the second metatarsal and the medial cuneiform (Figure 3). The wound was sutured, and the operation was concluded.

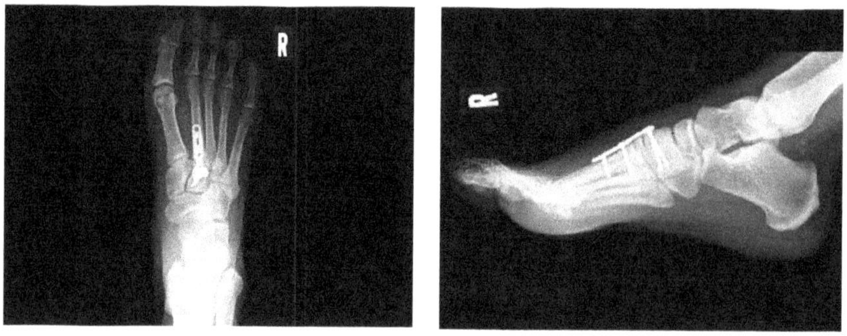


(a) (b)

Figure 3: Postoperative (a) anteroposterior and (b) lateral foot radiographs. The nonunion site was fixed using the bridging plate fixation technique with a locking plate, which was placed between the distal fragment of the second metatarsal and the medial cuneiform.

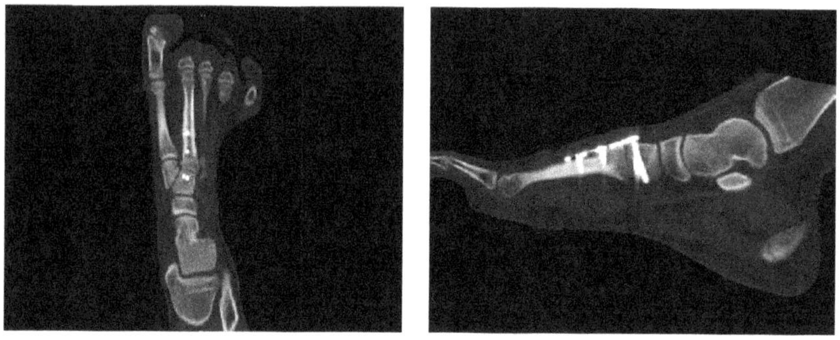

(a) (b)

Figure 4: At 12 weeks after the operation, CT demonstrated complete bone union at the fracture site on (a) coronal and (b) sagittal views.

Postoperatively, a nonweightbearing short leg splint was applied for 2 weeks, and when the splint was removed, active range of motion exercises of the ankle was initiated. Partial weightbearing was allowed at 4 weeks postoperatively and full weightbearing at 8 weeks postoperatively. At 4 months after the initial surgery, she was able to return to playing soccer at preinjury level without pain. She had no recurring symptoms and no refracture at 2 years postoperatively. AOFAS score improved to 100 points, and the patient was completely satisfied with the result. The locking plate was removed after confirming complete bone union on CT at 12 weeks after the operation (Figure 4).

## 4. Discussion

In this report, we have described a rare case of nonunion of a stress fracture at the base of the second metatarsal in a female soccer player who had persistent pain despite continued conservative treatment, then received operation. This athlete was able to return to playing soccer at preinjury level at 4 months after the operation using the bridging plate fixation technique, and no recurring symptoms nor refracture were present at the 2 years follow-up.

Stress fractures of the second metatarsal are common injuries due to overuse in athletes, and most of them occur at the shaft and the neck of the second metatarsal [8]. On the other hand, stress fractures at the base of the second metatarsal are relatively rare and account for less than 5% of all second metatarsal stress fractures [17]. It has been reported that most of the stress fractures at the second metatarsal base occur in classical ballet dancers. Previous reports demonstrated that anatomical factors and characteristics of classical ballet are involved in this fact. Anatomically, the second metatarsal base is surrounded by the first, second, and third cuneiform, constituting the mortise joint [17]. In addition, the extreme plantar flexion of the foot and ankle in the "en pointe" position is repeated in classical ballet dance. Due to the anatomical features and the characteristics of the competition, the base of the second metatarsal in classical ballet dancers easily undergoes repetitive stress. On the other hand, stress fractures of the second metatarsal base are extremely rare in nondancers. To our knowledge, there is only one report of stress fractures in nondancers, which involved 9 cases, all with underlying diseases with risk of stress fractures such as chronic steroid usage, calcium and phosphate metabolic disease, and female athlete triple triad [9]. However, there are no reports of stress fractures at the base of the second metatarsal in nondancers without underlying diseases.

In addition, several reports showed that cases with patients who have a short first metatarsal compared to the second metatarsal increases the risk of a second metatarsal stress fracture [11, 18]. These reports showed that the average length of the first metatarsal in patients with second proximal metatarsal stress fractures was approximately 80 to 82% of the second metatarsal [8, 11, 18].

There are several reports on treatments for stress fractures at the base of the second metatarsal. The optimal treatment is still under debate; however, conservative treatment including immobilization, restricted weight-bearing, and physical therapy is generally recommended as the initial treatment. Although a success rate of 75 to 100% have been reported for conservative treatment in previous literatures [11–14], treatment failures such as delayed union and nonunion can potentially occur [15]. Surgical treatment is generally indicated for these treatment failures [19]. There are only three previous reports on surgical treatment for nonunion of stress fractures at the base of the second metatarsal [9, 15, 16]. Plate fixation with bone grafting is one of the most common surgical methods with good results. Muscolo et al. [15] performed osteosynthesis between the proximal and distal fragment using a locking plate for a male ballet dancer who progressively returned to full-time dancing without symptoms at 3 months after surgery. Chuckpaiwong et al. [9] also performed plate fixation with allogeneic bone grafting for a female nondancer with diabetes and hypophosphatasia, and good union was obtained. In general, surgical outcomes with plate fixation generally achieve good results; however, in handling with small proximal fragment of second metatarsal, it might be difficult to fix both the distal and proximal fragments using a plate. To attain the bone fusion for small fracture fragment, the effectiveness of the bridging plate fixation technique has been reported [20, 21]. To our knowledge, there are no reports on surgical treatment using the bridging plate fixation technique for nonunion of stress fractures at the base of the second metatarsal.

The patient in this report was a soccer player in the defender position which indicated that she had a higher frequency of jumping than other players. For this reason, the base of the second metatarsal might have undertaken repetitive stress. In addition, the length of the first metatarsal was 79% of that of the second metatarsal, which is comparatively shorter than usual. Therefore, the morphologic abnormality of the first metatarsal was raised as a risk factor.

Operative treatment using the bridging plate fixation technique was performed since the proximal fragment was small. We suggest this technique to fix the nonunion site more easily in cases that the proximal fragment is small due to stress fractures at the base of the second metatarsal.

## 5. Conclusion

We reported a case of nonunion of a stress fracture at the base of the second metatarsal in a female soccer player without underlying diseases. In this case, we speculated that the stress fracture was caused by a playing style that involves a high frequency of jumping and a morphologic abnormality of a short first metatarsal. Furthermore, surgical treatment was indicated in this case, because the conservative treatment was ineffective for 6 months and led to nonunion. Osteosynthesis with the bridging plate fixation technique was a useful option for nonunion of a stress fracture at the base of the second metatarsal.

## Consent

Written informed consent was obtained from the patient for publication of this case report and any accompanying images. A copy of the written consent is available for review by the Editor-in-Chief of the Journal.

## Authors' Contributions

FM and SM contributed to the conception and design of the manuscript. All authors contributed to the data interpretation and preparation of the manuscript. The final version of the manuscript was approved by all authors.

## Acknowledgments

The authors thank Rebecca Imaizumi for their assistance in editing the English manuscript.

## References

[1] S. B. Behrens, M. E. Deren, A. Matson, P. D. Fadale, and K. O. Monchik, "Stress fractures of the pelvis and legs in athletes: a review," *Sports Health.*, vol. 5, no. 2, pp. 165–174, 2013.

[2] G. O. Matheson, D. B. Clement, D. C. McKenzie, J. E. Taunton, D. R. Lloyd-Smith, and J. G. MacIntyre, "Stress fractures in athletes. A study of 320 cases," *The American Journal of Sports Medicine*, vol. 15, pp. 46–58, 2016.

[3] A. Hulkko and S. Orava, "Stress fractures in athletes," *International Journal of Sports Medicine*, vol. 8, no. 3, pp. 221–226, 1987.

[4] J. Iwamoto and T. Takeda, "Stress fractures in athletes: review of 196 cases," *Journal of Orthopaedic Science*, vol. 8, no. 3, pp. 273–278, 2003.

[5] J. Iwamoto, Y. Sato, T. Takeda, and H. Matsumoto, "Analysis of stress fractures in athletes based on our clinical experience," *World Journal of Orthopedics*, vol. 2, no. 1, pp. 7–12, 2011.

[6] M. J. Welck, T. Hayes, P. Pastides, W. Khan, and B. Rudge, "Stress fractures of the foot and ankle," *Injury*, vol. 48, no. 8, pp. 1722–1726, 2017.

[7] E. Wilson and F. Katz, "Stress fractures an analysis of 250 consecutive cases," *Radiology*, vol. 92, no. 3, pp. 481–486, 1969.

[8] B. Chuckpaiwong, C. Cook, R. Pietrobon, and J. A. Nunley, "Second metatarsal stress fracture in sport: comparative risk factors between proximal and non-proximal locations," *British Journal of Sports Medicine*, vol. 41, no. 8, pp. 510–514, 2007.

[9] B. Chuckpaiwong, C. Cook, and J. A. Nunley, "Stress fractures of the second metatarsal base occur in nondancers," *Clinical*

*Orthopaedics and Related Research*, vol. 461, pp. 197–202, 2007.

[10] W. G. Raasch and D. J. Hergan, "Treatment of stress fractures: the fundamentals," *Clinics in Sports Medicine*, vol. 25, no. 1, pp. 29–36, 2006.

[11] M. J. O'Malley, W. G. Hamilton, J. Munyak, and M. J. DeFranco, "Stress fractures at the base of the second metatarsal in ballet dancers," *Foot & Ankle International*, vol. 17, no. 2, pp. 89–94, 1996.

[12] T. Harrington, K. J. Crichton, and I. F. Anderson, "Overuse ballet injury of the base of the second metatarsal: A diagnostic problem," *The American Journal of Sports Medicine*, vol. 21, no. 4, pp. 591–598, 1993.

[13] L. J. Micheli, R. S. Sohn, and R. Solomon, "Stress fractures of the second metatarsal involving Lisfranc's joint in ballet dancers. A new overuse injury of the foot," *The Journal of Bone and Joint Surgery. American Volume*, vol. 67, no. 9, pp. 1372–1375, 1985.

[14] M. Santi, D. Sartoris, and D. Resnick, "Diagnostic imaging of tarsal and metatarsal stress fractures. Part II," *Orthopedic Reviews*, vol. 18, no. 3, pp. 305–310, 1989.

[15] L. Muscolo, A. Migues, G. Slullitel, and M. Costa-Paz, "Stress fracture nonunion at the base of the second metatarsal in a ballet Dancer," *The American Journal of Sports Medicine*, vol. 32, no. 6, pp. 1535–1537, 2017.

[16] J. Sarimo, S. Orava, and J. Alanen, "Operative treatment of stress fractures of the proximal second metatarsal," *Scandinavian Journal of Medicine & Science in Sports*, vol. 17, no. 4, pp. 383–386, 2007.

[17] W. G. Hamilton and L. H. Hamilton, "Foot and ankle injuries in dancers," *Surgery of the Foot and Ankle, 7th edition*, M. J. Coughlin and R. A. Mann, Eds., pp. 1225–1256, St Louis: Mosby, 1999.

[18] D. J. Ogilvie-Harris, M. M. Carr, and P. J. Fleming, "The foot in ballet dancers: the importance of second toe length," *Foot & Ankle International*, vol. 16, no. 3, pp. 144–147, 2016.

[19] G. R. Matcuk, S. R. Mahanty, M. R. Skalski, D. B. Patel, E. A. White, and C. J. Gottsegen, "Stress fractures: pathophysiology, clinical presentation, imaging features, and treatment options," *Emergency Radiology*, vol. 23, no. 4, pp. 365–375, 2016.

[20] M. Charles, "Court brown fractures of the tibia and fibula," in *Rockwood & Wilkins Fractures in Adults*, W. B. Robert and C. B. Charles, Eds., Lippincott Williams & Wilkins, Philadelphia, 2006.

[21] C. Collinge, R. Sanders, and T. DiPasquale, "Treatment of complex tibial periarticular fractures using percutaneous techniques," *Clinical Orthopaedics and Related Research*, vol. 375, no. 1, pp. 69–77, 2000.

# Volar Dislocation of the Fourth and Fifth Carpometacarpal Joint Associated with Hamate Hook Fracture: A Case Report and Literature Review

**Natsumi Saka**,[1,2] **Hirotada Matsui**,[1] **and Hideki Tsuji**[1]

[1]*Orthopaedic Trauma Center, Sapporo Tokushukai Hospital, Sapporo, Hokkaido, Japan*
[2]*Department of Orthopaedics, Teikyo University School of Medicine, Tokyo, Japan*

Correspondence should be addressed to Natsumi Saka; natsumi613@gmail.com

Academic Editor: Kaan Erler

We report a case of volar fourth and fifth carpometacarpal (CMC) joint dislocation complicated by a hamate hook fracture. The CMC joint was reduced in a closed fashion and temporally fixed with Kirschner wires. Using intraoperative computed tomography, the displaced fracture of the hamate hook was reduced by open reduction and internal fixation and fixed with a screw. We suggest that this rare injury was caused by the over contraction of the flexor carpi ulnaris and avulsion force from the ligamentous structure around the pisiform, hamate, and metacarpal bones.

## 1. Introduction

Dislocation of the carpometacarpal (CMC) joint is a relatively rare injury, and volar dislocation of the CMC joint is less common than dorsal CMC joint dislocation. Nalebuff reported two types of volar dislocations of the fifth CMC joint: volar radial or volar ulnar, depending on the type of ruptured ligament [1]. Fracture of the hamate hook is also an uncommon injury, usually seen in athletes and caused by direct compression [2]. The purpose of this study was to present a case of volar dislocation of the fourth and fifth CMC joint with a hamate hook fracture and to discuss the mechanism of this injury. Careful assessment of radiographic findings is of paramount importance when considering the treatment strategy for this injury.

## 2. Case Report

A 60-year-old man fell from a staircase and landed on the floor with his right wrist hyperextended. He had no history of hand or wrist injury. He presented to the nearby clinic complaining of severe pain and swelling of the right hand. A diagnosis of fourth and fifth CMC joint dislocation was made by radiography (Figures 1(a) and 1(b)). Closed reduction was not successful, and he was referred to our clinic on the day after the injury. Physical examination revealed significant swelling of the hand. Sensation over the median and ulnar nerve area was intact, as was abductor pollicis brevis and interossei function. Computed tomography (CT) revealed a fracture of the hamate hook associated with volar ulnar dislocation of the fourth and fifth CMC joint, and the base of the dislocated metacarpal was incarcerated between the hook and body of the hamate (Figures 2(a)–2(c)). An avulsion fracture was noted between the base of the fourth and fifth metacarpal bones (Figure 2(d)).

Dislocation of the CMC joint was performed by longitudinal traction under sedation. The patient underwent open reduction and internal fixation of the hamate hook and percutaneous fixation of the CMC joint on the following day. The surgery was performed under general anesthesia. Surgical exposure was achieved with a longitudinal skin incision made between the hamate hook and pisiform, which was prolonged proximally by a palmer crease in a zigzag fashion. Guyon's canal was released for the exposure and protection of the ulnar artery and nerve. The pisiform and hamate hook was identified. The fracture site of the hamate hook was

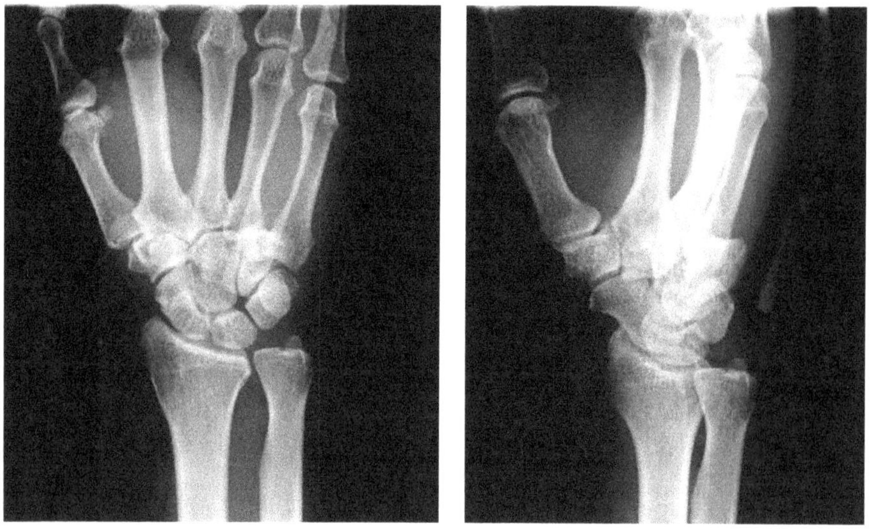

(a) (b)

Figure 1: Initial radiograph showing the proximal displacement of the fourth and fifth metacarpal bones. (a) Posteroanterior view. (b) Oblique semisupinated view.

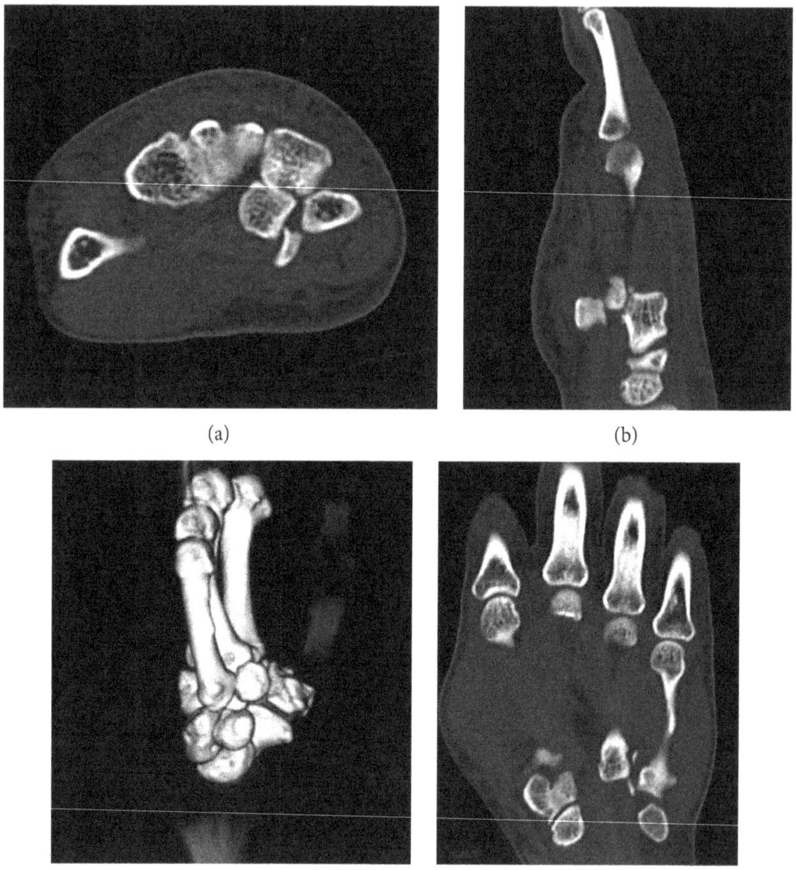

(a) (b) (c) (d)

Figure 2: CT scan showing the carpometacarpal bases incarcerated at the fracture gap of the hamate hook at the fracture site. (a) Axial view. (b) Sagittal view. (c) Three-dimensional view of the hand. (d) Coronal view of the CT scan also shows the avulsion fracture between the base of the fourth and fifth metacarpal bones.

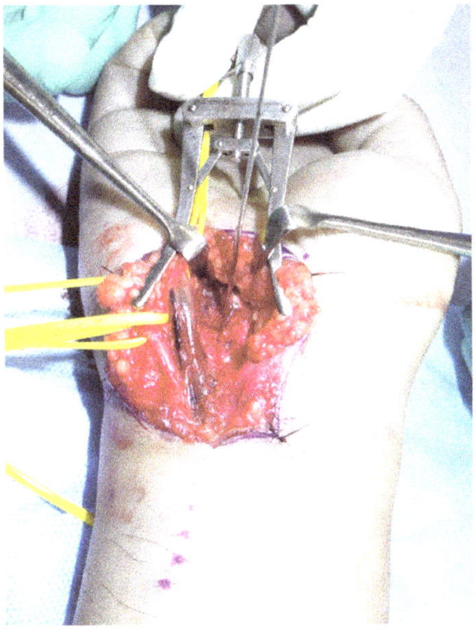

Figure 3: Intraoperative findings.

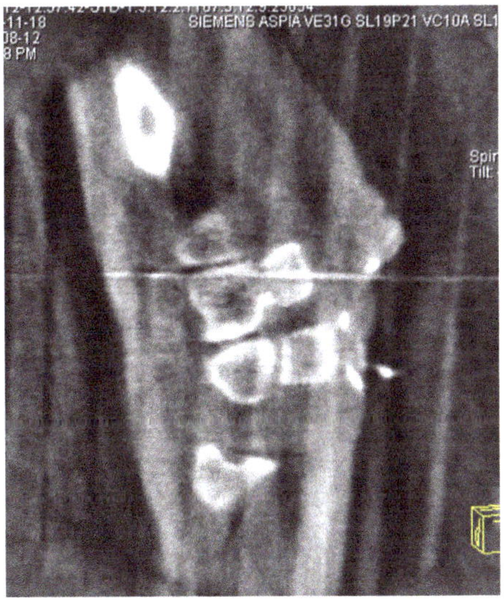


Figure 4: Intraoperative CT scan (sagittal view) showing the anatomical reduction of the hamate hook.

located using a longitudinal incision of the palmar carpal ligament (Figure 3). It was difficult to acquire good exposure of the fracture because of its depth in the surgical field. Therefore, to examine the reduction of the fracture, we used intraoperative CT after provisional fixation of the fracture site (Figure 4). After confirmation of the reduction, fixation was performed with a headless compression screw (Acutrak2 micro®, Acumed). The fourth and fifth CMC joint were temporally fixed percutaneously from the metacarpal bones to the carpal bones, respectively, using 1.5 mm Kirschner wires (K-wires; Figures 5(a) and 5(b)). Reduction and appropriate placement of the screw were confirmed postoperatively using CT (Figure 6). Immediate exercise of the fingers and wrist motion was allowed under a protective splint, and the K-wires were removed 7 weeks after surgery. A radiograph

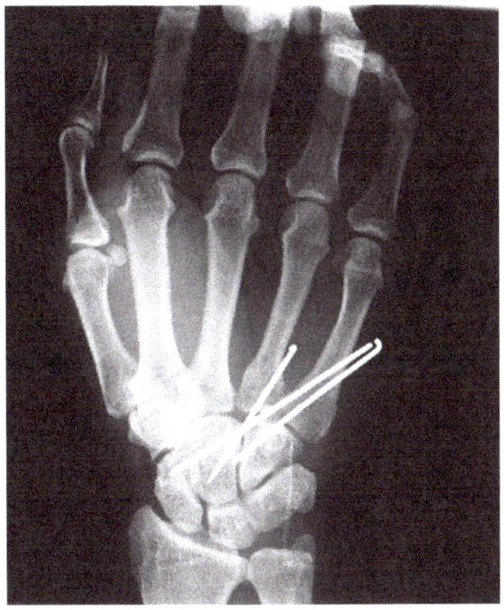

(a)

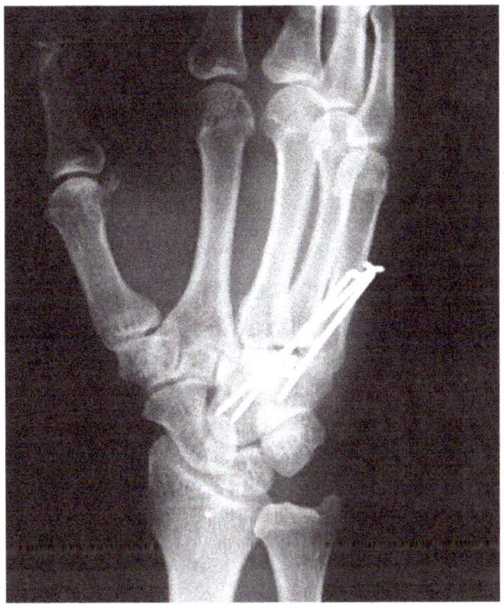

(b)

Figure 5: Postoperative radiograph. (a) Posteroanterior view. (b) Oblique semisupinated view.

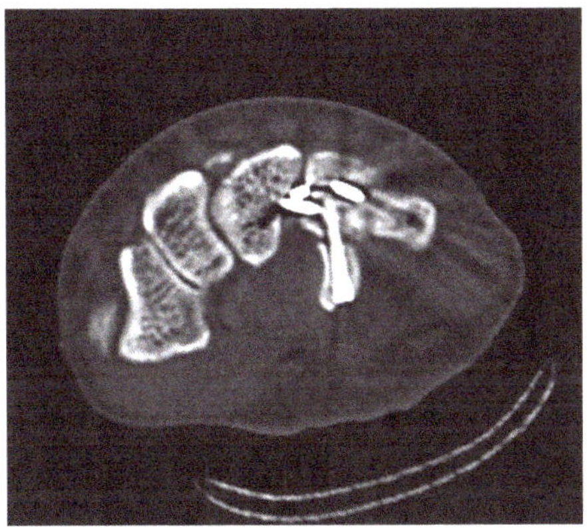

Figure 6: Postoperative CT scan showing the reduction and appropriate placement of the screw.

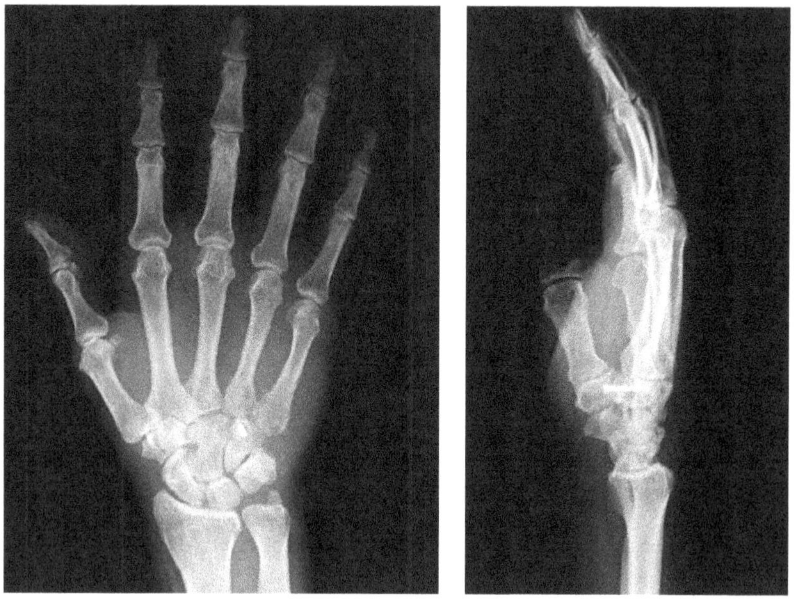

(a) (b)

FIGURE 7: Radiographs after the removal of the K-wires showing the maintenance of the reduction of CMC joint. (a) Posteroanterior view. (b) Oblique semisupinated view.

demonstrated the maintenance of the reduction after the removal of the K-wires (Figures 7(a) and 7(b)).

Three months after the operation, CT revealed a gap of the fracture site at the hamate hook (Figure 8). However, the patient did not have tenderness at the fracture site, and no secondary surgery was performed. Two years after the injury, the patient's active range of motion of the wrist was an extension of 75° and flexion of 60°. The Disability of the Arm, Shoulder, and Hand score was 0. He had no signs of rupture or irritation of the flexor digitorum profundus (Figure 9). The patient was informed that data from his case would be submitted for publication, and he provided consent.

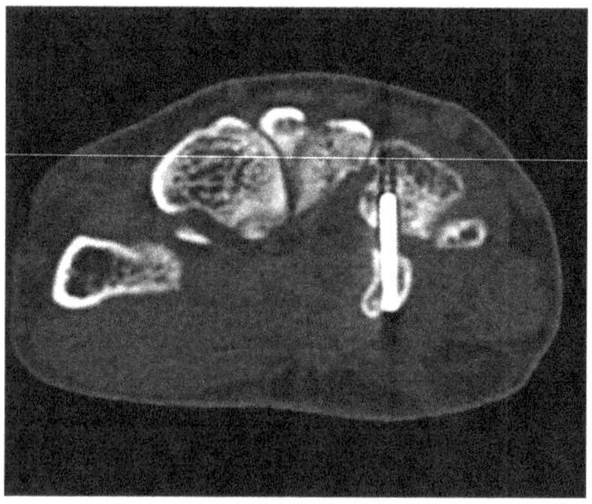

FIGURE 8: CT scan performed 3 months postoperatively showing the gap at the fracture site.

## 3. Discussion

Several studies have reported volar joint dislocation of the fifth CMC joint, mostly without accompanying fracture of the hamate hook [1, 3, 4]. Nalebuff reported two types of volar CMC joint dislocations of the fifth finger: volar radial or volar ulnar, according to the pattern of ligamentous injury [1]. The pisometacarpal, carpometacarpal (volar fifth metacarpal hook of the hamate ligament), and metacarpal interosseous ligaments (volar fourth metacarpal ulnar base–fifth metacarpal radial base ligament) are attached to the base of the fifth finger. Volar radial dislocation is accompanied by rupture of all three ligaments, whereas volar ulnar dislocation is accompanied by rupture of the CMC and metacarpal interosseous ligaments, leaving the pisometacarpal ligament intact.

In our case, the exact mechanism of the hamate hook fracture associated with the volar dislocation of the fourth and fifth CMC joint was unclear; however, we suggest that this injury was an avulsion injury, based on previously published studies. Garcia-Elias et al. reported a hamate hook fracture with volar dislocation of the fifth CMC joint and pointed out that this injury was caused as an avulsion injury from the ligamentous structure around the pisiform [5]. These authors suggested that the force from the flexor carpi ulnaris is transmitted distally to the pisohamate and pisometacarpal ligaments through the pisiform. They also indicated that tension on the pisohamate ligament causes an avulsion fracture of the hamate hook, and tension on the pisometacarpal ligament produces volar dislocation of the fifth CMC joint (Figure 10). Jackson et al. also reported a hamate hook fracture in an individual participating in clay shooting and suggested that the injury was caused by the avulsion force from the pisohamate ligament [6]. Our case is similar to the injury described by Garcia-Elias et al. but was accompanied by an additional fourth CMC joint dislocation and avulsion fracture between the base of the fourth and fifth metacarpal.

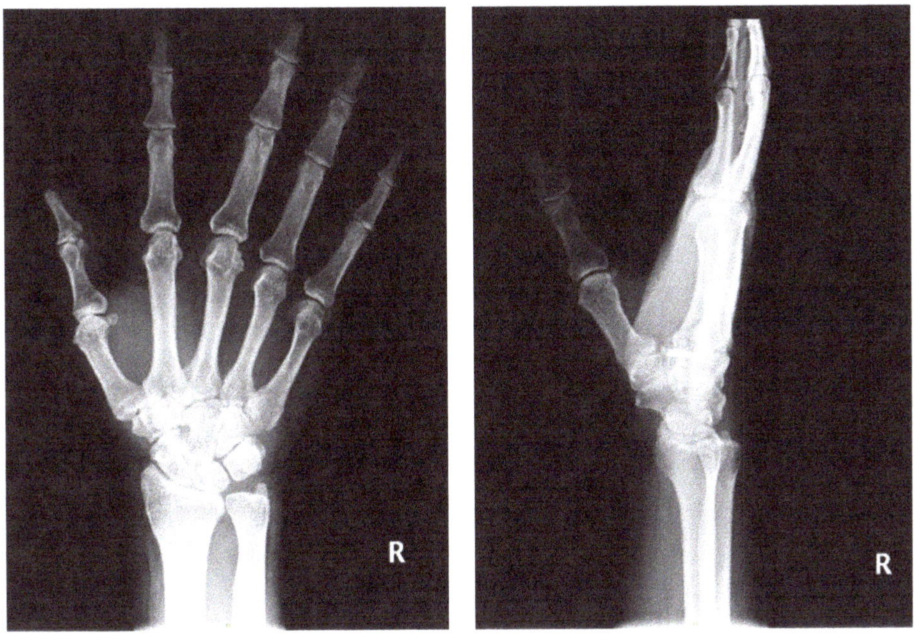


(a) (b)

FIGURE 9: Radiograph 2 years after the surgery. (a) Posteroanterior view. (b) Oblique semisupinated view.

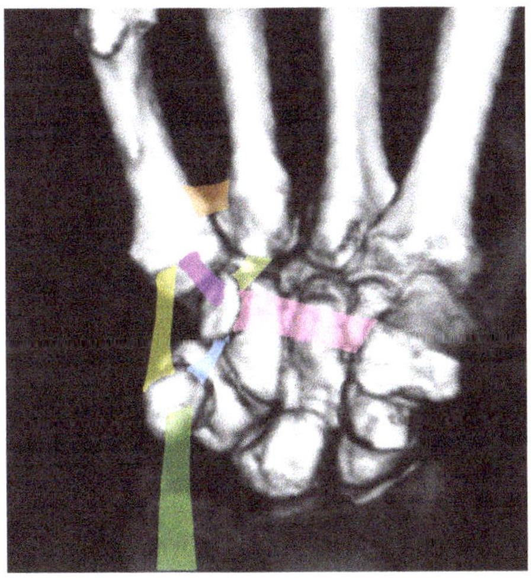

FIGURE 10: Ligamentous structure around the metacarpal bones, hamate hook, and pisiform. 1: flexor carpi ulnaris. 2: volar fifth metacarpal–pisiform ligament (pisometacarpal ligament). 3: volar fifth metacarpal–hamate hook ligament. 4: volar fourth metacarpal ulnar base–hamate hook ligament. 5: metacarpal interosseous ligament (volar fourth metacarpal ulnar base–fifth metacarpal radial base ligament). 6: pisohamate ligament. 7; transverse carpal ligament.

Therefore, we speculated that hamate hook fracture and volar fifth CMC dislocation were caused by the avulsion force to the pisohamate and pisometacarpal ligament, as suggested by Garcia-Elias et al. With regard to the fourth CMC joint dislocation, we speculated that it was caused by the traction from the volar fourth metacarpal ulnar base–hamate hook ligament (Figure 10).

To provide an anatomical and biomechanical background for this hypothesis, Pevny et al. showed that the pisohamate and pisometacarpal ligaments are much thicker and stronger than other soft-tissue attachments around the pisiform [7]. Rayan et al. proved that the pisometacarpal and pisohamate ligaments are the primary stabilizers of the pisiform [8]. Based on these anatomical studies, it can be speculated that avulsion force to the pisiform is transmitted to its primary stabilizer. Avulsion force by the pisometacarpal ligament leads to ulnar volar displacement of metacarpal, and avulsion force by the pisohamate ligament leads to the fracture of the hook of the hamate. Yoshida et al. conducted a biomechanical study using a cadaver to simulate a blow to the ulnar side of the hand with the wrist extended [9]. They showed that a fifth metacarpal volar base fracture and hamate hook fracture are attached to the volar fifth metacarpal–hamate hook ligament and concluded that the pathomechanical etiology of this injury is avulsion. This supports the hypothesis of our case, namely, that the metacarpal–hamate hook ligament caused the avulsion injury.

In terms of treatment of hamate hook fractures, most injuries of this type, which are typically caused by repetitive microtrauma or blunt trauma to the palm of the hand from playing golf or baseball, are treated by hook excision. In the report by Gunther et al., the fracture was left untreated, resulting in nonunion without symptoms [10]. Another report from Garcia-Elias et al. recommended open reduction and internal fixation of the hamate hook, which resulted in stabilization of the pisohamate ligament and pisiform [5]. The hook was successfully fixed with K-wires, and union was demonstrated on radiography.

In our case, open reduction and internal fixation of the fractured hook was performed, taking into account the mechanism of this injury. In contrast to the usual type of hamate hook fracture, we noted a gap between the hook and body of the hamate. An intraoperative three-dimensional CT scan was helpful for obtaining anatomical reduction of the fracture site. The fracture resulted in nonunion, which may have been related to the initial displacement and residual instability around the hamate hook, since the HCS screw length did not exceed the more than half of the hamate body.

This is the first report to describe volar dislocation of the fourth and fifth CMC dislocation with a hamate hook fracture and its relationship to the ligamentous structure around the hamate hook. Our case indicates the importance of traction force in the strategic treatment of this injury.

## Consent

Identifying information, including patients' names, initials, or hospital numbers, were not published in written descriptions, photographs, and pedigrees.

## Acknowledgments

The authors would like to thank Enago (http://www.enago.jp) for the English language review.

## References

[1] E. A. Nalebuff, "Isolated anterior carpometacarpal dislocation of the fifth finger: classification and case report," *The Journal of Trauma*, vol. 8, no. 6, pp. 1119–1123, 1968.

[2] N. Suh, E. T. Ek, and S. W. Wolfe, "Carpal fractures," *The Journal of Hand Surgery*, vol. 39, no. 4, pp. 785–791, 2014.

[3] P. M. Prokopis and A. J. Weiland, "Volar dislocation of the fourth and fifth carpometacarpal joints: a case report and review of the literature," *HSS Journal*, vol. 4, no. 2, pp. 138–142, 2008.

[4] M. Nakayama, Y. Horiuchi, and H. Kawashima, "Isolated volar dislocation of the fifth carpometacarpal joint: a case report," *Hand Surgery*, vol. 12, no. 3, pp. 165–168, 2007.

[5] M. Garcia-Elias, P. Rossignani, and M. Cots, "Combined fracture of the hook of the hamate and palmar dislocation of the fifth carpometacarpal joint," *Journal of Hand Surgery*, vol. 21, no. 4, pp. 446–450, 1996.

[6] T. Jackson and G. M. Rayan, "Avulsion fracture of the hamulus from clay gunshot sport: a case report," *The Journal of Hand Surgery*, vol. 30, no. 4, pp. 702–705, 2005.

[7] T. Pevny, G. M. Rayan, and D. Egle, "Ligamentous and tendinous support of the pisiform, anatomic and biomechanical study," *The Journal of Hand Surgery*, vol. 20, no. 2, pp. 299–304, 1995.

[8] G. M. Rayan, B. H. Jameson, and K. W. Chung, "The pisotriquetral joint: anatomic, biomechanical, and radiographic analysis," *The Journal of Hand Surgery*, vol. 30, no. 3, pp. 596–602, 2005.

[9] R. Yoshida, M. A. Shah, R. M. Patterson, W. L. Buford, J. Knighten, and S. F. Viegas, "Anatomy and pathomechanics of ring and small finger carpometacarpal joint injuries," vol. 28, no. 6, pp. 1035–1043, 2003.

[10] S. F. Gunther and P. D. Bruno, "Divergent dislocation of the carpometacarpal joints: a case report," *The Journal of Hand Surgery*, vol. 10, no. 2, pp. 197–201, 1985.

# Permissions

All chapters in this book were first published by Hindawi Publishing Corporation; hereby published with permission under the Creative Commons Attribution License or equivalent. Every chapter published in this book has been scrutinized by our experts. Their significance has been extensively debated. The topics covered herein carry significant findings which will fuel the growth of the discipline. They may even be implemented as practical applications or may be referred to as a beginning point for another development.

The contributors of this book come from diverse backgrounds, making this book a truly international effort. This book will bring forth new frontiers with its revolutionizing research information and detailed analysis of the nascent developments around the world.

We would like to thank all the contributing authors for lending their expertise to make the book truly unique. They have played a crucial role in the development of this book. Without their invaluable contributions this book wouldn't have been possible. They have made vital efforts to compile up to date information on the varied aspects of this subject to make this book a valuable addition to the collection of many professionals and students.

This book was conceptualized with the vision of imparting up-to-date information and advanced data in this field. To ensure the same, a matchless editorial board was set up. Every individual on the board went through rigorous rounds of assessment to prove their worth. After which they invested a large part of their time researching and compiling the most relevant data for our readers.

The editorial board has been involved in producing this book since its inception. They have spent rigorous hours researching and exploring the diverse topics which have resulted in the successful publishing of this book. They have passed on their knowledge of decades through this book. To expedite this challenging task, the publisher supported the team at every step. A small team of assistant editors was also appointed to further simplify the editing procedure and attain best results for the readers.

Apart from the editorial board, the designing team has also invested a significant amount of their time in understanding the subject and creating the most relevant covers. They scrutinized every image to scout for the most suitable representation of the subject and create an appropriate cover for the book.

The publishing team has been an ardent support to the editorial, designing and production team. Their endless efforts to recruit the best for this project, has resulted in the accomplishment of this book. They are a veteran in the field of academics and their pool of knowledge is as vast as their experience in printing. Their expertise and guidance has proved useful at every step. Their uncompromising quality standards have made this book an exceptional effort. Their encouragement from time to time has been an inspiration for everyone.

The publisher and the editorial board hope that this book will prove to be a valuable piece of knowledge for researchers, students, practitioners and scholars across the globe.

# List of Contributors

**Georgios Kalinterakis, Emmanouil Antonogiannakis, Ioannis Rampakakis, Evangelos Tsialogiannis and Miltiadis Ziogas**
First Department of Orthopedics, 401 General Military Hospital of Athens, Athens 11525, Greece

**Athanasios Syllaios**
First Department of Surgery, General Hospital of Athens "Laiko", National and Kapodistrian University of Athens, Athens 11527, Greece

**Danica D. Vance, Usama Qayyum and Charles M. Jobin**
The Center for Shoulder, Elbow and Sports Medicine, Columbia University Medical Center, New York, NY, USA

**Chelsea E. Minoughan and Adam P. Schumaier**
University of Cincinnati Department of Orthopaedics and Sports Medicine, Cincinnati, OH, USA

**Frank R. Avilucea**
Orlando Health Orthopedic Institute Orthopedic and Sports Medicine Group, Orlando, FL, USA

**Tommy Primeau, Philippe Beauchamp-Chalifour and Stéphane Pelet**
Centre de Recherche FRQS du CHU de Québec—Hôpital Enfant-Jésus, 1401, 18ème Rue, (Québec), Québec, Canada G1J 1Z4
Department of Orthopedic Surgery, CHU de Québec—Hôpital Enfant-Jésus, 1401, 18ème Rue, (Québec), Québec, Canada G1J 1Z4

**John G. Skedros, J. Hunter Marshall and John T. Cronin**
Utah Orthopaedic Specialists, Salt Lake City, Utah, USA

**Fumihiro Mukasa**
Department of Orthopedic Surgery, Tokyo Rosai Hospital, 4-13-21, Omori-minami, Ota-ku, Tokyo 143-0013, Japan
Department of Orthopedic Surgery, Juntendo University School of Medicine, 3-1-3, Hongo, Bunkyo-ku, Tokyo 113-8431, Japan

**Yoshimasa Tomita and Hideyuki Hirasawa**
Department of Orthopedic Surgery, Tokyo Rosai Hospital, 4-13-21, Omori-minami, Ota-ku, Tokyo 143-0013, Japan

**Kazuo Kaneko**
Department of Orthopedic Surgery, Juntendo University School of Medicine, 3-1-3, Hongo, Bunkyo-ku, Tokyo 113-8431, Japan

**Martine Christine Keuning and Wierd Pieter Zijlstra**
Department of Orthopaedic Surgery, Medical Center Leeuwarden, Leeuwarden, Netherlands

**Aziz Al Moujahid**
Center for Infectious Diseases Friesland, Izore, Leeuwarden, Netherlands

**WanYin Lim**
Dr Jones and Partners Medical Imaging, 226 Greenhill Road, Eastwood, South Australia 5063, Australia
Radiology Department, Royal Adelaide Hospital, 1 Port Rd, South Australia 5000, Australia

**Jonathan Heysen**
Dr Jones and Partners Medical Imaging, 226 Greenhill Road, Eastwood, South Australia 5063, Australia

**James Ilic**
Wakefield Sports and Exercise Medicine Clinic, Calvary Adelaide Hospital, South Australia, Australia

**Ben Beamond**
Radiology Department, Royal Adelaide Hospital, 1 Port Rd, South Australia 5000, Australia
Wakefield Orthopaedic Clinic, Calvary Adelaide Hospital, South Australia, Australia

**Steven Zadow**
Dr Jones and Partners Medical Imaging, 226 Greenhill Road, Eastwood, South Australia 5063, Australia
Flinders Medical Centre, South Australia, Australia

**Ismail Sahan and Konstantinos Anagnostakos**
Zentrum für Orthopädie und Unfallchirurgie, Städtisches Klinikum Saarbrücken, Saarbrücken, Germany

**Julie De Deken**
Klinik für Allgemein-, Viszeral-, Thorax- und Kinderchirurgie, Städtisches Klinikum Saarbrücken, Saarbrücken, Germany

**Abdul Rehman Arain, Muhammad Moral, Khusboo Desai and Khunwar Kalsa**
Department of Orthopedics, Albany Medical College, 1267 Washington Ave Suite 202, Albany, NY 12206, USA

**Saadia Shams**
Rawalpindi Medical College, Pakistan

**Paul Lecoanet, Mathias Blangis, Matthieu Garcia, Yohan Legallois and Thierry Fabre**
CHU de Bordeaux, Place Amélie Raba-Léon, 33000 Bordeaux, France

**Avinesh Agarwalla, Richard N. Puzzitiello and Brian Forsythe**
Midwest Orthopaedics at Rush, Rush University Medical Center, Chicago, IL, USA

**Natalie L. Leong**
Department of Orthopaedic Surgery, University of Maryland, College Park, MD, USA

**Alexander J. Johnson, Katharine D. Harper and Christopher Haydel**
Temple University Hospital Department of Orthopaedics and Sports Medicine, USA

**Rachel Michael, Nabil Ebraheim, Jacob Maier, Mina Tanios and Anthony Kouri**
University of Toledo Medical Center Department of Orthopaedic Surgery, 3000 Arlington Ave Toledo, OH 43614, USA

**Yoshinori Takashima, Shingo Hashimoto, Tomoyuki Kamenaga, Masanori Tsubosaka, Yuichi Kuroda, Kazuhiro Takeuchi, Koji Takayama, Shinya Hayashi, Ryosuke Kuroda and Tomoyuki Matsumoto**
Department of Orthopaedic Surgery, Kobe University Graduate School of Medicine, Kobe, 7-5-1, Kusunoki-cho, Chuo-ku, Kobe 650-0017, Japan

**Dane Gary Maimin**
Madadeni Hospital, Newcastle, South Africa

**Livan Meneses-Turino**
Madadeni Hospital, Newcastle, South Africa 2HOD Orthopaedics Northdale Hospital, Pietermaritzburg, South Africa

**T. M. Gause II, T.E. Moran, J.B. Carr and D. N. Deal**
Department of Orthopedic Surgery, University of Virginia Health System, Charlottesville, VA, USA

**Mark K. Lyons, Matthew T. Neal, Naresh P. Patel and Holenarasipur R. Vikram**
Department of Neurological Surgery, Mayo Clinic Arizona, 5777 East Mayo Boulevard, Phoenix, AZ 85054, USA

**Arash Calafi**
University of Washington Department of Orthopaedics and Sports Medicine, 1959 N.E. Pacific St., Seattle, WA 98195, USA

**Alton W. Skaggs**
School of Medicine at University of California at Davis, Sacramento, CA 95817, USA

**Trevor J. Shelton**
Department of Orthopaedic Surgery, University of California at Davis, 4860 Y Street, Suite 3800, Sacramento, CA 95829, USA

**Brian M. Haus**
Department of Orthopaedic Surgery, University of California at Davis, 4860 Y Street, Suite 3800, Sacramento, CA 95829, USA
Shriners Hospital for Children, Northern California, 2425 Stockton Blvd., Sacramento, CA 95817, USA

**Kazunobu Kida, Toshikazu Tani and Tateo Kawazoe**
Department of Orthopaedic Surgery, Kubokawa Hospital, 902-1 Mitsuke, Shimanto-cho, Takaoka-gun, Kochi 786-0002, Japan

**Michio Toda**
Department of Orthopaedic Surgery, Kurashiki Medical Center, 250 Bakuro-cho, Kurashiki City, Okayama 710-8522, Japan

**Joseph Maalouly, Dany Aouad, Elias Saidy and Chawki Cortbawi**
Department of Orthopedic Surgery and Traumatology, Saint Georges University Medical Center, Balamand University, Achrafieh, Beirut 1100 2807, Lebanon

**Antonios Tawk**
Saint Georges University Medical Center, Balamand University, Achra ieh, Beirut 1100 2807, Lebanon

**Georges Baaklini**
Department of Vascular Surgery, Saint Georges University Medical Center, Balamand University, Achrafieh, Beirut 1100 2807, Lebanon

**John F. Dankert and Mandeep S. Virk**
Department of Orthopedic Surgery, NYU Langone Health, New York, New York, USA

**Charles C. Pitts, Walter R. Smith and Michael J. Conklin**
Department of Orthopaedic Surgery, University of Alabama at Birmingham, USA

**Matthew T. Neal, Maziyar A. Kalani and Mark K. Lyons**
Department of Neurologic Surgery, Mayo Clinic College of Medicine and Science, 5777 East Mayo Boulevard, Phoenix, AZ 85054, USA

**Futoshi Morio, Tomokazu Fukui, Makoto Kanto, Kenta Amai and Toshiya Tachibana**
Department of Orthopaedic Surgery, Hyogo College of Medicine, Japan

**Shinichi Yoshiya and Shigeo Fukunishi**
Nishinomiya Kaisei Hospital, Japan

**Haruka Maehara**
Department of Orthopaedic Surgery, Kochi Prefectural Hata Kenmin Hospital, 3-1 Yoshina, Yamana-cho, Sukumo, Kochi 788-0785, Japan
Department of Orthopaedic Surgery, Susaki Kuroshio Hospital, 4–30, Midorimachi, Susaki, Kochi 785-0036, Japan

**Toshihiro Sano, Yuki Yanagawa and Kyuichi Hashimoto**
Department of Orthopaedic Surgery, Kochi Prefectural Hata Kenmin Hospital, 3-1 Yoshina, Yamana-cho, Sukumo, Kochi 788-0785, Japan

**Nobuaki Tadokoro**
Department of Orthopaedic Surgery, Kochi Medical School, 185-1 Kohasu, Oko-cho, Nankoku, Kochi 783-8505, Japan

**Karen Nishikawa**
Hirosaki University School of Medicine, 5 Zaifu-cho, Hirosaki, Aomori, Japan

**Yuka Kimura, Daisuke Chiba, Norihiro Sasaki, Shizuka Sasaki and Yasuyuki Ishibashi**
Department of Orthopaedic Surgery, Hirosaki University Graduate School of Medicine, 5 Zaifu-cho, Hirosaki, Aomori, Japan

**Shinji Nishikawa**
Nishikawa Hand Surgery Orthopaedic Clinic, 2-2-12 Waseda, Hirosaki, Aomori, Japan

**George El Rassi, Nabil Dib, Joseph Maalouly and Dany Aouad**
Department of Orthopedic Surgery and Traumatology, Saint Georges University Medical Center, Balamand University, 166378, Achrafieh, Beirut 1100 2807, Lebanon

**Rita Moukarzel**
Medical School, Lebanese American University Medical Center, Lebanese American University, Chouran, Beirut 1102 2801, Lebanon

**Adam Kurland, Brian Batko and Jeremy Hreha**
Department of Orthopaedic Surgery, Rutgers New Jersey Medical School, New Jersey, USA

**Ashley Ignatiuk**
Department of Surgery, Plastic & Reconstructive Surgery Division, Rutgers New Jersey Medical School, New Jersey, USA

**Petros Ismailidis, Corina Nüesch and Annegret Mündermann**
Department of Orthopaedics and Traumatology, University Hospital Basel, Spitalstrasse 21, 4031 Basel, Switzerland
Department of Biomedical Engineering, University of Basel, Gewerbestrasse 14, 4123 Allschwil, Switzerland
Department of Clinical Research, University of Basel, Schanzenstrasse 55, 4056 Basel, Switzerland

**Rolf Kernen**
Clinic for Orthopedics "Claraortho", Claragraben 82 4058 Basel, Switzerland

**Christian Egloff and Sebastian Andreas Müller**
Department of Orthopaedics and Traumatology, University Hospital Basel, Spitalstrasse 21, 4031 Basel, Switzerland

**Kyriakos Papavasiliou, Sousana Panagiotidou, Panagiotis Kakoulidis and Eleftherios Tsiridis**
Academic Orthopaedic Department, Papageorgiou General Hospital, Aristotle University Medical School, Thessaloniki Ring Road, 56403 Nea Efkarpia, Greece

**Antonia Bintoudi**
Department of Radiology, Papageorgiou General Hospital, Thessaloniki Ring Road, 56403 Nea Efkarpia, Greece

**Kostoula Arvaniti**
Intensive Care Unit, Infection Control and AMS Unit, Papageorgiou General Hospital, Thessaloniki Ring Road, 56403 Nea Efkarpia, Greece

**Mason Uvodich**
Mayo Clinic Department of Orthopaedic Surgery, USA

**Ross Barman**
Mayo Clinic Department of Anesthesiology and Perioperative Medicine, USA

**Adam Reitz**
Kentucky College of Osteopathic Medicine, USA

**Matthew Sexton**
Department of Critical Care Medicine, USA

**R. Jansen, A. T. Besselaar, J. J. Tolk and F. van Rooijen**
Máxima MC, Department of Orthopaedic Surgery and Trauma, 5600 PD Eindhoven, Netherlands

**J. P. Toirkens**
Máxima MC, Department of Radiology, 90052, 5600 PD Eindhoven, Netherlands

**Sean Mc Millan**
Department of Orthopedics, Virtua Health System, 2103 Burlington-Mount Holly Rd, Burlington, NJ 08016, USA

**Danielle Thorn**
Department of Orthopedics, Virtua Health System, Burlington, NJ, USA

**Elizabeth Ford**
Department of Orthopedics, Inspira Health System, Vineland, NJ, USA

**Truong Nguyen Khanh Hung**
College of Medicine, Taipei Medical University, Taipei City, Taiwan
Orthopedic and Trauma Department, ChoRay Hospital, Ho Chi Minh City, Vietnam

**Tran Binh Duong, Tran Phuoc Binh, Dao Thanh Tu, Huynh Phuoc Hau and Le Van Tuan**
Orthopedic and Trauma Department, ChoRay Hospital, Ho Chi Minh City, Vietnam

**Truong Trong Tin and Cao Thi**
Orthopedic and Rehabilitation Department, University of Medicine and Pharmacy at Ho Chi Minh City, Ho Chi Minh City, Vietnam

**Ichiro Tonogai and Koichi Sairyo**
Department of Orthopedics, Institute of Biomedical Science, Tokushima University Graduate School, 3-18-15 Kuramoto, Tokushima, Tokushima 770-8503, Japan

**Mohammad A. Alsofyani**
Department of Spinal Surgery Unit, Bordeaux University, Bordeaux University Hospital, C.H.U Tripode Pellegrin, Place Amélie Raba Léon, 33076 Bordeaux, France
Orthopedic Department, College of Medicine and University Hospital, University of Hail, 2440, Hail City, Saudi Arabia

**Soufiane Ghailane, Sreenath Jakinapally, Louis Boissière, Ibrahim Obeid and Jean-Marc Vital**
Department of Spinal Surgery Unit, Bordeaux University, Bordeaux University Hospital, C.H.U Tripode Pellegrin, Place Amélie Raba Léon, 33076 Bordeaux, France

**Sultan Alsalmi**
Department of Neurosurgery, Amiens University Medical Center, Amiens University, Amiens, France
Department of Neurosurgery, Imam Abdulrahman Bin Faisal University, Dammam City, Saudi Arabia

**Llano Lionel, Jorge D. Barla, Campelo Diego, Taype Danilo, Carlos F. Sancineto and Guido Carabelli**
Instituto de Ortopedia y Traumatología "Carlos E. Ottolenghi", Hospital Italiano de Buenos Aires, Argentina

**Yuji Maenohara, Ryutaro Takeda, Song Ho Chang, Yasunori Omata, Sakae Tanaka and Takumi Matsumoto**
Department of Orthopaedic Surgery, Faculty of Medicine, The University of Tokyo, 7-3-1 Hongo, Bunkyo-ku, Tokyo 113-8655, Japan

**Brody W. King**
University of Utah School of Medicine, Salt Lake City, Utah, USA

**John G. Skedros**
Utah Orthopaedic Specialists, Salt Lake City, Utah, USA
Intermountain Medical Center, Salt Lake City, Utah, USA

**Robert E. Glasgow**
University of Utah Department of Surgery, Salt Lake City, Utah, USA

**D. Glen Morrell**
Tanner Clinic, Layton, Utah, USA

**Halle E. K. Burley**
Seattle Science Foundation, Seattle, Washington, USA
Western University of Health Sciences, College of Osteopathic Medicine of the Pacific-Northwest, 200 Mullins Dr., Lebanon OR 97355, USA

**Darius S. Ansari**
Seattle Science Foundation, Seattle, Washington, USA
University of Illinois College of Medicine, 1835 W Polk St., Chicago, IL 60612, USA

**Alexander von Glinski**
Seattle Science Foundation, Seattle, Washington, USA
Swedish Neuroscience Institute, Swedish Medical Center, Seattle, Washington, USA
Department of Trauma Surgery, BG University Hospital Bergmannsheil, Ruhr University Bochum, Bochum, Germany
Hansjörg Wyss Hip and Pelvic Center, Swedish Hospital, Seattle, Washington, USA

**Ryan Goodmanson, Benjamin Schell, Jens R. Chapman and Rod J. Oskouian**
Seattle Science Foundation, Seattle, Washington, USA
Swedish Neuroscience Institute, Swedish Medical Center, Seattle, Washington, USA

**Shuhei Mizobuchi, Nobuaki Tadokoro, Shogo Takaya, Katsuhito Kiyasu, Ryuichi Takemasa and Masahiko Ikeuchi**
Department of Orthopaedic Surgery, Kochi Medical School, Kochi University, Kohasu, Oko-cho, Nankoku 783-8505, Japan

**Isamu Miura and Oji Momosaki**
Department of Spinal Surgery, Kameda Medical Center, 929 Higashi-cho, Kamogawa-shi, Chiba 296-8602, Japan
Department of Neurosurgery, Tokyo Women's Medical University, 8-1 Kawada-cho, Shinjuku-ku, Tokyo 162-8666, Japan

**Motoo Kubota and Masahito Yuzurihara**
Department of Spinal Surgery, Kameda Medical Center, 929 Higashi-cho, Kamogawa-shi, Chiba 296-8602, Japan

**Kento Takebayashi and Takakazu Kawamata**
Department of Neurosurgery, Tokyo Women's Medical University, 8-1 Kawada-cho, Shinjuku-ku, Tokyo 162-8666, Japan

**Mariko Kamiya, Gen Sasaki, Kensuke Ikuta, Hideaki Miyamoto, Michio Kimura and Hirotaka Kawano**
Department of Orthopaedic Surgery, Teikyo University School of Medicine, 2-11-1 Kaga, Itabashi-ku, Tokyo 173-8606, Japan

**Futoshi Morio, Shota Morimoto, Shintaro Onishi, Toshiya Tachibana and Tomoya Iseki**
Department of Orthopedic Surgery, Hyogo College of Medicine, 663-8501, 1-1 Mukogawa-cho, Nishinomiya City, Hyogo, Japan

**Natsumi Saka**
Orthopaedic Trauma Center, Sapporo Tokushukai Hospital, Sapporo, Hokkaido, Japan
Department of Orthopaedics, Teikyo University School of Medicine, Tokyo, Japan

**Hirotada Matsui and Hideki Tsuji**
Orthopaedic Trauma Center, Sapporo Tokushukai Hospital, Sapporo, Hokkaido, Japan

# Index